Experimental Pharmaceutics

fourth edition

Eugene L. Parrott
University of Iowa, Iowa City

Witold Saski
University of Nebraska Medical Center, Omaha

Alpha Editions
A Division of Burgess International Group, Inc.

ISBN 0-8087-9015-3
Printed in the United States of America.

Burgess International Group Inc. / ALPHA EDITIONS
7110 Ohms Lane
Minneapolis, Minnesota 55435

30 29 28

Previous editions entitled *Experimental Pharmaceutical Technology*

PREFACE

Pharmaceutics quantitatively correlates physicochemical theories with the characterization, design, development, evaluation, and preparation of dosage forms. Specifically, the area of pharmaceutics is concerned with properties and means of classifying properties of drugs, absorption, dosage forms, extraction, chemical kinetics, solubility, polyphasic systems, preservation, formulation, patient acceptance, sterilization, packaging and stability, and the physiological availability of the medicinal substance from the dosage form.

It is a purpose of this manual to aid in establishing pharmacy on a more mathematical and scientific basis. With this underlying purpose, pharmaceutics will acquaint the student with the characteristics of pharmaceutical systems, will teach the student skills and techniques, will familiarize the student with equipment used in pharmaceutical processes, will acquaint the student with scientific and and technical terminology, will let the student know and apply scientific principles to solving pharmaceutical problems, will give the student judgement in evaluating pharmaceutical products and problems, and will aid in the development of logical and creative thinking.

Another purpose of this manual is to aid the beginning student to obtain an overall concept of a dosage form. He should appreciate a pharmaceutical product not only from the viewpoint of skills and techniques of preparation, packaging, and stability, but also from the viewpoint of patient utilization and physiological availability of the drug from the dosage form. The pharmacist uses his knowledge and appreciation of biological sciences to safeguard the public health by evaluation of the dose of a drug and its interactions with excipients and other medication.

The exercises on the compressed tablet can be used as an example of this philosophy and means of presentation. The section on the manufacture of a compressed tablet is arranged so that the student will prepare a compressed tablet, which he will in subsequent exercises evaluate and coat. The evaluation of the tablet includes not only traditional *in vitro* tests, but also a dissolution test and the urinary recovery technique by which the student determines the biological availability of the drug from his tablet. The tablet is then enteric coated, and the effectiveness of the coating is evaluated by *in vitro* tests and through a urinary recovery technique by a comparison of the biological availability of the drug from the tablet to that from the coated tablet. Thus, the student acquires a total appreciation of the most commonly prescribed dosage form, the compressed tablet. His comprehension includes: the skills and techniques of weighing, blending, milling, and granulation; the familiarization with the equipment used in tabletting; the specifications of tablets and their physical testing; and the *in vivo* evaluation of the bioavailability of the drug from his tablet as it will be used by the patient. By coating the tablets and by *in vitro* and *in vivo* evaluation of the effectiveness of the coating his overall comprehension of the tablet is further expanded.

Sufficient exercises are available so that selections may be made according to the requirements of the individual college. For example, the instructor may use the section on the manufacture of a compressed tablet and the section on suppositories to provide the student with experience in comparing oral and rectal absorption. Or if the instructor prefers, he may use the section on suppositories to demonstrate the effect of the vehicle or base on the release of the medication from a dosage form.

The use of this manual does not presuppose a background in calculus or physical chemistry. A logical outline of presentation is followed according to physical state: solids, solutions, polyphasic systems, and plastic systems. Preparations, as such, are not stressed; however, the traditional pharmaceutical classes are given consideration within their classification by physical state to show their fundamental relationships and similarities.

Laboratory instructions are maintained at a minimum to permit the student to reason, experiment, and apply his theoretical knowledge. When feasible, each exercise has a practical formulation to be developed by the student applying facts or skills gained in previous exercises.

Experience has shown that mathematics are often forgotten by the time a student enters professional training. As an aid to the student, the appendix includes a concise review of the simpler mathematics utilized in the manual. Differentiation is discussed in the appendix with the hope that the concept of a rate of change of a function and limits will be gained by the student.

Spring 1977

E. L. P.
W. S.

CONTENTS

METROLOGY

1. CHARACTERISTICS OF THE PRESCRIPTION BALANCE

Although the mortar and pestle are commonly used as a symbol of pharmacy, the ever-present prescription balance could as appropriately represent pharmacy. As the prescription balance is used daily to weigh vital medicinals, it is imperative that the pharmacist completely understands its characteristics and correct usage.

Balances must meet standards set forth by the National Bureau of Standards. The Class A prescription balance has a sensitivity requirement of 6 mg with no load and with a load of 10 g on each pan. Most Class A balances have a capacity of 120 g and bear a statement to that effect. If no information is given, the nominal capacity of a Class A is assumed to be 15.5 g. The Class A balance should be used for all the weighing operations required in prescription compounding. In order to avoid errors of 5% or more which might be due to the limit of accuracy of the Class A prescription balance, no less than 120 mg of any substance should be weighed.

The Class B Balance has a sensitivity requirement of 30 mg. It is used for weighing larger amounts of drugs but nothing less than 648 mg.

Every prescription counter must have a Class A balance, but the Class B balance is optional and is becoming of less use to the modern practitioner.

PROCEDURE. The Class A prescription balance meets the four tests using metric weights described in the National Formulary, which require that set of analytical weights meet the National Bureau of Standards requirements. Test weights consist of two 20-g, two 10-g, one 1-g, one 500-mg, one 20-mg, one 10-mg, and one 6-mg weights.

Before weighing or testing the balance, level the balance by means of the thumbscrews and adjust the balance to obtain equal swings of the pointer to the right and left or up and down (depending on the type of indicator) or to obtain stoppage or rest with exact alignment of the double pointers. The rider on the graduated beam must be at its zero position at all times during operations, unless otherwise specified.

A. SENSITIVITY REQUIREMENT. The sensitivity requirement is the maximum change in load that will cause a specified change in the position of rest of the indicating element, or elements, of the balance. The smaller the weight required to move the indicator one division, the more sensitive is the balance. The National Formulary calls for a sensitivity requirement of 6 mg for a Class A prescription balance.

1. Level the balance and determine the rest point. The balance lid is to be closed to prevent drafts from affecting the oscillations.
2. Place a 6-mg weight on the right pan. The rest point should not shift less than one division on the indicator scale.
3. Level the balance and determine the rest point with a 10-g weight in the center of each pan.
4. Place a 6-mg weight on the right pan. The rest point should not be shifted less than one division.

Since few, if any, Class C sets of weights include a mass of less than 10 mg, the following practical procedure is suggested:

1. Record the number of scale divisions the index pointer is shifted by a 30-mg, a 20-mg, and a 10-mg weight.
2. Plot the weight against the number of scale divisions shifted by each weight.
3. Draw a straight line through the points, and from the straight line read the weight that will cause a shift of one scale division.
4. Repeat with a 10-g weight on each pan.

B. **ARM RATIO TEST.** The arm ratio test detects errors in the equality of length of the two arms of the balance.

1. Determine the rest point of the balance without any weights on the pans.
2. Place a 30-g weight in the center of each pan and determine the rest point.
3. If the two rest points are different, place a 20-mg weight on the lighter side. If the rest point does not move back to the original place on the index plate or farther, the arm lengths are incorrect and the balance should be repaired.

C. **SHIFT TEST.** The shift test reveals improper arm and lever components of a balance. This series of tests is particularly useful when there has been some abuse of the balance. A balance that does not pass this test should be factory repaired.

1. Determine the rest point without any weights on the pans.
2. Place a 10-g weight in the center of the left pan and another 10-g weight successively toward the right, left, front, and back of the right pan, noting the rest point in each case. If the rest point differs from the rest point without weights, add a 10-mg weight to the lighter side; this should cause the rest point to shift back to the rest point or farther.
3. Place a 10-g weight in the center of the right pan, and place a 10-g weight successively toward the right, left, front, and back of the left pan noting the rest point in each case. If the rest point differs from the rest point without weights, the difference should be overcome by the addition of the 10-mg weight to the lighter side.
4. Make several observations in which both weights are simultaneously shifted to off-center position on their pans, both toward the outside, both toward the inside, one toward the outside and the other toward the inside, both toward the back, and so on until all combinations have been checked. The addition of a 10-mg weight should correct any variation of the rest point from the rest point with no weights on the pan.

D. **RIDER AND GRADUATED BEAM TEST.** The rider and graduated beam test detects improper weighbeam graduations or an improper rider.

1. Determine the rest point for the balance with no weight on the pans.
2. Place a 500-mg weight on the left pan and move the rider to the 500-mg mark. Determine the rest point. If this rest point is different than the rest point with no weights, a 6-mg weight added to the lighter side should bring the rest point back to its original position or farther.
3. Place a 1-g weight on the left pan and move the rider to the 1-g position. If the rest point is different than the rest point with no weights on the pan, it should be brought back to at least zero rest point by the addition of a 6-mg weight to the lighter pan.

REFERENCES

Goldstein, S. W. and A. M. Mattocks. 1967. Professional equilibrium and compounding accuracy. American Pharmaceutical Association, Washington, D.C.

The National Formulary, 14th ed. 1975, p. 1036.

National Bureau of Standards Handbook 44. 4th ed. 1971. U.S. Government Printing Office, Washington, D.C.

Characteristics of the Prescription Balance

Data and Conclusions Balance No.____

1. Sensitivity Requirement.

   How many divisions is the rest point shifted by 6 mg with no load?

   How many divisions is the rest point shifted by 6 mg with a 10 g load?

   What is the sensitivity requirement of the balance?

   If the alternative procedure was followed, do the two curves coincide?

2. Arm Ratio Test.

   Does 20 mg overcome the rest point difference?

3. Shift Test.

   Does 10 mg overcome the rest point difference when:

   a. the right weight is shifted?

   b. the left weight is shifted?

   c. both weights are shifted?

4. Rider and Weighbeam Test.

   Does 6 mg overcome the rest point difference with:

   a. 500 mg?

   b. 1 g?

2. USE OF THE PRESCRIPTION BALANCE

The pharmacist must not only maintain a proper prescription balance, but he must employ the correct weighing technique and be conscious of the limitations of the balance for the particular quantity of drug to be weighed.

Medicinal substances are weighed on powder papers. The paper protects the pans from chemical action and eliminates the need for repeated washing of the pans. A new paper for each item prevents contamination. Another advantage to utilizing a paper is that it serves as a transfer funnel.

Weighing papers should have a glazed surface so that no appreciable amount of the drug will adhere to the paper. This is especially important when small quantities are to be weighed. A paper should be chosen so it is of reasonable size giving a maximum weighing area without touching any part of the balance except the pan. The papers should be creased diagonally from each corner to the opposite corner and then flattened before placing on the pans. If desired, tared watch glasses may be used on the balance pans instead of papers.

WEIGHING TECHNIQUE. Place the creased papers on the balance pans and adjust the balance by means of the leveling screws so the index pointer is at zero. It is an inviolable rule that before compounding any prescription the balance must be adjusted in this manner. Powder papers taken from the same box can vary in weight by as much as 65 mg. If equilibrium is not established after the papers are placed on the pans, an error of more than 30% can result in weighing 200 mg of material.

With the balance arrested, open the balance lid and place the desired weights on the right pan and/or the weighbeam. Place the material to be weighed on the left pan, then unlock the balance to observe if too little or too much material was deposited. Using a spatula, remove or add material, arresting the balance each time a transfer is made. When equilibrium is established, the balance should be arrested, the lid closed, and the arrest released to check the equilibrium. The arresting knob is most conveniently operated by the left hand.

When a substance is stated to have weighed a certain quantity, this includes not only the true weight but also the possible excessive or deficient weight by virtue of the sensitivity of the balance. Knowing the sensitivity of the balance, one may calculate the percent of possible error for a given amount to be weighed.

Assuming 5 mg produce a change of one index plate division in the rest point and 200 mg of drug is to be weighed, the actual weight could be between 195-205 mg. The percentage of possible error is calculated by the ratio

$$\frac{5 \text{ mg}}{200 \text{ mg}} = \frac{x\%}{100\%}$$

$$x = 2.5\%$$

Thus, the inherent percentage of error for any given situation may be expressed

$$\text{Percentage of Error} = \frac{\text{Sensitivity Requirement} \times 100}{\text{Quantity Desired}}$$

The same relationship may be used to calculate the smallest amount that can be weighed within a particular permissible percentage of error. Assuming the sensitivity requirement of a balance is 5 mg and the permissible percentage of error is 5%, one may calculate the smallest quantity that can be weighed within this limit of error. A ratio is set up as before

$$\frac{5 \text{ mg}}{x \text{ mg}} = \frac{5\%}{100\%}$$

$$x = 100 \text{ mg}$$

Thus, the smallest amount that can be weighed with a certain permissible percent of error may be expressed

$$\text{Smallest Quantity to be Weighed} = \frac{\text{Sensitivity Requirement} \times 100}{\text{Permissible Percent of Error}}$$

In order to achieve 99% accuracy, that is, to permit a 1% error, the amount weighed must be at least 100 times as great as the sensitivity requirement of the balance: To achieve 90% accuracy or to allow a 10% error, one must weigh at least 10 times as much as the sensitivity requirement of the balance.

ALIQUOT METHOD. An aliquot part may be defined as any part that is contained a whole number of times in a quantity; e.g., 2 is an aliquot part of 10. When the amount of drug is too small to be weighed directly on the balance, the aliquot method of weighing is used. The aliquot method consists of weighing a multiple of the amount desired, of diluting the multiple amount, and of weighing an aliquot of the dilution.

Using a balance with a sensitivity requirement of 5 mg to weigh 15 mg of atropine sulfate with 95% accuracy with lactose as a diluent, one would first select the multiple quantity. Calculate the smallest quantity of the substance that can be weighed with the required accuracy. To ensure an error no greater than 5%, an amount at least 20 times the sensitivity of the balance must be weighed.

$$5 \text{ mg} \times 20 = 100 \text{ mg}$$

This amount is not convenient since 100 divided by 15 is not a whole number; therefore, 14 is arbitrarily chosen as a multiple for convenience and to aid in lowering the total error

$$15 \text{ mg} \times 14 = 210 \text{ mg}$$

Thus, an amount 42 times the sensitivity requirement of the balance is to be weighed. The size of this multiple quantity is determined by the accuracy desired, the convenience of the multiple, the availability of weights, and the cost of the substance.

The amount of inert diluent to be added must be a quantity large enough to be weighed within the desired limit of error. The weight of the aliquot must be at least as much as the multiple quantity, and to reduce the error its weight should usually be somewhat greater. Here the multiple quantity weighs 210 mg, so the aliquot must weigh at least 210 mg. If 500 mg is selected as the aliquot, it is multiplied by the multiple quantity

$$500 \text{ mg} \times 14 = 7{,}000 \text{ mg}$$

Knowing that the total dilution of 7,000 mg will contain 210 mg of atropine sulfate, one can calculate that 6,790 mg of lactose must be added to form the dilution.

Since the total trituration weighing 7,000 mg contains 210 mg of atropine sulfate, a 500-mg aliquot will contain the desired weight of atropine sulfate

$$\frac{210 \text{ mg of atropine sulfate}}{7{,}000 \text{ mg of trituration}} = \frac{x \text{ mg of atropine sulfate}}{500 \text{ mg of trituration}}$$

$$x = 15 \text{ mg}$$

PROCEDURE. When mixing a small amount of a drug with a large amount of a second ingredient, the drug present in the smaller amount is placed in the mortar with an equal bulk of the other ingredient. The two ingredients are triturated until intimately mixed. Then, an equal bulk of the second ingredient is added to the mixture, and the powders are triturated until intimately mixed. This procedure is repeated until all of the powders have been added and thoroughly mixed. Using this procedure, prepare in a glass mortar and submit to the instructor the following triturations:

A. Five grams of a trituration containing 25 mg of charcoal prepared with 95% accuracy. Charcoal has been selected to give visual appreciation of the accuracy of weighing and mixing. Lactose is to be used as a diluent.

B. Weigh 6 mg of amaranth or another colorant assigned by the instructor, using lactose as a diluent so that a 90% accuracy is maintained. Add sufficient lactose so that the final trituration will weigh 6 g.

REFERENCES

Lesshafft, C. T., Jr. 1965. The development and use of equations for determining the percentage of error in compounding. Am. J. Pharm. Ed. 29:125.

Lindstrom, R. E. 1971. Compounding accuracy. In Dispensing of medication, E. W. Martin, Ed., 7th ed., Chap. 2. Mack Publishing Company, Easton, Pa. p. 47.

Lowenthal, W. and S. W. Goldstein. 1975. Weighing and measuring. In Remington's Pharmaceutical sciences, 15th ed., Chap. 9. Mack Publishing Company, Easton, Pa. p. 83.

Plein, E. M. 1970. Aliquot method of weighing and measuring. In Prescription pharmacy, J. B. Sprowls, Ed., 2nd ed., J. B. Lippincott Co., Philadelphia. p. 21.

Rowles, B. 1974. The pharmacist as compounder and consultant. Drug Intelligence and Clinical Pharmacy, 8:242.

Stoklosa, M. J. 1974. Pharmaceutical calculations, 6th ed., Lea and Febiger, Philadelphia. p. 34.

Wertheimer, A. I., C. Ritchko, and D. W. Dougherty. 1973. Prescription accuracy: Room for improvement. Medical Care, 11:68.

Use of the Prescription Balance

Data and Conclusions

1. Show the calculations made in preparing the charcoal trituration.

2. Show calculations for B.

3. Why is lactose the most commonly used diluent in aliquots, divided powders, and capsules?

4. Why is the balance arrested at each transfer during the process of weighing?

5. Why was a glass mortar and pestle used in A?

6. To achieve 95% accuracy the amount to be weighed must be how many times as great as the sensitivity requirement of the balance?

7. Is the aliquot method used only with dry ingredients?

8. What is the smallest quantity that can be weighed with a potential error of not more than 4% on a balance with a sensitivity requirement of 2 mg?

9. A pharmacist attempts to weigh 10 mg of atropine on a balance having a sensitivity requirement of 30 mg. Calculate the error involved and comment.

10. Using a balance with a sensitivity requirement of 10 mg, show calculations made to compound the prescription with 95% accuracy.

Rx	Digitoxin		0.002
	Lactose	q. s.	0.300

Make powders. Send such doses X

3. MEASUREMENT OF PHARMACEUTICAL LIQUIDS

To accurately and rapidly measure liquids the pharmacist should have graduates, burets, and graduated pipets from which to select the proper measuring vessel.

Cylindrical graduates are preferred to conical graduates, for the smaller the diameter at the measuring point, the greater the degree of accuracy obtained. The National Conference on Weights and Measures developed the following specifications for pharmaceutical graduates:

1. Graduates of a capacity of 4 drams and less may be graduated in only one scale – English or metric, not both.
2. A graduate of 1/2-ounce capacity (4 drams) or less, must be cylindrical in shape. Graduates larger than 1/2 ounce may be cylindrical or conical in shape.
3. The initial graduation (lowest graduation marking) on all graduates must be not less than 1/5 or more than 1/4 of the nominal capacity of the graduate.
4. The metric graduates will more closely follow a true metric volume system. There will be 25-, 50-, and 100-ml graduates instead of the obsolete 30-, 60-, and 125-ml graduate.

The portions of graduated cylinders that should not be used for measuring based upon a deviation of ±1 mm from the mark with allowable errors of 2.5 and 5%, are given in the following table.

Size of Cylinder, cc	Internal Diameter, cm	Deviation, cc	Min. Vol. Giving 2.5% Error, cc	Part of Cylinder not Useful, %	Min. Vol. Giving 5% Error, cc	Part of Cylinder not Useful, %
5	0.98	0.075	3.00	60	1.50	30
10	1.18	0.109	4.36	44	2.18	22
25	1.94	0.296	11.84	48	5.92	24
50	2.24	0.394	15.76	32	7.88	16
100	2.58	0.522	20.88	22	10.44	11
250	3.40	0.908	36.32	16	18.16	7
500	4.60	1.660	66.40	9	33.20	7

(From Goldstein, S. W. and A. M. Mattocks. 1967. Professional equilibrium and compounding accuracy. American Pharmaceutical Association, Washington, D.C. p. 13.)

The proper choice of a vessel is the first factor to consider in measuring a liquid; obviously a fraction of a milliliter cannot be correctly measured in a graduate. The vessel must be the correct type, be clean, and have the correct graduation.

The liquid will contribute to an error in measuring when the surface tension and density are different than that of water as the meniscus volume is altered. The volume above the horizontal tangent touching the lowest point of the surface is the meniscus volume. With an opaque liquid, difficulty may be experienced in reading the lowest point of the surface. Viscous liquids have a longer drainage time, and the liquid clinging to the surface of the measure will produce considerable error.

Errors in measuring may be made by the operator if he tilts the measure or fails to align the graduation mark and the bottom of the meniscus (parallax effect). Failure to perceive the true bottom of the meniscus is a common source of error when the meniscus is viewed against a uniformly lighted background. Under these circumstances the surface becomes almost imperceptible and the lower edge of a band reflection may be mistaken for the bottom of the meniscus although it is, in fact, well above this level. This phenomenon may cause a 5% error when measuring 60 minims of water in a 2-dram conical graduate. A suitable background consists of a broad black band on a piece of white painted board or a card affixed to the prescription counter at eye level. The surface of the liquid reflects the darker surface and enables the true bottom of the meniscus to be clearly seen.

For measuring volumes which are too small to be measured in a graduate, 1-ml pipets graduated in 0.01 and 0.1 ml increments are useful. If a small volume of liquid is to be measured in a pharmacy where no pipet is available, one may calibrate a dropper for measuring small volumes. The calibration is done by counting the drops added to a graduate until a measurable volume has accumulated in the graduate. Although adequate, this method is tedious; procurement of a pipet would save valuable time, both in measuring and in washing the equipment.

The pharmacopeial medicine dropper is constricted at the delivery end to a round opening having an external diameter of 3 mm. A vertically positioned pharmacopeial medicine dropper delivers a drop of water weighing between 45 and 55 mg. In using droppers the pharmacist must realize that a drop is not a unit of volume as the volume of a drop delivered from the same dropper depends on the liquid. For a given dropper, the volume of a drop varies as a function of the pressure applied and the temperature, and as the function of the density, viscosity, and surface tension of the liquid delivered.

PROCEDURE. Prescriptions consisting of several liquids should not be compounded in prescription bottles, but they must be accurately measured in a suitable graduate. To avoid the use of the inaccurate graduations on prescription bottles, it is desirable to use ungraduated prescription bottles.

A. Fill a 3-ounce prescription bottle with water to the 90-ml mark. Transfer the contents of the bottle to a 100-ml cylindrical graduate. Record the volume.

B. Observe the parallax effect with the graduate containing water. Read the measuring level against a uniformly lighted background. Compare this with the reading against the black band on a white paper placed just below the meniscus.

C. Holding a medicine dropper vertically, count the number of drops required to fill a 10-ml cylindrical graduate to the 3-ml mark.

D. Repeat C, holding the dropper at a 20° angle.

E. Holding a medicine dropper vertically, count the number of drops of alcohol required to fill a 10-ml cylindrical graduate to the 3-ml mark.

F. Prepare a 1% solution of the sodium lauryl sulfate or the surfactant provided. Holding the dropper vertically, count the number of drops required to fill a 10-ml cylindrical graduate to the 3-ml mark.

G. Heat the surfactant solution to 70°. Using this warm solution, repeat F.

H. Dispense the following using a 10-ml and a 100-ml cylindrical graduate.

Gentian Violet Solution	0.25 ml
Distilled water qs ad	90 ml

REFERENCES

Capper, K. R., D. B. Cowell, and J. A. Thomas. 1955. The measurement of liquids—An examination of some causes of error. Pharm. J. 175:241.

Freeman, L. A. 1955. The optical properties of the meniscus. Pharm. J. 175:256.

Lesshafft, C. T., Jr. and L. E. Sykes. 1965. Determining the volume deviation in measuring. J. Am. Pharm. Assoc., NS 5:643.

National Bureau of Standards Circular 602. April, 1959.

Scattergood, G. M. 1958. Standards for Rx glassware. J. Am. Pharm. Assoc., Pract. Ed. 19:36.

The National Formulary, 14th ed. 1975. Mack Publishing Co., Easton, Pa., p. 1037.

The United States Pharmacopeia, 19th rev. 1975. Mack Publishing Co., Easton, Pa., p. 694.

Measurement of Pharmaceutical Liquids

Data and Conclusions

1. When measured in a proper graduate, what volume did the 3-ounce prescription bottle actually hold at the 90-ml mark?

2. By means of a diagram, explain what is meant by "parallax effect."

3. Compare the meniscus reading with a uniformly lighted background versus a background of a black band on a white paper.

4. For ______________ dropper complete the following table:
(type of)

Procedure	Number of Drops in 3 ml
Water, vertical dropper	
Water, oblique dropper	
Alcohol, vertical dropper	
1%____________________solution	
1%____________________solution at 70°	

5. Briefly, how should surface tension, temperature, and position of the dropping tube affect the size of a drop delivered from a particular dropper? Compare with experimental results.

6. Show the calculations by which you obtained the desired amount of gentian violet solution by the aliquot method using a 10-ml and 100-ml graduate in H.

7. Calculate the smallest amount of liquid one could measure in a 100-ml cylindrical graduate with an allowable error of ±5%. The internal diameter of the cylinder is 2.58 cm. Assume the true meniscus can be read with a deviation of ± 1 mm. Compare your calculation with the table on page 12.

SOLIDS

4. CHARACTERISTICS OF PARTICLES

The reduction of particle size of drugs is important in pharmacy. Not only do small particles of various solid drugs mix to form a more uniform dose than larger particles, but properties of the drug itself are modified by a reduction in particle size.

As the particles of a drug are reduced in size there is a more rapid release of the drug from the solid, because with smaller particle size there is a greater specific surface area. The dissolution of a given weight of a drug is directly proportional to the surface area. Thus, an increase in area causes more rapid solution, which is followed by increased absorption from the gastrointestinal tract. This is especially important with sparingly soluble drugs, such as the corticosteroid and sulfa drugs. Microcrystalline sulfadiazine given orally appears more rapidly and in higher concentrations in the blood than ordinary sulfadiazine powder. The experimental results shown in Figure 1 are actually due to an increase in exposed surface. It has been demonstrated that 0.5 g of microcrystalline griseofulvin produced blood concentrations equal to or higher than 1.0 g doses of regular griseofulvin. A high fat diet administered with microcrystalline griseofulvin will more than double the blood concentration.

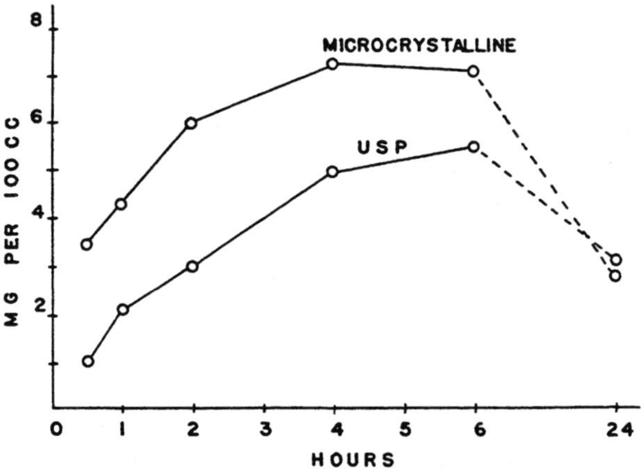

Figure 1 — Serum levels of sulfadiazine and microcrystalline sulfadiazine after oral administration of 3 g to humans, showing that a higher serum level is obtained when the drug has a smaller particle size (J. G. Reinhold, F. J. Phillips, H. F. Flippin, and L. Pollack: Am. J. Med. Sci., 210, 141, 1945).

The effect of particle size on plasma concentration of phenacetin is shown in Figure 2 for fine (< 75 μm), medium (150-180 μm), and coarse (> 250 μm) particles. The fine particles produce the greatest plasma concentration followed in decreasing order by medium and coarse particles. The addition of 0.1% Polysorbate 80 to the fine particles increased the plasma concentration of phenacetin presumably due to the surface-active agent wetting the particles to provide a greater effective surface from which dissolution could occur.

The plasma concentration of phenacetin at any time is the resultant of the simultaneous processes of dissolution, absorption, tissue equilibrium and metabolism by the hepatic microsomal enzymes since negligible phenacetin appears in the urine. The major metabolite of phenacetin is N-acetyl-p-aminophenol. Although the concentration of N-acetyl-p-aminophenol in the plasma indicates a less marked difference between the fine, medium and coarse particles, the plasma concentrations as shown in Figure 3 are related in the same order to the size of the particles as the unmetabolized drug.

The effect of particle size upon solution and absorption has also been demonstrated with novobiocin. When the crystalline acid form of novobiocin is given orally, practically no absorption occurs as indicated by blood levels. If this antibiotic is micronized or precipitated in a finely divided, amorphous form, it becomes an orally effective drug. As the sodium and calcium salts of novobiocin are water soluble and have a rapid dissolution rate, their particle size does not significantly influence plasma concentration.

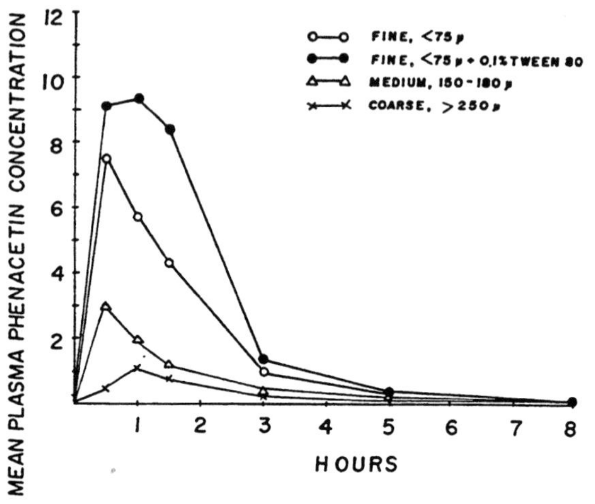

Figure 2 — Mean concentration in μg/ml of phenacetin in plasma of six adult volunteers following the administration of 1.5 g doses of phenacetin in different ranges of particle size (L. F. Prescott, R. F. Steel, and W. R. Ferrier: Clin. Pharmacol. Ther., 11, 496, 1970).

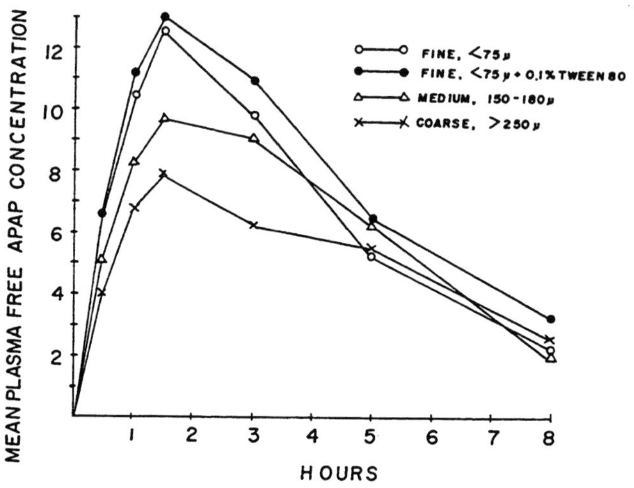

Figure 3 — Mean concentration in μg/ml of N-acetyl-p-aminophenol in plasma of six volunteers receiving 1.5 g doses of phenacetin in different ranges of particle size (L. F. Prescott, R. F. Steel, and W. R. Ferrier: Clin. Pharmacol. Ther., 11, 496, 1970).

The dissolution of a sparingly soluble drug is the rate determining step in drug absorption, and it is proportional to the product of the surface area and the solubility of the drug. In the intelligent formulation of solid dosage forms it is important that the pharmacist mill the medicinal compound to the optimum size and that for weak acids and bases he select an appropriate salt of the drug or blend the drug with buffer adjuvants.

A drug should not be micronized unless there is a reason for micronization. Nitrofurantoin may produce nausea and vomiting when administered orally. Capsules containing macrocrystals of nitrofurantoin were administered to 112 patients, who had experienced nausea and vomiting after the administration of tablets prepared using fine crystals. No symptoms of gastric upset occurred in 89 patients receiving the macrocrystals. Nitrofurantoin in macrocrystalline form is absorbed slower than the finer crystals. There is an optimum crystal size (approximately 150 μm), which reduces emesis, while still permitting ample urinary excretion for therapeutic efficacy.

Under controlled conditions insulin and zinc react to form a complex used in insulin suspensions for subcutaneous injection. The size of the particles of the complex may be controlled by the pH at which complexation occurs. Commercial products available contain large or small sized particles, which provide a slow onset and prolonged activity or a fast onset and a shorter period of activity, respectively.

The outstanding characteristic arising from reduction of particle size is the tremendous increase in surface area. A cube with an edge of 1 cm, when cut in half in three directions, will form eight cubes, each having an edge of 0.5 cm and a total surface of 12 cm^2. If such a cube were cut into 1000 cubes with an edge of 1 mm, the total surface area would be 60 cm^2. If the size of the cubes could be reduced to an edge of 1 micron, the total surface would be 60,000 cm^2 or 6 m^2. It is this large surface area which imparts special properties.

Thermodynamic calculations based on surface energy of particles indicate that by reducing particle size, the solubility may be increased. If d_2 is the diameter of a small particle and d_1 is the diameter of a large particle, the relative solubility of the two particles may be expressed

$$(1 - \alpha + n\alpha)\frac{RT}{M}\ln\frac{S_2}{S_1} = \frac{4\sigma}{\rho}\left(\frac{1}{d_2} - \frac{1}{d_1}\right)$$

where α is the degree of dissociation, n the number of ions from one molecule of molecular weight M, R the gas constant (8.31×10^7 erg deg^{-1} $mole^{-1}$), T the absolute temperature, ρ the density, and σ the surface energy (erg cm^{-2}).

Consider at room temperature a nondissociating substance with a molecular weight of 150 g $mole^{-1}$ and a density of 2.3 g cc^{-1}. If a particle with a diameter of 10^{-4} cm has a surface energy of erg cm^{-2}, one may calculate the reduction in particle size necessary to increase the solubility 10%. As no dissociation occurs the relationship becomes

$$2.3 \frac{RT}{M} \log \frac{S_2}{S_1} = \frac{4\sigma}{\rho} \left(\frac{1}{d_2} - \frac{1}{d_1} \right)$$

Substituting, one obtains

$$\frac{2.3 \times 8.31 \times 10^7 \times 298}{150} \log 1.1 = \frac{4 \times 50}{2.3} \left(\frac{1}{d_2} - \frac{1}{10^{-4}} \right)$$

which contains only one unknown d_2, which can be readily calculated.

A particle of 10^{-4} cm has a small surface energy; a particle must be in the order of 10^{-6} cm before it has appreciable surface energy. As the reality of this phenomenon is evident only in the colloidal range, for practical purposes solubility remains unchanged with a change in particle size.

Color may be affected by particle size. Upon prolonged trituration in a mortar, red mercury oxide is reduced in size to yellow mercury oxide. Hyperfine zinc oxide is red in color and has a diameter of 0.02 μm. A dental cement composed of red zinc oxide and eugenol sets much faster than other cements because of the enhanced activity resulting from the huge specific surface area.

The practicing pharmacist commonly uses sieves for making certain that the particle size has been properly reduced. The size of the sieve is expressed in mesh which refers to the number of openings per linear inch. Obviously the size of the openings varies with the diameter of the wire composing the screen; therefore, specifications for the U. S. Standard Sieves have been established by the National Bureau of Standards (see Appendix: Standard Sieves).

PROCEDURE. The particles of a powdered substance may appear of uniform size to the naked eye, yet there is a wide variation in the size of the particles. Most of the particles will fall within a narrow range about the average particle size, but there will be some much larger and some much smaller. The percent frequencies of the various particles plotted against the mean of a group size forms a "size frequency" curve. By examining such a curve, one can determine if a pharmaceutical unit, such as an injectable suspension, has been reduced to the proper state of subdivision. An average of the particles would not indicate if the particles were adequately reduced, as there could be an equal number of very large particles and very small particles which would produce the desired average size, yet the size would not be clinically acceptable.

Complex and varied means have been employed to obtain size-frequency curves. A simple method employing U. S. Standard Sieves may be used to obtain a weight-size distribution curve and to permit calculation of the average particle size.

When fine material is passed through two sieves, the size of the material retained on the sieve with the smaller openings is usually taken as the arithmetic or geometric mean of the openings of the two screens. Actually the material varies as to size, and the arithmetic or geometric mean of the openings does not indicate the true mean size of the material. Particles of a given size may be found on several sieves. However, by using a uniform procedure and treatment of data, a valid distribution curve may be obtained as the particles are actually classified in subgroups with a limited range of size. It is important that the size of the openings upon which the diameter of the particle is based be defined, such as the opening of the smaller size, as the arithmetic mean or as the geometric mean of two adjacent sieves.

A. Triturate 100 g of granular boric acid in a mortar for exactly one minute. Place the material in the upper sieve of a Tyler or Cenco-Meinzer Sieve Shaker, which will provide a vibratory motion that is most efficient for passing material through a sieve. Allow the powder to be classified for five minutes. Quantitatively remove, weigh, and record the amount of powder retained on each sieve.

B. Using the same shaker, repeat the above procedure after triturating the powder exactly ten minutes. A uniform shaking for the same period of time should be used throughout both procedures.

For larger particles the most rapid and simplest method of determining particle-size distribution is sieving. The sieve analysis can be completed in a short time and does not involve any special skill on the part of the operator. The sieve method is limited to particles larger than 50 microns because of the difficulty of weaving wire cloth having uniform openings of such small sizes. With the recent available micromesh sieves, the range of sieve analysis may be extended as low as 10 microns.

For subsieve particles a sedimentation method may be used to obtain a weight-size distribution curve and to permit calculation of the average particle size. The sedimentation method is based on the dependence of the velocity of sedimentation on size of the particles as expressed by the Stokes equation

$$v = \frac{x}{t} = \frac{d^2 (\rho - \rho_0) g}{18 \eta}$$

or

$$d = \sqrt{\frac{18 \eta \quad x}{(\rho - \rho_0) g \, t}}$$

where v is the velocity of sedimentation in cm sec^{-1}, x is the distance of fall in cm in time t in sec, d is the mean diameter in cm of the particle based on velocity of sedimentation, ρ is the density of the particle, ρ_0 is the density of the dispersion medium, g is the acceleration of gravity, and η is the viscosity in poises of the dispersion medium. The Stokes equation is applicable to free-falling spheres that are falling at a constant rate. If the concentration of the suspension does not exceed 2%, the particles do not interact and fall independent of one another.

Measurement of subsieve size may be carried out in an Andreasen pipet, shown in Figure 4. The apparatus consists of a 550-ml glass cylinder graduated from 0 to 20 cm. The cylinder is provided with a ground-glass stopper through which a pipet stem passes. The tip of the 10-ml pipet is at the level of the zero mark on the scale. The pipet is provided with a 2-way stopcock through which a 10-ml sample may be slowly aspirated and then drained into a tared evaporating vessel.

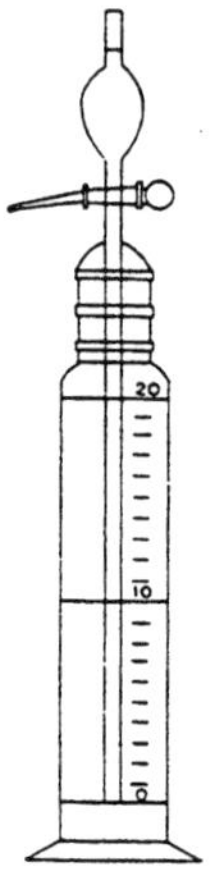

Figure 4 — Andreasen pipet for determination of particle size by a sedimentation technique.

The powder to be analyzed is weighed on an analytical balance, placed in the cylinder, shaken with the dispersion medium, and brought to the 20-cm mark. The apparatus is shaken for 2 minutes and placed in a position in which it will not be disturbed. Ten-milliliter samples are withdrawn at given time intervals without distrubing the suspension. The samples are evaporated to dryness and weighed. Approximately 20 seconds are required for withdrawing each sample.

The particle diameter corresponding to each time interval is calculated from the Stokes equation, with x being the height of the liquid above the lower end of the pipet at time t when each sample is removed. From the weight of the dried sample the percentage by weight of the initial suspension is calculated for particles having sizes smaller that the size calculated by the Stokes equation for that time. The weight of each sample residue is called the weight undersize. It may be expressed as weight or percent of total weight of the final sediment. On a probability scale the cumulative percents by weight undersize may be plotted against particle diameters on a logarithmic scale, and statistical diameters may be calculated by use of the Hatch-Choate equations.

C. Determine the size frequency distribution of magnesium hydroxide or another powder assigned by the instructor by use of the Andreasen pipet. For each time period record the height of the liquid above the lower end of the pipet and the weight of the residue from each sample after it has been dried.

D. Place 1 g lump alum or cupric sulfate in a bottle. Add 90 ml of water and stopper. Observe the time it requires for complete solution. Agitate the solution in a uniform manner by inverting the bottle every minute until solution is complete.

E. Triturate some alum or cupric sulfate to a fine powder. Weigh 1 g and place in a bottle; add 90 ml of water and stopper. Agitate and observe the time required for complete solution.

It is desirable to have free-flowing particles in many pharmaceutical processes and products. A dusting powder should be free-flowing so that it will readily spread when it is applied. Tablet granulations should be free-flowing so that they will uniformly flow from the hopper to the die cavity of the tablet machine and will produce tablets of constant weight. A tablet lubricant is often added to facilitate such a flow. Powders with high interparticular friction cannot be filled into containers by automatic filling devices.

The flowability of a powder depends on the number of points of contact or the frictional forces between the particles. With rough and irregular particles the frictional force is increased and the powder does not flow as readily. Flowability is also a function of particle size. The frictional force may be expressed in terms of the angle of repose. The angle of repose is the maximum angle possible between the surface of a pile of powder and the horizontal plane. Figure 5 shows an apparatus used to measure the angle of repose. The powder or granulation is placed in the funnel centered over a fixed circular vessel, e.g., a shallow petri dish of known radius r. The powder is discharged from the funnel until the circumference of the circular vessel is touched by the pile of powder formed. At this point the height, h, from the apex of the conical pile to the horizontal surface, is measured. Knowing these two values, the angle of repose may be calculated (see Appendix: Trigonometric Terms).

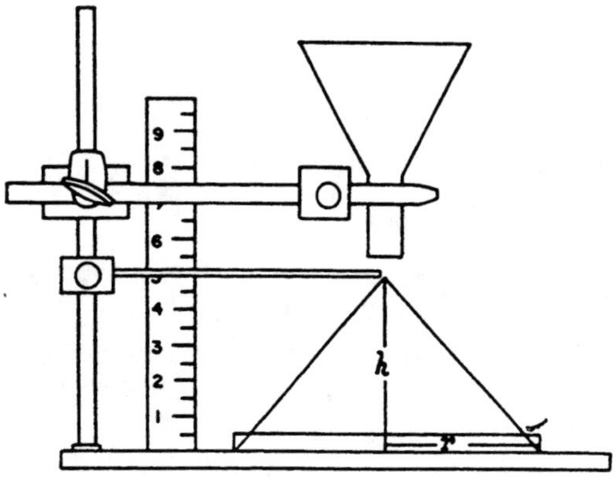

Figure 5 – Apparatus for measuring the angle of repose.

$$\tan \phi = \frac{h}{r}$$

The flowability of a powder or granulation may be expressed as a rate of flow. Since pharmaceutical processes are concerned with the actual movement of particulate systems in mechanical equipment, the rate of flow is more meaningful than the static property characterized by the angle of repose. Figure 6 shows a simple apparatus used to measure rate of flow. The flowmeter consists of a stainless steel column with a circular orifice from 3/8" to 1/2" in diameter. A shutter is held in position in the guide track by means of a spring. When the shutter is pulled, the material flows from the orifice into a tared vessel. The interval that the shutter is open is timed. The material that has flowed in this interval is weighed. The rate of flow is expressed in g sec^{-1}.

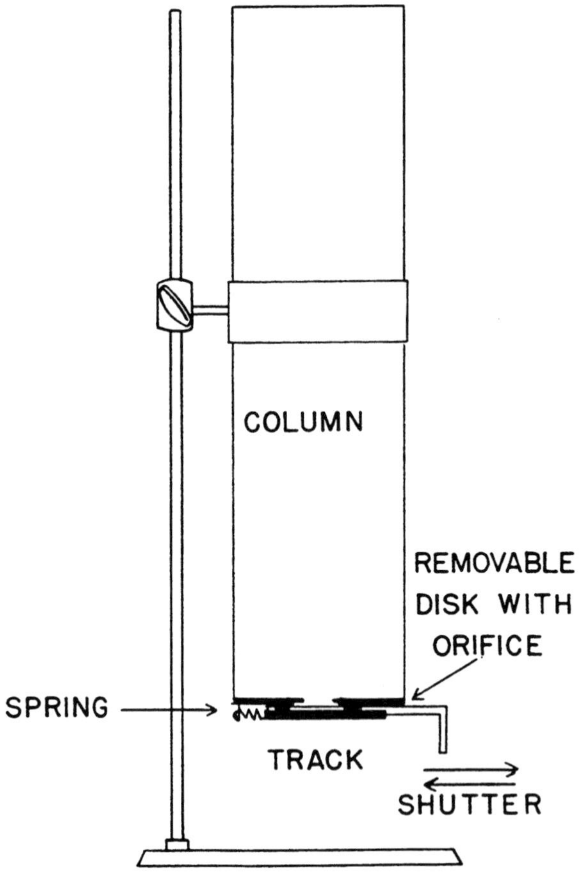

Figure 6 — Flowmeter for measuring rate of flow of powders and granules.

F. Measure and record the angle of repose and the rate of flow of a larger particle (10/20) and a smaller particle (100/140). Clean the equipment after each measurement.

G. Measure and record the angle of repose and the rate of flow of a powder or granulation provided by the instructor. Measure and record the angle of repose and the rate of flow of the same powder or granulation in which 1% magnesium stearate has been blended by the instructor. Clean the equipment after each measurement.

If a powder is placed in a cylindrical graduate, the volume occupied is defined as the bulk volume V_b. If the powder is nonporous (has no internal pores or capillary space), the bulk volume consists of the true volume of the solid particles plus the volume of the void between the particles. The percent porosity of the powder is defined as

$$\text{Porosity} = 100\left(\frac{V_b - V}{V_b}\right) = 100\left(1 - \frac{V}{V_b}\right)$$

The determination of the volume of particles containing internal pores, capillary spaces and microscopic cracks is difficult. The true density ρ is the weight per unit volume excluding the entire pore volume larger than the spacings of molecular or atomic dimensions that exist in the crystal lattice of the solid. The apparent or bulk density ρ_a is obtained by dividing the weight of the sample by the bulk volume. Substituting the densities into the above equation,

$$\text{Porosity} = 100\left(1 - \frac{\rho_a}{\rho}\right)$$

H. Determine the porosity of magnesium carbonate or talc. Weigh a sample of the drug having a volume of approximately 90 ml. Place the sample in a 100-ml graduated cylinder and drop the cylinder onto a wood surface three times from a height of approximately 2 cm. Record the volume and the weight of the sample. Calculate the apparent density of the powder.

REFERENCES

Cole, E. T., P. H. Elworthy, and H. Sucker. 1974. Determination of the flow properties of powders by means of a flow balance. J. Pharm. Pharmacol., 26, Suppl., 57P.

Conn, J., W. Humphrey, J. Magee, and W. Wallace. 1956. Zinc oxide hyperfine: Preparation and properties. J. Am. Pharm. Assoc., Sci. Ed. 45:311.

Dallavalle, J. M. 1948. Micromeritics, 2nd ed. Pitman Publishing Co., New York. Chap. 5 and 12.

Danish, F. Q. and E. L. Parrott. 1971. Flow rates of some solid particulate pharmaceuticals. J. Pharm. Sci. 60:548.

Edmundson, I. C. 1967. Particle-size analysis. In H. S. Bean, A. H. Beckett, and J. E. Carless, Advances in pharmaceutical sciences, Vol. 2. Academic Press, Inc., New York. p. 95.

Fincher, J. H. 1968. Particle size of drugs and its relationship to absorption and activity. J. Pharm. Sci. 57:1825.

Haleblian, J. and W. McCrone. 1969. Pharmaceutical applications of polymorphism. J. Pharm. Sci., 58:911.

Harwood, C. F. and N. Pilpel. 1968. Rotational viscometer for powder and granules. Laboratory Practice, 17:1236.

Irani, R. R. and C. F. Callis. 1963. Particle size: Measurement, interpretation, and application. John Wiley & Sons, Inc., New York.

Kelly, J. J. 1970. The kinetic angle of repose of powders. J. Soc. Cosm. Chem., 21:37.

Martin, A. N., J. Swarbrick, and A. Cammarata. 1969. Physical pharmacy, 2nd ed. Lea and Febiger, Philadelphia. Chap. 17.

Nelson, E. 1955. Measurement of the repose angle of a tablet granulation. J. Am. Pharm. Assoc., Sci. Ed. 44:435.

Neumann, B. S. 1967. The flow properties of powders. In Advances in pharmaceutical sciences, H. S. Bean, A. H. Beckett, and J. B. Carless, Eds., Vol. 2. Academic Press, Inc., New York. p. 181.

Notari, R. E. 1976. Biopharmaceutics and pharmacokinetics, 2nd ed. Marcel Dekker, Inc. New York.

Parrott, E. L. 1966. Student experiments in pharmaceutical technology. II. Flowability of powders. Am. J. Pharm. Ed. 30:205.

Parrott, E. L. 1975. Influence of particle size on rectal absorption of aspirin. J. Pharm. Sci., 64:878.

Parrott, E. L. and A. M. Salpekar. 1966. Student experiments in pharmaceutical technology. I. Particle size distribution measurements. Am. J. Pharm. Educ. 30:196.

Parrott, E. L., D. E. Wurster, and T. Higuchi. 1955. Some factors influencing the dissolution rate. J. Am. Pharm. Assoc., Sci. Ed. 44:269.

Paul, H. E., K. J. Hayes, M. F. Paul, and A. R. Borgmann. 1967. Laboratory studies with nitrofurantoin: Relationship between crystal size, urinary excretion in the rat and man, and emesis in dogs. J. Pharm. Sci., 56:882.

Prescott, L. F., R. F. Steel, and W. R. Ferrier. 1970. The effects of particle size on the absorption of phenacetin in man. Clinical Pharmacology and Therapeutics, 11:496.

Reinhold, J. G., F. J. Phillips, H. F. Flippin, and L. Pollack. 1945. Comparison of the behavior of microcrystalline sulfadiazine with that of ordinary sulfadiazine. Am. J. Med. Sci. 210:141.

Simond, A., K. Linquist, F. Tendick, and R. Rowe. 1950. The effect of crystal size on the estrogenic activity of theelin. J. Am. Pharm. Assoc., Sci. Ed. 39:52.

Smith, E. A. 1970. Very fine particles. J. Soc. Cosm. Chem., 21:563.

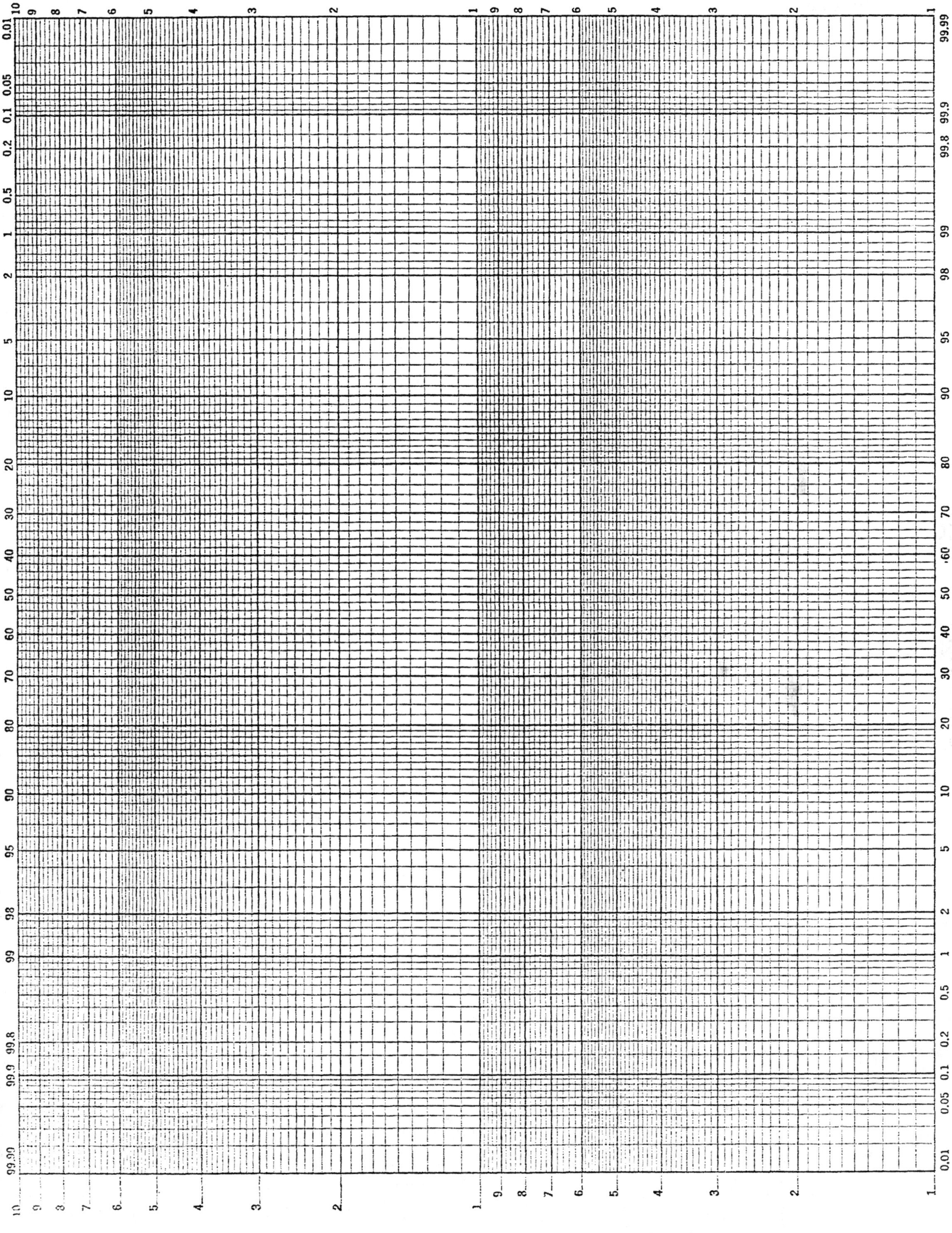

0.01 0.05 0.1 0.2 0.5 1 2 5 10 20 30 40 50 60 70 80 90 95 98 99 99.8 99.9 99.99
99.99 99.9 99.8 99 98 95 90 80 70 60 50 40 30 20 10 5 2 1 0.5 0.2 0.1 0.05 0.01
10 9 8 7 6 5 4 3 2 1 9 8 7 6 5 4 3 2 1

Characteristics of Particles

Data and Conclusions

1. Complete the following table:

Sieve Number (Passed/Retained)	Particle Size, μm	Weight Retained, g	Per Cent Retained	Cumulative Per Cent
A.				
B.				

2. Calculate the average diameter of the entire powder in A and B (see Appendix: Particle Size).

$$\text{Average Diameter} = \frac{\Sigma\ (\text{Percent Retained} \times \text{Average Size})}{100} = \frac{\Sigma\ (\text{Weight Size})}{100}$$

3. Plot the percent retained as the ordinate versus the mean arithmetic particle size for each group.

4. By graphic means determine the median particle size of the powder in A and B.

5. Is a size frequency distribution or an average diameter more valuable in characterizing solid particles in a pharmaceutical? Why?

6. Explain the difference in time required to dissolve a given weight of alum or cupric sulfate in lumps and in powdered form.

7. Record the following data for C and give a sample calculation:

Density of the dispersion medium: | Density of solid:

Viscosity of the dispersion medium: | Temperature:

Initial concentration of suspension:

Time, sec	Height, cm	Weight of Pan and Residue, g	Weight of Pan, g	Weight of Residue, g	Weight Per Cent Residue of Initial Suspension	Stokes Diameter, μm

8. Plot the percentages by weight smaller than the stated size on the ordinate axis versus the particle size calculated using the Stokes equation. What is the median diameter?

9. On logarithm-probability paper plot the percentage smaller than the stated size versus the particle size. Give the values for the geometric mean diameter and the standard deviation.

10. Terramycin Oral Pediatric Drops consist of a vial containing a dry powder to which a certain amount of water is added to form a solution. Of what importance is the particle size of such a product?

11. Inhalation therapy is the administration by the respiratory system of medicinals which are in the form of fine solid or liquid particles. How is the clinical usefulness affected by the size of the particles?

12. Explain the difference in duration of action of Semi-Lente Iletin, Ultra-Lente Iletin, and Lente Iletin.

13. Record the angle of repose and rate of flow of the small and the large particles in F. What effect did the particle size have on the angle of repose and rate of flow?

14. In G compare the angle of repose and the rate of flow of the material before and after the addition of the magnesium stearate. What does this comparison indicate in terms of the flowability of the powder?

15. Define apparent density. What is the apparent density of the powder in H?

16. Calculate the porosity of the powder in H.

5. REDUCTION OF PARTICLE SIZE

The practicing pharmacist commonly reduces particle size by triturating a substance in a mortar with a pestle. Although small mills may be obtained, they generally are not available to the community pharmacist.

After primary cutting or crushing, mechanical subdivision is accomplished industrially by hammer, attrition, or high-speed mills. The hammer mill consists of a number of rigid or swinging hammers which by impact break up the particles. The attrition mill consists of two grinding plates which rotate in opposite directions or one which rotates against a stationary plate. The grinding chamber of a high-speed impact mill consists of a high-speed rotor, which by centrifugal force advances the material toward the periphery, where by impact against various beaters and teeth on the grinding rings of the inner face of the mill, the particle size is rapidly reduced.

Drugs to be used in the solid state for insufflation, parenteral, or ophthalmic use, such as antibiotics and steroids, must be of very fine size ranging from 1-5 microns. Comminution may be carried out at low temperatures to facilitate fracture and passage of the particles; proteins and methylcellulose are reduced in size at low temperatures.

Minute particle size has been attained experimentally by various applications of spray drying, freeze drying, ultrasonic, and impingement techniques; however, these methods have as yet found only limited acceptance commercially.

PROCEDURE. Dusting powders are very fine medicinal powders intended to be dusted on the skin by means of a sifter box. Not only will the active ingredient treat a certain dermatological condition, but the basic powder protects the skin from irritation and friction. Powders absorb secretions exerting a drying and cooling effect as the fluid is absorbed on the great surface and increased evaporation from the large surface facilitates the removal of heat from the irritated area.

Dusting powders are prepared by trituration of a substance in a mortar with a pestle and are subsequently passed through a 60-mesh sieve. All dusting powders must be sifted, as any irregular crystals applied would be irritating to any already traumatic area. Reduction of particle size is occasionally aided by the addition of a substance which will be removed after the reduction has been complete; this is referred to as pulverization by intervention.

A. Prepare 30 g of the following:

Camphor	100 g
Starch	600 g
Zinc oxide	300 g

Weigh the camphor and place it in a mortar. Try to pulverize the camphor with a pestle. Add a few drops of alcohol and pulverize. Gradually add the starch and zinc oxide previously mixed to the camphor. Triturate until uniformly mixed. Pass through a 60-mesh sieve. Dust and rub the powder on the back of your hand, and then answer Question 1.

B. Divided powders are individual doses of medicinal substances in powdered form, each wrapped in paper. In preparing divided powders, the powdered ingredients are triturated in a mortar until the mixture is uniform. The finished blend of medicinals is then divided into the prescribed number of doses and folded into appropriate papers. In dividing the individual doses, the correct quantity of powder is weighed on counterbalanced papers on a balance and transferred to the paper in which it is to be wrapped. Folding is done in the following steps:

1. Fold over about 1/2 inch of the long edge of the paper. Several folds should be made at once to save time and to obtain a uniform fold.
2. With the fold distal, lay the powder papers side by side so they overlap slightly.
3. Place the weighed powder in the center of the paper.
4. Bring the lower edge up and fit it into the top fold.
5. Pull the top fold toward you until it divides the remainder of the paper approximately in half.
6. Pick up the folded paper with the thumb and index finger of each hand and fold the ends over a powder box so that the finished paper will just fit into the box.

Compound the following:

Rx Magnesium trisilicate
Tribasic calcium phosphate
Activated charcoal aa 0.1 g
M. F. Pulv. D. T. D. No. xii
Sig: t i d p c

If difficulty is experienced in folding powder papers to a correct height, the following procedure is suggested:

1. Using the box as a guide, measure a distance twice the depth of the box on the paper; a slight crease will clearly indicate the correct distances.
2. Fold over the upper edge of the paper so that it divides the remaining portion of the paper into thirds and crease.
3. Place the weighed powder in the center of the paper.
4. Bring the lower edge up and fit it into the top fold.
5. Pull the top fold toward you, folding under exactly the width of the powder paper marked by the first crease.
6. Continue folding as described in the other method.

REFERENCES

Felmeister, A. 1975. Powders. Particle-size reduction, classification, measurement, mixing powders as a dosage form. In Remington's Pharmaceutical sciences, 15th ed., Mack Publishing Company, Chap. 88, p. 1554.
Parrott, E. L. 1975. Milling of pharmaceutical solids, J. Pharm. Sci., 63:813.
Parrott, E. L. 1976. Milling. In The theory and practice of industrial pharmacy, 2nd ed., L. Lachman, H. A. Lieberman, and J. L. Kanig, Eds. Chap. 15, Lea and Febiger, Philadelphia, p. 466.
Temperley, H. N. V. and G. E. K. Blythe. 1968. Mills which grind to micron size without moving parts. Nature, 219:1218.
The United States Pharmacopeia, 19th rev. 1975. Powder fineness, pp. 655-656.

Reduction of Particle Size

Data and Conclusions

1. After rubbing the powder prepared in A on the back of your hand, do you consider reduction of a solid to a 60-mesh size adequate to eliminate grittiness?

2. Discuss the factors that influence the milling (mechanical size reduction) of solid medicinal compounds.

3. Define specific surface. What is the relationship between specific surface and particle size?

4. In the laboratory how would you determine the porosity of a powder?

5. How is a divided powder administered?

6. BLENDING OF SOLIDS

All dosage forms must be uniformly mixed to ensure that the proper dose of medication is given to the patient. If the initial drugs are markedly different in size, they should be reduced to approximately the same size before mixing as it is difficult to uniformly mix particles of considerable difference of size. The drug present in the smallest amount is placed in a mortar, and an equal volume of the next most potent substance is added; the two drugs are triturated until finely divided and intimately mixed. This procedure is repeated until all of the material has been added and thoroughly mixed. This is known as mixing by geometric dilution because each portion added is equal in bulk to the material already in the mortar.

V-blenders, double conical and ribbon blenders are used in pharmaceutical industry to blend up to several tons of powders. The effectiveness of a blender depends on the powders to be mixed, the time of mixing, the number of rotations of the mixer and other factors which may be characterized by complex mathematical relationship.

PROCEDURE. Bulk powders are used for a variety of purposes such as dusting powders, oral use, insufflation, and douches.

A. Prepare 30 g of the following:

Rx	Belladonna extract	0.25 g
	Phenobarbital	0.4 g
	Bismuth subnitrate	24.0 g
	Kaolin	45.0 g
	Peppermint oil	0.12 ml

Mix and make powder.
S. ʒ i a. c. until diarrhea subsides.

B. The aliquot method of weighing small quantities often is used in compounding prescriptions. Using proper pharmaceutical procedure, compound the following:

Rx	Atropine sulfate	0.02 mg
	Hyoscyamine sulfate	0.10 mg
	Phenobarbital	0.015 g
	Lactose q. s.	

Give of such doses 12 powders.
S. Contents of a powder p. r. n.

C. A twin shell V-blender is available. Observe the mixing action of this type of blender by making a blend of 1/2% charcoal with magnesium oxide.

D. In a 15-cm test tube place approximately 10 g of aspirin granulation (20-mesh). Add approximately 1 g of calamine as a layer on top of the aspirin granulation. Stopper the test tube and attach it in a vertical position to the arm of a Tyler sieve shaker or a similar vibrating apparatus and shake for 20–30 minutes. Observe the distribution of the particles.

E. Capsules are gelatin shells which generally enclose powdered drugs, although semisolid masses and liquids may be dispensed in capsules. At the prescription counter capsules are usually filled by the "punching" method.

The properly triturated powder is placed on a powder paper and smoothed with a spatula to a height approximately equal to half the length of the body of the capsule. The open end of the body of the capsule is held vertically and is repeatedly pushed into the powder until the capsule is filled; the cap is then replaced to close the capsule. Each filled capsule is weighed, using an empty capsule as a counter-poise. Powder is added or removed until the correct weight has been placed in the capsule. The filled capsule is tapped so that the powder will fill the cap.

In order to produce capsules that are free from fingerprints, the hands must be clean and dry. After the capsules are filled, any powder that may cling to the outside may be removed by rubbing them in the folds of a clean, dry towel.

1. In preparing the following prescription, weigh enough of the ingredients for 25 capsules. Mix the powdered substances in the order of ascending weights. Fill the capsules by hand, weigh each one, and adjust its weight to the proper value.

Rx Aspirin	0.15 g
Phenacetin	0.12 g
Citrated caffeine	0.03 g

   Misce et ft. capsula una.
   Mitte tales numero xxiv.
   Sig: One capsule every three hours.

2. The particles of some powders do not cohere nor adhere to the capsule when they are being packed. Sliding the capsule horizontally into the powder appears to be the best method for filling such substances. These capsules are to be saved and coated at a future time.

   Rx Methenamine
   Ammonium chloride aa 0.2 g

   M. Ft. Cap. D. T. D. No. xii
   S. One q. h.

3. Several small manually operated capsule-filling machines with a capacity of 20–36 capsules are available such as Eastman, Ideal, Universal, and Cap-Fill. Familiarity with the operation of such capsule-filling apparatus will be gained by using those provided to fill the following:

   Rx Quinine sulfate 0.3 g

   Make 20 such capsules
   Label. For my office.

4. Place two capsules which you have filled in a beaker containing approximately 350 ml of water at body temperature. Determine the time required before the drug is released from the gelatin capsule.

REFERENCES

Parrott, E. L. 1974. Precision solid-solid blending. Drug and Cosm. Ind., 115:42.
Rippie, E. G. 1976. Mixing. In The theory and practice of industrial pharmacy, 2nd ed., L. Lachman, H. A. Lieberman, and J. L. Kanig, Eds., Lea and Febiger, Philadelphia. Chap. 16, p. 486.
Train, D. 1960. Pharmaceutical aspects of mixing solids. The Pharm. J., 185, 4th series, 131:129.

Blending of Solids

Data and Conclusions

1. How is the peppermint oil correctly measured and incorporated in A?

2. Show the calculations and total weight of each powder compounded in B.

3. Does the V-blender appear to be an effective type of blender? Does the V-blender reduce particle size?

4. After the 24 capsules in the prescription in E1 were filled, how many milligrams of powder remained?

5. If the physician wished to replace the caffeine citrate in E 1 with an equivalent amount of caffeine, how much caffeine would you use?

6. A certain size of a powder paper weighs 0.48 g with a maximum variation of 65 mg between any two papers. A size O capsule weighs 90 mg with a 15% variation between any two capsules. One-half gram of a powdered drug is to be filled into each dosage form. In filling the capsule, an empty capsule may be correctly used as a tare for checking the accuracy of fill. In filling a powder paper, the powder is weighed always on a counter-poise paper and then transferred to the paper into which it will be folded. By means of the data supplied, show by calculations the validity of these accepted procedures.

7. How long does a gelatin capsule shell delay the release of the medication to an aqueous environment?

8. Record your observation in D. During processing, what effect might the vibration of mechanical equipment have on the uniformity of blend of a dry mixture? How may this be minimized?

7. SOME PROPERTIES OF SOLIDS

The informed pharmacist must know not only the chemistry of the drugs he is compounding, but he must know the equally important physical properties of the drugs. Chemically, sodium sulfate offers no problems in dispensing, yet the pharmacist must be aware that sodium sulfate contains 10 units of water of hydration; thus, the salt effloresces in air and liquefies in its water of hydration at 33°. Other physical properties important to the pharmacist are discussed in this exercise.

Drugs may exist in more than a single crystal lattice arrangement. Each crystalline form is known as a polymorph, which usually displays a different x-ray diffraction pattern, infrared spectrum, density, melting point and solubility from other polymorphic forms. The difference in solubility may result in the more soluble polymorph being more readily bioavailable and consequently more effective therapeutically. Only one polymorphic form is stable at a given temperature and pressure, and in time other forms will convert to the stable form.

Adsorption is a process caused by the interaction of the unsatisfied physical or chemical forces at any solid surface and the molecules which strike the surface. If the interaction is chemical and irreversible, it is known as chemisorption. Physical adsorption involves a weak and reversible interaction between a solid and the adsorbate. Molecules may be adsorbed unto the surface of a solid from a vapor phase or from a solution. The use of charcoal as a nonspecific antidote in poisoning is based on its adsorbent property. Bacteriostatic and fungistatic agents used in parenterals may be adsorbed by the rubber stopper of the multidose vial. Aluminum hydroxide, kaolin and talc may adsorb drugs administered concurrently to the extent that absorption is greatly reduced.

PROCEDURE. A hygroscopic drug is one which readily adsorbs and becomes coated with moisture. If the attraction of a hygroscopic drug for moisture is so great that the solid liquefies due to the solution of the drug in the adsorbed water, the drug is said to be deliquescent.

In preparing powders containing a hygroscopic drug, dry chemicals and utensils must be used. It has been the custom to double-wrap such divided powders, using waxed paper for the inner paper. A simpler and more effective means of excluding moisture in dispensing hygroscopic drugs is to enclose them in a sealed cellophane envelope. Sealing of the cellophane envelope is done in the following steps:

1. The correct weight of medicament is placed into the cellophane envelope, using the weighing paper as a funnel and taking care that no powder collects at the open end of the envelope. As the envelopes are filled, they are set upright.
2. Fold the open end over about 1/2 inch and crease sharply.
3. Lay the folded envelope on a pill tile and rapidly pass a heated spatula or a small photographic iron over the fold, fusing a seal.

A. Compound the following and dispense in cellophane envelopes:

Rx Ferric ammonium citrate	0.5 g
Sodium bromide	0.3 g
Pepsin	0.2 g

Make 12 powders.
Sig: One q. i. d.

B. Compare the efficiency of double-wrapped papers and cellophane envelopes in stabilizing a hygroscopic powder by compounding the following prescription. Dispense half in envelopes and half in double-wrapped papers. Examine several times during a two-week period.

Rx Sodium sulfocyanate	0.25 g

M. and Ft. Pulv. No. xii
S. *i* t. i. d. and h. s.

Certain crystalline materials, e.g., uneffloresced sodium sulfate, change on the surface or throughout to a whitish, mealy, or crystalline powder from the loss of water on exposure to air. They are said to be efflorescent substances.

Relative humidity is the ratio of the amount of water vapor actually present and that which the air could hold if saturated at the same temperature. Solids exposed to the atmosphere may adsorb water vapor on their surfaces. The amount of water of hygroscopicity is a function of the relative humidity.

In an atmosphere with a high relative humidity, a hygroscopic drug will adsorb a high percent of water. As the relative humidity decreases, less water is adsorbed. With very low relative humidity, water will not be adsorbed to any significant extent, and a crystalline hydrate may lose part or all of its water of hydration.

C. Compare the effect of relative humidity on dried starch, choline chloride, citric acid monohydrate and talc at room temperature. Relative humidity chambers at approximately 0, 20, 45, 70, and 90% relative humidity are provided by the instructor. Pass each of the drugs to be used through a 100-mesh sieve. Place approximately 2 g (accurately weighed on an analytical balance) of the powder in a tared aluminum foil container or a weighing bottle so that the loosely spread powder is less than 0.5 cm deep. Record the weight of the container and the container with the powder. Place the sample in each of the relative humidity chambers provided. After one week remove, quickly weigh, and record the weight of each sample at the various humidities.

Impurities added to a chemically pure compound will, for the most part, lower the melting point of that substance. If the melting points of such mixtures are high, this phenomenon offers no problem to the pharmacist. However, many drugs used in medicine have a low melting point, and when mixed intimately with other drugs, the lowered mixed melting point becomes less than room temperature and the mixture melts. An instance in which two or more drugs are mixed and become liquid is known as a "pharmaceutical eutectic."

An eutectic may be anticipated with crystalline substances having low intermolecular attractive forces such as phenolic, aldehydic, and ketonic compounds.

Liquefaction of powders upon mixing is sometimes desirable in pharmacy. For example, the eutectic liquid resulting from mixing equal parts of cocaine, phenol and menthol (Bonain's solution) is applied to the tympanic membrane. A blend of sulfathiazole and urea may be melted, congealed and milled to a fine powder. When placed in water, the very soluble urea rapidly dissolves and extremely fine particles of sulfathiazole are released. The large specific surface of the fine particles speeds dissolution of the relatively insoluble sulfathiazole. When administered orally to humans higher serum concentrations of sulfathiazole are obtained than by administration of ordinary sulfathiazole.

Considering atmospheric pressure constant, the particular state that a mixture of pure substances exists in is primarily a function of temperature and composition of the mixture. Since in pharmacy medicinals are prepared to be stable at room temperature, temperature is not a variable and all our considerations are at room temperature. The important factor remaining then is the composition of the mixture.

D. Determine the melting point-composition curve for Drug A and Drug B, which will be supplied. Using a conventional melting-point determination apparatus, find the melting point of pure Drug A and Drug B.

Prepare mixtures of 20, 40, 60, and 80% Drug A with Drug B. Place the mixture in a small beaker and immerse in warm water until just melted. Slowly cool the melt with agitation until it solidifies. Determine the melting point of each mixture.

For more precise determinations a Beckmann molecular weight apparatus, as described in *Colligative Properties of Solutions,* page 132, may be used for determining the freezing points of the mixtures.

To avoid liquefaction of a mixture of several eutectic substances, an inert, high melting-point substance is generally added to surround or coat the drugs, preventing them from coming into contact. If the liquid has been formed, it may be taken up in the pores and on the surface of an inert substance to produce a satisfactory preparation.

E. The effectiveness of various inert powders in this respect may be determined for the following prepared by Methods I and II using 0.2 g of inert ingredient per powder.

Rx Camphor	0.06 g
Salol	0.20 g

Make such powders No. 3

In Method I the camphor is triturated with part of the adsorbent, the salol is triturated with the remainder, and the two resulting powders are mixed with light trituration. In Method II the salol and camphor are triturated to form a pasty mass, the adsorbing agent is added, and the mixture is triturated lightly.

Using both methods, determine and tabulate the effectiveness of the following inert ingredients: light magnesium oxide, magnesium carbonate, corn starch, and kaolin. The following abbreviations are suggested for tabulating the results:

L = soft mass or liquid
P = dry powder
D = damp powder
SD = slightly damp powder
CM = cementlike mass

The minimum weight W in grams of an inert protective agent required to coat all particles of an eutectically interacting drug in a formulation may be calculated by use of the equation

$$W = \frac{4\,W_d r \rho}{r_d \rho_d}$$

where r and ρ are the radius and density of the protective agent, and W_d, r_d and ρ_d are the weight in grams, the radius and the density of the drug, respectively.

REFERENCES

Chemical Rubber Publishing Co. 1969-1970. Handbook of chemistry and physics, 50th ed., "Constant humidity" and "Constant humidity with sulfuric acid solutions." Cleveland. p. E-40.

Clements, J. A. and D. Stanski. 1971. Dissolution studies on some polymorphs of phenobarbitone, Canad. J. Pharm. Sci., 6:9.

Decker, W. J., H. F. Combs, and D. G. Corby. 1968. Adsorption of drugs and poisons by activated charcoal. Toxicology and Applied Pharmacology, 13:454.

Gibaldi, M. 1976. Biopharmaceutics. In The theory and practice of industrial pharmacy. L. Lachman, H. A. Lieberman, and J. L. Kanig, Eds. 2nd ed., Lea and Febiger, Philadelphia. Chap. 3, p. 103.

Kolthoff, I. M. and E. B. Sandell. 1952. Water in solids. Efflorescence and deliquescence. Preparation of hydrates with a definite amount of water of crystallization. Adsorption of water vapor. Essential and nonessential water. In Textbook of quantitative inorganic analysis, 3rd ed., The Macmillan Co. New York, Chap. IX. p. 138.

Levy, G. and T. Tsuchiya. 1972. Effect of activated charcoal on aspirin absorption in man. Part I. Clinical Pharmacology and Therapeutics, 13:317.

Monkhouse, D. C. and J. L. Lach. 1972. Use of adsorbents in enhancement of drug dissolution I and II. J. Pharm. Sci., 61:1430 and 1435.

Nogami, H., T. Nagai, E. Fukuoka, and H. Uchida. 1968. Physico-chemical approach to biopharmaceutical phenomena. I. Adsorption of tryptophan from aqueous solution. Chem. Phar. Bull., 16:2248.

Parrott, E. L. 1966. Student experiments in pharmaceutical technology. III. Humidity. Am. J. Pharm. Ed., 30:470.

Parrott, E. L. 1970. Properties of solids. In Pharmaceutical technology. Fundamental pharmaceutics, Burgess Publishing Co., Minneapolis. Chap. 4, p. 107.

Patel, N. K. 1970. Experiments in physical pharmacy. IV. Pharmaceutical eutectic mixtures. Am. J. Pharm. Ed., 34:47.

Saski, W. 1963. Adsorption of sorbic acid by plastic cellulose acetates. J. Pharm. Sci., 52:264.

Sekiguchi, K. and N. Obi. 1961. Studies on absorption of eutectic mixture. I. A comparison of the behavior of eutectic mixture of sulfathiazole and that of ordinary sulfathiazole in man. Chem. Pharm. Bull., 9:866.

Sorby, D. L. 1968. Effect of adsorbent on drug absorption: Importance of preequilibrating drug and adsorbent. J. Pharm. Sci., 57:1604.

Strickland, W. A. 1962. Study of water vapor sorption by pharmaceutical powders. J. Pharm. Sci., 51:310.

Some Properties of Solids

Data and Conclusions

1. Complete the following table with data from C:

	Percent Relative Humidity				
Drug:	0	20	45	70	90
A. Initial					
Weight of pan and drug Weight of pan Weight of drug					
B. One-Week Exposure					
Weight of pan, drug, and any vapor sorbed Weight of pan Weight of drug and any vapor sorbed Weight of water vapor sorbed per g of drug					
Drug:					
A. Initial					
Weight of pan and drug Weight of pan Weight of drug					
B. One-Week Exposure					
Weight of pan, drug, and any vapor sorbed Weight of pan Weight of drug and any vapor sorbed Weight of water vapor sorbed per g of drug					

	Percent Relative Humidity				
Drug:	0	20	45	70	90
A. Initial					
Weight of pan and drug					
Weight of pan					
Weight of drug					
B. One-Week Exposure					
Weight of pan, drug, and any vapor sorbed					
Weight of pan					
Weight of drug and any vapor sorbed					
Weight of water vapor sorbed per g of drug					
Drug:					
A. Initial					
Weight of pan and drug					
Weight of pan					
Weight of drug					
B. One-Week Exposure					
Weight of pan, drug, and any vapor sorbed					
Weight of pan					
Weight of drug and any vapor sorbed					
Weight of water vapor sorbed per g of drug					

2. For each drug, plot the milligrams of water sorbed per gram of drug as the ordinate and the relative humidity as the abscissa.

3. What effect does the relative humidity have on each of the drugs?

4. If the particle size of the drugs had been larger or smaller, how might this have affected the amount of water vapor sorbed?

5. How can a constant humidity be maintained in a closed vessel? Give some examples.

6. Did you find double-wrapped papers or cellophane envelopes more effective in dispensing hygroscopic drugs?

7. Complete the following table for D:

Percent Composition	Melting Point

8. Plot the melting point as the ordinate and the percent composition as the abscissa. What is the eutectic point of this mixture? Indicate the phases existing in each portion of the curve.

9. Complete the following table:

Adsorbent	Immediately After Mixing		Effect After One Week	
	Method I	Method II	Method I	Method II

10. What conclusions can you make from the chart in Question 9 as to the methods and inert adsorbents used?

11. Explain what occurs when parachlorophenol and camphor are triturated together.

12. Epsom salt, which had lost 50% of its water of hydration, was sold over the counter. If the consumer took 15 g of the salt, how much of an overdose was administered? Show your calculations.

8. GRANULATIONS

Granulations are small grainlike particles; they are prepared as a convenience for packaging, as a more stable product due to less surface exposure, and as a popular dosage form.

Dietary supplements such as Somagen and Granulestin are often prepared in a granular form. Laxatives in granular form are Bassoran, Imbicoll with Cascara and Siblin.

The effervescent granulation is popular with the laity perhaps due to its taste and psychological impression. Bromo-Seltzer, Citrocarbonate, and Salicionyl are examples of such preparations. Usually the medication is combined with sodium bicarbonate and citric or tartaric acid, which when placed in water effervesces as carbon dioxide is liberated.

The formulation of an effervescent granulation can be illustrated with the preparation of twenty-four 1-g doses of effervescent sodium bromide. A heaping teaspoonful of an effervescent salt weighs about 5 g. The weight depends on the densities of the ingredients and the size of the granules. The effervescent sodium bromide would be made up of 24 g of sodium bromide and 96 g of granulation base to make a total of 120 g of finished granulation.

It is arbitrarily decided that citric acid and tartaric acid are to be used in the ratio of 1:2, respectively. The amount of sodium bicarbonate to be used may be calculated from the equation of the reaction,

$$\underset{(3 \times 84)}{3\,NaHCO_3} + \underset{210}{HO{-}\overset{\displaystyle CH_2{-}COOH}{\underset{\displaystyle CH_2{-}COOH}{C}}{-}COOH \cdot H_2O} \longrightarrow 4\,H_2O + 3\,CO_2 + HO{-}\overset{\displaystyle CH_2{-}COONa}{\underset{\displaystyle CH_2{-}COONa}{C}}{-}COONa$$

Setting up a proportion to determine the amount of sodium bicarbonate that will react with 1 g of citric acid, one has,

$$\frac{1.0}{210} = \frac{x}{3 \times 84}$$

$x = 1.2$ g of sodium bicarbonate to react with 1.0 g of citric acid.

Similar calculations show that 2.24 g of sodium bicarbonate react with 2 g of tartaric acid. Thus, with the acids in a ratio of 1:2, it has been calculated that 3.44 g of sodium bicarbonate is necessary to react stoichiometrically with the 3 g of combined acids.

To enhance the flavor, the amount of sodium bicarbonate may be reduced to 3.4 g to allow for a tart taste.

Ninety-six grams of the effervescent base is to be prepared in the ratio,

citric acid	1
tartaric acid	2
sodium bicarbonate	3.4
	6.4

By proportion, the amount of tartaric acid to be used may be determined

$$\frac{2}{6.4} = \frac{x}{96}$$

$$x = 30 \text{ g of tartaric acid.}$$

Similarly, the amounts of citric acid and sodium bicarbonate may be calculated. The final formula is then

sodium bromide	24 g
sodium bicarbonate	51 g
tartaric acid	30 g
citric acid	15 g
	120 g

PROCEDURE. The citric acid should be uneffloresced and powdered just prior to use. The sodium bicarbonate should be powdered and dry. Other ingredients should be dried at 100° until they cease to lose weight. All ingredients should pass through a 60-mesh sieve. The ingredients are mixed with the citric acid and granulated.

A. Prepare 50 g of Effervescent Sodium Phosphate N. F.

Dried sodium phosphate	200 g	10
Sodium bicarbonate	477 g	23.85
Tartaric acid	252 g	12.6
Citric acid monohydrate	162 g	8.1

Powder the citric acid, mix it intimately with the dried sodium phosphate and tartaric acid, and thoroughly incorporate the sodium bicarbonate.

Place the mixture in a beaker immersed in a vigorously boiling water bath. In a few minutes the heat causes the water of crystallization to be released and to slightly moisten the powder.

Force the warm, slightly pasty mass with an acid-resistant spatula through a 6-mesh sieve. Dry the granulation and package in a tight container.

B. Formulate and prepare by the wet method 24 doses of an effervescent granulation containing in each teaspoonful 300 mg of sodium salicylate.

The powder is moistened with a liquid which exerts only slight solvent action. Alcohol is usually satisfactory for this purpose. The powders are placed in a suitable dish and alcohol is gradually added with stirring until the mass coheres as small granular lumps. A paste should not be made. The granules are formed entirely by the cohesiveness of the moist mass under the influence of kneading.

It is best to pass the moistened mass through a 6-mesh sieve. The granulation is dried in the air to remove the alcohol. All effervescent preparations must be packaged in an air-tight container.

C. The biological availability of salicylate from an effervescent granulation may be determined by the administration of two teaspoonfuls, each containing 300 mg of sodium salicylate, and the collection of urine specimens at 2-hour intervals.

On the day preceding the laboratory period the student voids his or her bladder upon arising and collects a urine specimen to be used as a blank. Two teaspoonfuls of the granulation are immediately taken with a minimum of 250 ml of water. Food may be ingested as desired, but no salicylates should be ingested. Urine specimens are collected every two hours for fourteen hours. The volumes of the urine specimens are measured and recorded, and aliquots are retained in test tubes for analysis in the laboratory. The 14- to 24-hours urine specimens are pooled, the volume is measured, and the specimen is analyzed.

Each aliquot of urine specimen is diluted with water so the salicylate concentration is from 0.1 to 0.5 mg per ml. The dilution depends on the volume of urine, but it is usually from 2- to 5-fold.

To 1.0 ml of diluted urine specimen 5.0 ml of color reagent is added. In each 100 ml of aqueous solution the color reagent contains 4 g of ferric nitrate [$Fe(NO_3)_3 \cdot 9H_2O$], 4 g of mercuric chloride and 12 ml of N hydrochloric acid. The clear, supernatant liquid is placed in a cuvette and the absorbance is determined using a spectrophotometer at 540 nm. The urine specimen which was collected upon arising is diluted in the same manner, and 1.0 ml of the diluted specimen is mixed with 5.0 ml of the color reagent to provide a blank for each analysis. A standard absorption curve relating the absorbance to concentration of salicylate is provided by the instructor.

Record the time interval of the specimen collected, the volume of each specimen, the absorbance, and milligrams of salicylate in each sample analyzed. Calculate the milligrams of salicylate excreted per time interval. Plot the cumulative amount excreted against time. Plot the amount excreted per time interval against time. This data will be used in a future exercise.

REFERENCES

Gibaldi, M. and D. Perrier. 1975. Pharmacokinetics. Marcel Dekker, Inc., N.Y. pp. 6-11.

Leeling, J. L., B. M. Phillips, T. L. Kowalski, and R. L. Kowalski. 1976. Influence of aspirin formulation and dose on concentration of total salicylate in rat kidney. J. Pharm. Sci., 65:447.

Granulations

Data and Conclusions

1. Show the equation and calculations for determining the amount of citric acid to be used in the effervescent sodium salicylate granulation.

2. Record the data from C. Show a sample calculation.

Time Interval	Ml of Urine	Dilution	Absorbance	Concentration	Mg Excreted

3. Assuming that all the salicylate is excreted within 24 hours after administration, calculate the fraction of the orally administered dose recovered in the urine.

4. The amount of drug remaining in the body at any time is equal to the total excretable drug minus the amount excreted to that time. Using the data from C, plot the logarithm of the unexcreted salicylate against time. Express an equation for the urinary elimination of the salicylate. Calculate the biological half-life.

5. What is your opinion about dispensing potent drugs as granulations?

9. MOLDED SOLIDS: TABLET TRITURATES

In addition to being administered as powders and granulations, solid drugs may be formed into solid dosage forms. Tablets are prepared by compression using high forces; other solid dosage forms such as the tablet triturate, pill, and troche are commonly molded or formed without high compressional forces.

Tablet triturates are really powder triturates made into tablets for convenience. Molded tablets consist of fine powders, usually lactose or sucrose together with the medicament, molded into shape while moist. A tablet triturate is readily soluble and disintegrates almost instantaneously.

The hypodermic tablet is a special, completely soluble tablet triturate, which after being dissolved in sterile water is used for parenteral injection. Beta-lactose is generally used as a base due to its greater solubility than other forms of lactose.

PROCEDURE. Although tablet triturate molds are assigned a capacity by the manufacturer, the mold must be calibrated for each formulation due to the variation in density and porosity of different tablets.

A tablet triturate mold is best calibrated as follows:

1. Mix the active ingredient with an amount of diluent known to be insufficient to fill the prescribed number of cavities in the mold.
2. Moisten the mixture with 50% alcohol until the powders are dampened but not pasty.
3. By use of a spatula, pack the moistened mass into the holes of the tablet mold.
4. Moisten an additional portion of the diluent and completely fill the cavities of the mold.
5. Punch out the tablets, crush, mix intimately, moisten again if necessary, and fill into the die again.

A. Prepare 50 of the following molded tablets.

Rx	Atropine sulfate	30 mg
	Lactose	q. s.

Mix the fine powders in a glass mortar by the geometric dilution method. Carefully add 50% alcohol until the powders are moist enough to adhere but not pasty; as a guide to the novice, 0.8 ml of alcohol is sufficient to moisten 4 g of lactose. The excipient may be added by means of a dropper, pipet, or nebulizer.

Lay the die or upper plate of the mold on a pill tile and force the mass into the holes with a spatula. Exert firm pressure while moving the spatula in a circular manner on the die so the tablets will be smooth and flat. Inspect both sides of the die to ensure complete filling of the cavities.

After a minute or two, place the die with the beveled edge downward on the matching pegs of the base or lower plate and gently press down, forcing the tablets out of the mold. Allow the tablets to remain on the pegs for two minutes, remove, and let them dry on a clean gauze for at least an hour.

B. Devise a method for and prepare the following tablet triturates.

Rx Belladonna tincture	0.6 ml
Lactose	q. s.
D. T. D. No. xx	

C. Test the disintegration time and the complete solubility of the commercial nitroglycerin hypodermic tablet provided by the instructor. Place the tablet in a test tube about 15 mm in diameter containing 2.5 ml of purified water. Shake the test tube with a moderate sidewise motion for two minutes. To be satisfactory each tablet should dissolve completely without effervescence to give a clear solution.

REFERENCES

The United States Pharmacopeia, 19th rev. 1975. Preparation of molded tablets. p. 705.

Molded Solids: Tablet Triturates

Data and Conclusions

1. Name several tablet triturate bases used in addition to lactose.

2. How did you prepare the belladonna tincture tablet triturate?

3. Name five drugs that are marketed as hypodermic tablets.

4. What is the difference between powdered sugar as purchased in the market and pulverized sugar?

5. How does the solubility of the active ingredient affect the choice of an excipient?

6. What are the requirements for the packaging and labeling of nitroglycerin tablets?

10. COMPRESSED TABLETS

Without question, the compressed tablet is the most popular dosage form today. There are approximately 380 official tablets, and about one half of the prescriptions dispensed are for tablets.

Usually one considers a compressed tablet as an oral medication; however, compressed tablets have many other uses. The sublingual tablet, the pellet, the wafer, the dental cone, the troche, and the vaginal insert are manufactured by the same procedure as an oral tablet.

PROCEDURE. There are three methods of making compressed tablets. In the direct compression method, a compressible vehicle is blended with the medicinal compound, and if necessary, with a lubricant and a disintegrating agent, and then the blend is compressed. Substances that have been suggested as directly compressible vehicles are: anhydrous and spray dried lactose, dicalcium phosphate dihydrate (Emcompress), granulated mannitol, microcrystalline cellulose (Avicel), compressible sugar (Di-Pac), starch (Sta-Rx 1500), hydrolyzed starch (Celutab), and a blend of sugar, invert sugar, starch and magnesium stearate (Nutab).

In the slugging method the ingredients in the formulation are intimately mixed and precompressed on heavy-duty tablet machines. The slug which is formed is ground to a uniform size and compressed into the finished tablet.

The wet granulation method has more operational manipulations and is more time-consuming than the other methods: however, it is widely used. The wet granulation method cannot be used for drugs which are thermolabile or are degraded by the liquid binder. The wet granulation procedure is done in the following steps:

1. The granulating solution or binder is prepared.
2. The powdered ingredients are weighed and mixed intimately.
3. The powders are granulated by adding an appropriate amount of binding solution and are kneaded to the proper consistency.
4. The wet granulation is forced through a screen or wet granulator.
5. The granules are dried in an oven.
6. The dried granules are ground to the final and suitable size for compression.
7. A lubricant and a disintegrating agent are mixed with the granulation.
8. The granulation is compressed into the finished tablet.

A. By manual means, prepare 500 tablets containing 250 mg of sulfadiazine per tablet.

	mg per tablet
Sulfadiazine, powdered	250
Starch	18
Lactose	60
Magnesium stearate	2

In a tared container prepare a 10% w/w starch paste by first making a slurry with 25 g of starch and 25 g of purified water. Add 200 g of boiling purified water to the slurry and stir. A translucent gel is formed.

In a mortar blend the sulfadiazine and lactose. Gradually, with kneading and mixing add 90 g of the starch paste. The wet granulation balls and sticks together when squeezed, but it does not become sticky or gummy.

Pass this mass through a 10-mesh screen and collect on a tray lined with paper. Dry the wet granulation in an oven at 55°.

After the granulation is dried, pass it through a 20-mesh screen. Weigh the dried granulation and calculate the proper weight of magnesium stearate to be added. Add the magnesium stearate to the granulation and blend in a V-blender or by tumbling.

Using a 13/32-inch standard concave punch and die set, compress the finished tablet to a hardness of 6 to 8 kg. Save the sulfadiazine tablets for a future exercise.

B. By manual means, prepare 500 tablets containing 300 mg of sodium salicylate per tablet.

	mg per tablet
Sodium salicylate, powdered	300.0
Lactose	65.0
Gelatin	9.2
Starch	10.0
Magnesium stearate	7.8

In a tared container prepare a 20% w/w gelatin solution by first soaking 20 g of gelatin with 80 g of distilled water. Then heat at 60° on a water bath until a clear solution is produced.

In a mortar blend the sodium salicylate and the lactose. Gradually, with kneading and mixing, add 23 g of the gelatin solution. The wet granulation balls and sticks together when squeezed, but it does not become sticky or gummy.

Pass this mass through a 14-mesh screen and collect on a tray lined with paper. Dry the wet granulation overnight in an oven at 65°. It is essential that the granulation be dry in order to prevent sticking during compression.

After the granulation is dried, it is weighed. Calculate the proper weight of starch and magnesium stearate to be added. Add the starch and magnesium stearate to the granulation and blend in a V-blender or by tumbling.

Using a 13/32-inch standard concave punch and die set, compress the finished tablets to a hardness of 3 to 5 kg. Save the sodium salicylate tablets for a future exercise.

C. Chewable tablets are compressed tablets that are pleasantly flavored and dissolve in the mouth in approximately one minute. They may be chewed, sucked, or swallowed whole. Chewable tablets are recommended for pediatric use.

Prepare 500 chewable, pediatric aspirin tablets.

	mg per tablet
Aspirin, 20-mesh	81.0
Mannitol	97.0
Saccharin sodium	1.0
Acacia	4.5
Starch	11.0
Talc	8.0
Dry orange flavor	7.0
Stearic acid, spray dried	0.4

Prepare a 20% w/w acacia mucilage by adding the warm purified water to powdered acacia in a mortar and triturating until it is dispersed. The acacia mucilage should be strained through muslin before incorporation.

Blend the mannitol and the saccharin sodium. Add the acacia mucilage and knead to the proper consistency. Pass the wet mass through an 8-mesh screen. Dry the granulation at 45°. After the granulation is dried, pass it through a 20-mesh screen.

The aspirin is mixed with the dried mannitol granulation. The dry orange flavor is added to the starch and mixed thoroughly. The talc and the stearic acid are blended with the flavor mixture. This blend is then added and mixed with the mannitol-aspirin mixture.

The tablets are compressed to a hardness of 4 to 6 kg using a 11/32-inch standard concave punch and die set.

D. By direct compression prepare 500 tablets containing 50 mg of ascorbic acid per tablet.

	mg per tablet
Ascorbic acid	50.0
Compressible sugar U.S.P.	63.5
Calcium stearate	1.0

Blend all ingredients for five minutes in a suitable blender. Compress using a ¼-inch flat punch and die set.

REFERENCES

Cooper, J. 1971. In Advances in pharmaceutical sciences, Vol. 3, H. S. Bean and J. E. Carless, Eds. Academic Press, London and New York, p. 1.

Cooper, J. and J. E. Rees. 1972. Tableting research and technology, J. Pharm. Sci., 61:1511.

Gunsel, W. C. and J. L. Kanig. 1976. Tablets. In The theory and practice of industrial pharmacy, 2nd ed., L. Lachman, H. A. Lieberman, and J. L. Kanig, Eds. Lea and Febiger, Philadelphia. Chap. 11, p. 321.

Khan, K. A. and C. T. Rhodes. 1973. The production of tablets by direct compression. Canad. J. Pharm. Sci., 8:1.

King, R. E. 1975. Tablets, capsules, and pills. In Remington's Pharmaceutical sciences, 15th ed., Mack Publishing Company, Easton, Pa. Chap. 89, p. 1576.

The United States Pharmacopeia, 19th rev. 1975. Tablets. pp. 704-706.

Compressed Tablets

Data and Conclusions

1. Give the reasons for the popularity of the compressed tablet.

2. For what type of tablets are the following abbreviations employed?

C. T.	D. A. T.
D. T.	E. C. T.
T. T.	S. A. T.
S. C. T.	

3. Can all drugs be satisfactorily tabletted? Explain your answer.

4. What relationship does the force of compression have to the density and the porosity of a compressed tablet?

5. What relationship does the force of compression have to the hardness and disintegration time of a tablet?

6. Troches may be made by compression. What is done in such a product so that the troche will dissolve slowly?

7. Drug A is thermolabile and is rapidly hydrolyzed in the presence of moisture. You are to formulate a 125-mg tablet containing 25 mg of Drug A. The tablet is to disintegrate within 15 minutes. Give your formulation and method of preparation.

11. EVALUATION OF COMPRESSED TABLETS

One of the important duties of the pharmacist is to provide an accurate dose of the drug in a form which will provide the desired release of the drug in the body. During the manufacture of a dosage form, the product is carefully controlled and analyzed in all steps of the procedure to ensure that an active drug in the correct amount is present. These analytical procedures fall within the realm of the pharmaceutical chemist and are not discussed here.

The final appearance and characteristics of the tablet must be evaluated. The tablet must appear attractive and uniform with no chipping. A tablet should be hard enough to withstand transportation within professional channels as well as the movement of the consumer, and yet it must disintegrate readily into primary particles which dissolve readily. Numerous tests have been developed for such evaluations.

PROCEDURE. Hardness is not a fundamental property but may be defined as the resistance of a solid to attrition or breakage. It has been used in characterizing tablets as it is simple and convenient to measure. The Strong Cobb, Pfizer, and the Stokes hardness testers are used in the pharmaceutical industry. Although the instruments give different hardness values for a given set of tablets, it has been reported that a constant ratio of hardness results with the Strong Cobb Tester, giving results 1.6 times those of the Stokes Tester.

Oral tablets normally have a hardness of 4 to 6 kg; however, hypodermic tablets are much softer and some sustained-release tablets are much harder.

There appears to be a linear relationship between the tablet hardness and the logarithm of the compressional force. One would anticipate that as a tablet becomes more dense, its hardness would increase. It has been shown that hardness varies in a linear manner with density of the tablet.

The amount of solid in a tablet is determined by the depth of the die cavity. Even with proper granulation, a volume fill is not as accurate as a fill based on weight. The resulting variations in the weight of finished tablets must fall within certain specifications.

A. Determine the weight variation of the sodium salicylate or sulfadiazine tablets you manufactured. Weigh twenty tablets and calculate the average weight. The weights of not more than two tablets should differ from the average weight by more than the following percentages, and no tablet should be more than double the percentage,

Average Weight, mg	Percentage Difference
130 or less	10
From 130 to 324	7.5
More than 324	5

B. Visually inspect the sodium salicylate or sulfadiazine tablets you manufactured.

C. Using a hardness tester, determine the hardness of ten tablets you manufactured.

When a powdered drug is granulated and compressed into a tablet, the effective surface area of the medicinal compound is decreased. A tablet must break up or disintegrate in the gastrointestinal fluids into granules, and then the granules must disintegrate into primary particles. The medicinal compound must dissolve from the primary particles before the molecules or ions of the medicinal compound can be absorbed by the gastrointestinal mucosa.

Improperly formulated and improperly processed compressed tablets may retard drug release with a decrease in physiological availability. If a tablet does not disintegrate, the surface available for dissolution is restricted to the surface area of the tablet. The disintegration of the tablet, but not of the granules, provides a larger surface than that of the intact tablet; however, this surface is considerably smaller than the surface provided by the disintegration of the granules.

Disintegrating agents are substances which facilitate or hasten the breakdown of the tablet in the gastrointestinal tract. Starch, agar, algin products, and other vegetable substances are commonly used as they absorb water and swell, pushing the tablet apart. No one agent is the universal disintegrating agent, and numerous formulations are required to determine which agent is best for a particular tablet.

D. Using a U. S. P. disintegration apparatus and procedure, determine and record the disintegration time of a tablet containing 250 mg of sulfadiazine in distilled water at 37°C.

E. Repeat D for tablet containing 300 mg of sodium salicylate.

Disintegration time specification is a useful tool for production control, but disintegration of a tablet does not imply that the drug has dissolved. A tablet may pass a disintegration test and yet the drug may be biologically unavailable. Although the disintegration time of a tablet may influence the rate of drug release to the body, the dissolution rate of the drug from the primary particle is fundamentally important because dissolution of the drug is essential for absorption to occur. Dissolution is a function of the effective surface area of the particles, the intrinsic dissolution rate of the medicinal compound, and the properties of the dissolving fluid.

The tablet formulation and the manufacturing procedure affect dissolution; therefore, the biological availability of drugs from chemically equivalent tablets may be different. As shown in Figure 7, the administration of 12 g of sodium para-aminosalicylate in two formulations of a tablet does not provide the same blood concentration at given times or the same total amount of drug in the blood.

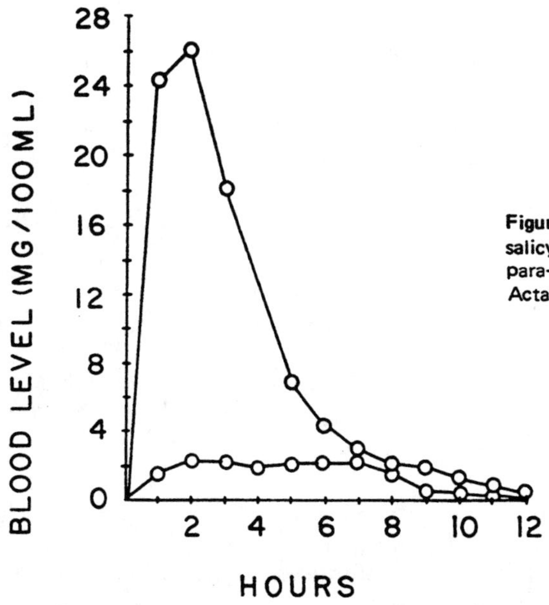

Figure 7 — The mean concentration of free para-aminosalicylate acid in blood after a single 12 g dose of sodium para-aminosalicylate in two tablet formulations (S. Frostad: Acta tuberc. pneumol. scand., 41, 68, 1961).

There is extreme specificity in the presence or absence of a correlation between disintegration time and absorption. In general, the dissolution profile is more indicative of absorption rate than the disintegration time. The correlation of *in vitro* dissolution rate with blood levels or clinical response has become an accepted technique in product development. A correlation between dissolution rate and biological availability for griseofulvin is shown in Figure 8. There is a linear relationship between the logarithm of amount dissolved in simulated intestinal fluid in thirty minutes and the mean plasma level for a twenty-four hour period after the oral administration of 500 mg of griseofulvin.

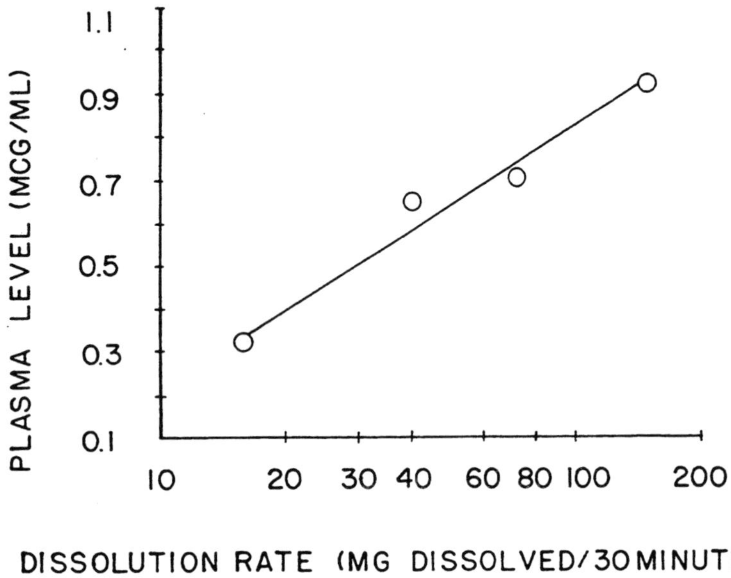

Figure 8 – Correlation of dissolution rate and mean griseofulvin plasma level. (B. Katchen and S. Symchowicz: J. Pharm. Sci., 56, 1108, 1967. Reproduced with permission of the copyright owner.)

F. Using the U. S. P. dissolution apparatus and procedure, determine the amount of sulfadiazine dissolved in simulated gastric fluid without pepsin at 15, 30, 45, and 60 minutes.

Place one tablet containing 250 mg of sulfadiazine in the dissolution apparatus and immerse in 900 ml of fluid at 37°. At each time interval withdraw a 1.0-ml sample of the solution by a pipet fitted with a filter and transfer to a 100-ml volumetric flask. Add 5.0 ml of 0.5 N hydrochloric acid and 5.0 ml of 0.1% sodium nitrite solution. Allow to stand for three minutes. Add 5.0 ml of 0.5% ammonium sulfamate solution. Add 5.0 ml of 0.1% N-(1-naphthyl)-ethylenediamine dihydrochloride solution and adjust the volume to 100 ml with purified water. Within 15 minutes read the absorbance of the solution with a spectrophotometer at 545 nm using a reagent blank. A standard curve relating the absorbance to the amount of sulfadiazine is supplied by the instructor. Record the absorbance and the milligrams of sulfadiazine in the sample. Then calculate the amount of sulfadiazine dissolved in 900 ml of the dissolving fluid.

Plot the cumulative per cent of sulfadiazine dissolved from the tablet against time.

G. Using the U. S. P. dissolution apparatus and procedure, determine the amount of sodium salicylate dissolved in simulated gastric fluid without pepsin. A sample is removed at 5, 10, 15, and 30 minutes.

Place one tablet containing 300 mg of sodium salicylate in the dissolution apparatus and immerse in 900 ml of fluid at 37°. At each time interval withdraw a 5.0-ml sample of the solution by a pipet fitted with a filter and transfer to a 50-ml volumetric flask. Adjust the volume to 50 ml by the addition of 0.1 N hydrochloric acid. Measure the absorbance of the solution with a spectrophotometer at 302 nm, using 0.1 N hydrochloric acid as a blank. A standard curve relating the absorbance to the amount of sodium salicylate is supplied by the instructor. Record the absorbance and the milligrams of sodium salicylate in the sample. Then calculate the amount of sodium salicylate dissolved in 900 ml of the dissolving fluid.

Plot the cumulative per cent of sodium salicylate dissolved from tablet in gastric fluid against time

H. The biological availability of salicylate from a compressed tablet is determined by the administration of two tablets, each containing 300 mg of sodium salicylate, and the collection of urine specimens at 2-hour intervals.

On the day preceding the laboratory period the student voids his or her bladder upon arising and collects a urine specimen to be used as a blank. Two tablets are immediately taken with a minimum of 250 ml of water. Food may be ingested as desired, but no salicylates should be ingested. Urine specimens are collected every two hours for fourteen hours. The volumes of the urine specimens are measured and recorded, and aliquots are retained in test tubes for analysis in the laboratory. The 14- to 24-hours urine specimens are pooled, the volume is measured, and the specimen is analyzed.

Each aliquot of urine specimen is diluted with water so the salicylate concentration is from 0.1 to 0.5 mg per ml. The dilution depends on the volume of urine, but it is usually from 2- to 5-fold.

To 1.0 ml of diluted urine specimen 5.0 ml of color reagent is added. In each 100 ml of aqueous solution the color reagent contains 4 g of ferric nitrate $[Fe(NO_3)_3 \cdot 9H_2O]$, 4 g of mercuric chloride and 12 ml of N hydrochloric acid. The clear, supernatant liquid is placed in a cuvette and the absorbance is determined using a spectrophotometer at 540 nm. The urine specimen which was collected upon arising is diluted in the same manner, and 1.0 ml of the diluted specimen is mixed with 5.0 ml of the color reagent to provide a blank for each analysis. A standard absorption curve relating the absorbance to concentration of salicylate is provided by the instructor.

Record the time interval of the specimen collected, the volume of each specimen, the absorbance, and milligrams of salicylate in each sample analyzed. Calculate the milligrams of salicylate excreted per time interval. Plot the cumulative amount excreted against time. Plot the amount excreted per time interval against time. This data will be used in a future exercise.

REFERENCES

Alam, A. S. and E. L. Parrott. 1971. Effect of aging on some physical properties of hydrochlorothiazide tablets. J. Pharm. Sci., 60:263.

Brook, D. and K. Marshall. 1968. "Crushing-strength" of compressed tablets I. Comparison of testers. J. Pharm. Sci., 57:481.

Ceschel, G. S. and C. Mazzonetto. 1970. Evaluation of the dissolution rate of drugs from solid pharmaceutical forms. Il Farmaco. Ed. Pratica, 25:700.

Frostad, S. 1961. Continued studies in concentrations of para-aminosalicylic acid (PAS) in the blood. Acta Tuberc. Pneumol. Scand., 41:68.

Katchen, B. and S. Symchowicz. 1967. Correlation of dissolution rate and griseofulvin absorption in man. J. Pharm. Sci., 56:1108.

Lachman, L. and P. De Luca. 1976. Physical stability. Tablets. In The theory and practice of industrial pharmacy, 2nd ed. L. Lachman, H. A. Lieberman, and J. L. Kanig, Eds. Lea and Febiger, Philadelphia. Chap. 2. pp. 64-65.

Leeson, L. J. and J. T. Carstensen, Eds. 1974. Dissolution technology. Academy of Pharmaceutical Sciences, Washington, D.C.

Levy, G. 1967. Effect of dissolution rate on absorption, metabolism and pharmacologic activity of drugs. J. Mond. Pharm. 3:237.

Levy, G. 1970. Biopharmaceutical considerations in dosage form design and evaluation. In Prescription pharmacy, 2nd ed. J. B. Sprowls, Jr., Ed., J. B. Lippincott Company, Philadelphia. Chap. 2, p. 36.

Lowenthal, W. and J. H. Wood. 1973. Mechanism of action of starch as a tablet disintegrant. VI. Location and structure of starch in tablets. J. Pharm. Sci. 62:287.

Martin, B. K. 1971. The formulation of aspirin. In Advances in pharmaceutical sciences. H. S. Bean, A. H. Beckett, and J. E. Carless. Vol. 3. Academic Press, London and New York. p. 107.

Morrison, A. B. and J. A. Campbell. 1965. Tablet disintegration and physiological availability of drugs. J. Pharm. Sci. 54:1.

Parrott, E. L. 1967. Student experiments in pharmaceutical technology. VI. Evaluation of dosage forms by urinary excretion. Am. J. Pharm. Ed., 31:154.

Ritschel, W. A. 1972. Biological half-lives and their clinical applications. In Perspectives in clinical pharmacy. D. E. Francke and H. A. K. Whitney, Jr., Eds. Drug Intelligence Publications, Hamilton, Illinois. Chap. 16, p. 286.

Shafer, E., E. Wollish, and C. Engel. 1956. The "Roche" friabilator. J. Am. Pharm. Assoc., Sci. Ed., 45:114.

Swintosky, J. V., M. J. Robinson, and E. L. Foltz. 1957. Sulfaethylthiadiazole. II. Distribution and disappearance from the tissues following intravenous injection. J. Am. Pharm. Assoc., Sci. Ed., 46:403.

Symchowicz, S. and B. Katchen. 1968. Griseofulvin absorption in man after single and repeated treatments and its correlation with dissolution rates. J. Pharm. Sci., 57:1383.

The United States Pharmacopeia, 19th Rev. 1975. Content uniformity, p. 648, Disintegration, p. 650, Dissolution, p. 651.

Wagner, J. G. 1971. Biopharmaceutics and relevant pharmacokinetics. Drug Intelligence Publications, Hamilton, Illinois.

Evaluation of Compressed Tablets

Data and Conclusions

1. Record the weight of twenty tablets in A. Calculate the average weight. Do your tablets meet U. S. P. specifications?

2. Record the hardness of ten tablets in C. What is the average and the range of hardness?

3. What is the relationship of hardness to porosity of a tablet?

4. Record the disintegration time in D of the sulfadiazine tablet in water at 37° C. What is the acceptable disintegration time for sulfadiazine tablets?

5. Record the disintegration time in E of the sodium salicylate tablet. What is the acceptable disintegration time for sodium salicylate tablets?

6. If the ingredients of a tablet are soluble, is a disintegrating agent necessary in the formulation of a tablet? Explain your answer.

7. If a tablet meets the specifications of a disintegration test, does this guarantee the drug is available for absorption? What is the usefulness of a disintegration test?

8. Describe the Content Uniformity Test for tablets.

9. Describe the U. S. P. dissolution test.

10. Record the data in F for the dissolution of a sulfadiazine tablet in simulated gastric fluid without pepsin at 37°. Show a sample calculation.

Time, Min	Absorbance	Mg in Sample	Mg Dissolved from Tablet	Percent Drug Dissolved

11. Give the equations for the chemical reactions that occur in the assay for sulfadiazine.

12. Record the data in G for the dissolution of a sodium salicylate tablet in simulated gastric fluid without pepsin at 37°.

Time, Min	Absorbance	Mg in Sample	Mg Dissolved from Tablet	Percent Drug Dissolved

13. Since the sodium salicylate and sulfadiazine tablets have essentially the same formulation, how do you explain the difference found in comparing their disintegration and dissolution?

14. Record the data from H. Show a sample calculation.

Time Interval	Ml of Urine	Dilution	Absorbance	Concentration	Mg Excreted

15. Assuming that all of the salicylate is excreted within 24 hours after administration, calculate the fraction of the orally administered dose recovered in the urine.

16. Sketch the gastrointestinal tract. Label its segments and indicate the pH and enzymes present in each segment.

17. The amount of drug remaining in the body at any time is equal to the total excretable drug minus the amount excreted to that time. Using the data from H, plot the logarithm of the unexcreted salicylate against time. Express an equation for the urinary elimination of the salicylate. Calculate the biological half-life. (See article by J. V. Swintosky, M. J. Robinson, and E. L. Foltz in J. Amer. Pharm. Assoc., Sci. Ed., 46, 403, 1957.)

18. Compare your data (17) with the analogous data obtained with the effervescent granulation of sodium salicylate in Chapter 8, Item C.

12. COATING OF SOLIDS

An enteric coating is one which does not disintegrate in the stomach but rapidly disintegrates or dissolves in the intestine. Enteric coatings usually are formulated with ingredients which have acidic groups and are consequently insoluble in the low pH of the stomach, but they are more soluble in the higher pH of the intestine.

The enteric substance may also be hydrolyzed by enzymes of the intestine and emulsified and dispersed by the bile salts. Time-disintegration coating utilizes a waxy base blended with a hygroscopic substance which absorbs moisture, swells, and ruptures the enteric coating.

PROCEDURE. Many formulas have been suggested for the extemporaneous coating of pills and capsules; however, none have been completely satisfactory.

A. Coat the hexamethylenetetramine and ammonium chloride capsules previously prepared with the following coating:

n-butyl stearate	45 g
Carnauba wax	30 g
Stearic acid	25 g

Fuse the mixture in a water bath at 75° and keep at this temperature during the coating process. Hold the capsule by means of a forceps and dip it into the molten mixture. Withdraw the capsule and gently touch its end to the lip of the beaker to remove the excess coating. Allow the coating to congeal, reverse the capsule, and repeat the operation.

B. With the above enteric coating, coat eight sodium salicylate tablets which you prepared.

C. A 10% cellulose acetate phthalate solution will be supplied by the instructor. Coat eight sodium salicylate tablets with cellulose acetate phthalate. Place 25-30 ml of the solution in a small beaker and drop in a tablet. Remove the tablet immediately with a forceps, allowing the excess coating to drain away. Place the tablet on a paper and allow it to dry. When the tablet is dry, repeat the process until a continuous coat has been applied.

D. Using a U.S.P. disintegration apparatus, test the disintegration time of the two types of enteric coating applied to the sodium salicylate tablets.

Immerse the basket containing six coated sodium salicylate tablets in simulated gastric fluid T.S. at 37° and operate the apparatus for one hour. A properly enteric coated tablet will show no distinct evidence of dissolution or disintegration.

Replace the simulated gastric fluid with simulated intestinal fluid T. S. and operate the apparatus for one hour at 37° using six tablets that have withstood exposure to the gastric fluid. At the end of this time, the coatings of all six tablets must be broken and the contents dissolved or softened so that all material remaining on the screen is soft.

In vitro test methods may indicate that a dosage form possesses the desired characteristics of drug release, but ultimately the pattern of availability of a drug must be determined in humans. The resistance of an enteric formulation to simulated gastric fluid in a U. S. P. disintegration apparatus strongly suggests an enteric coating is satisfactory; however, only by administration to humans can one be certain the coating is successful. Clinical tests, in addition to determining that the enteric coating delays the release of the drug until the dosage form has passed from the stomach, show that the total amount of the drug available is comparable to the total drug available from a nonenteric form of the drug. If any interaction between the drug and the ingredients of the coating occurs, this comparison will demonstrate the interference of the interaction with the availability of the drug. When an *in vitro* test is correlated with clinical behavior, one has a control test for manufacturing operations and a useful screening test for new formulations.

E. The effectiveness of one of the enteric coatings above is evaluated *in vivo* by the administration of two coated tablets, each containing 300 mg of sodium salicylate, and the collection of urine specimens at two-hour intervals. The procedure and the analytical method are described in H of *Evaluation of Compressed Tablets.*

Record the time interval of the specimen collected, the volume of each specimen, the absorbance and milligrams of salicylate in each sample analyzed. Calculate the milligrams of salicylate excreted per time interval. Plot the cumulative amount excreted against time. On the same graph, plot the cumulative amount of salicylate against time after the oral administration of two tablets containing 300 mg of sodium salicylate.

REFERENCES

Ellis, J. R., E. B. Prillig, and A. H. Amann. 1976. Tablet coating. In The theory and practice of industrial pharmacy, 2nd ed., L. Lachman, H. A. Lieberman, and J. L. Kanig, Eds. Lea and Febiger, Philadelphia. Chap. 12, p. 359.

Parrott, E. L. 1961. An extemporaneous coating. J. Am. Pharm. Assoc., NS1. p. 158.

Parrott, E. L. 1967. Student experiments in pharmaceutical technology. IV. Coating of solids. Am. J. Pharm. Ed. 31:1.

Windheuser, J. and J. Cooper. 1956. The pharmaceutics of coating by compression. J. Am. Pharm. Assoc., Sci. Ed. 45:542.

Wurster, D. E. 1960. Preparation of compressed tablet granulations by air-suspension technique. J. Am. Pharm. Assoc., Sci. Ed. 49:82.

Partial translation of Les enrobages modernes des dragées et des pilules. 1958. Distillation Products Industries, Rochester, N.Y.

Coating of Solids

Data and Conclusions

1. Give the formula for simulated gastric fluid T. S. and simulated intestinal fluid T. S.

2. Did the enteric coatings on the sodium salicylate tablets meet official specifications?

3. What is the procedure to follow if the enteric coating ruptured on two tablets during the first hour in gastric fluid?

4. What is the disintegration procedure for plain coated tablets?

5. Record the data from E. Show a sample calculation.

Time Interval	Ml of Urine	Dilution	Absorbance	Concentration	Mg Excreted

6. Plot the cumulative amount of salicylate excreted against time for the enteric-coated tablets. On the same graph plot the cumulative amount of salicylate excreted against time for the administration of the same weight of salicylate in uncoated tablets (see H of *Evaluation of Compressed Tablets*). How many hours did the enteric coating delay the release of the sodium salicylate? In the twenty-four hour period, how much salicylate is available from the uncoated and the coated tablets?

7. Explain the mechanism by which the waxy enteric coat of A is removed in the gastrointestinal tract.

8. Give the structure of cellulose acetate phthalate. Explain the mechanism by which a cellulose acetate phthalate coat is removed in the gastrointestinal tract.

9. Give some applications and advantages of press coating of tablets.

SOLUTIONS

13. SATURATED SOLUTIONS

A phase is a definite homogeneous part of a system and is physically separated from other phases by distinct boundaries. The solubility of a substance at a given temperature is defined as the concentration of solute in solution which is in equilibrium with the solute phase.

Solubility is an equilibrium phenomenon. In a saturated solution in contact with undissolved solute, the rate of dissolution of the solute is equal to the rate at which the solute returns to the solute phase. Theoretically at a given temperature, the solubility or the concentration of solute in solution is a constant but due to the dynamic situation the identical molecules or ions of the solute may not necessarily perpetually exist in the dissolved state. This may be expressed as an equilibrium reaction

$$\text{Solute}_{(\text{solid phase})} \underset{k_c}{\overset{k_s}{\rightleftharpoons}} \text{Solute}_{(\text{solution phase})}$$

where k_s is the rate constant of the process of dissolution and k_c is the rate constant of the process of return to the solid phase. The solubility is the ratio at equilibrium of the rate constants.

Solubilities are expressed in various ways, such as g of solute per 100 g of solvent, g of solute per 100 ml of solvent, g of solute per 100 ml of solution, or g of solute per 100 g of solution. If the respective densities are known, interconversion of these values is simple.

Solubilities for physicochemical work are often expressed as mole fractions, because the properties of the solutions are then expressed in terms of the relative numbers of molecules. Mole fraction, N, of a substance in solution is the number of moles of that substance divided by the total number of moles of all substances comprising the solution.

PROCEDURE. Aromatic waters are saturated aqueous solutions of volatile oils or other aromatic or volatile substances. If a large amount of water-soluble drug is added to an aromatic water, there may be a separation of an insoluble layer at the top. If this layer is taken with the first dose of medication, a burning taste will be experienced. This separation may be looked on as a competitive process in which the molecules of the water-soluble drug have more attraction for the solvent molecules of water than the volatile oil molecules, and the associated water molecules were pulled away from the volatile oil molecules so they were no longer held in solution.

Aromatic waters are prepared by three officially recognized methods—distillation, solution, and alternative solution. Distillation is a universal method but is not practical or economical in most cases; however, it is the only method for preparing Stronger Rose Water and Orange Flower Water.

In the solution method 2 ml or 2 g of the volatile substance is agitated for 15 minutes with sufficient water to make 1000 ml of solution, is set aside for 12 hours, and filtered. It is difficult to obtain a clear solution in this time-consuming method.

The alternative solution is the most expedient means of preparing waters. The volatile substance is thoroughly mixed with 15 g of an inert adsorptive agent. A liter of purified water is added and agitated for 10 minutes. The solution is filtered until a clear filtrate is obtained and enough purified water is added to make the product measure 1000 ml. The volatile substance is adsorbed on the inert ingredient, increasing the total area of volatile substance exposed to the water, thus facilitating the formation of a saturated solution. The adsorptive agent also acts as a clarifier in filtrations as the undissolved volatile material remains adsorbed and does not pass through the filter.

A. Using recently boiled and cooled purified water, prepare 200 ml of Peppermint Water N. F., using talc as an adsorbing agent in the alternative solution method. Examine your produce for clarity, intensity of odor, and taste. By means of short-range pHydrion paper, determine the pH of the water. To 5 ml of Peppermint Water in a test tube add 1 g of sodium bromide and record your observation.

B. Repeat A using light magnesium carbonate.

C. Repeat A using charcoal.

The solubility of a very slightly soluble electrolyte may be expressed as a solubility product. When the solute phase is composed of two more definite ionic species, the solubility may be expressed as the product of the concentrations of the ions in a saturated solution, each concentration, expressed in g ions liter^{-1}, being raised to the power corresponding to the number of each species of ion produced. In the saturated solution if

$$C_nA_{m(\text{solid})} \rightleftharpoons C_nA_{m(\text{solution})} \rightleftharpoons nC^+ + mA^-$$

the solubility product, S, is

$$S = c_{C^+}^{n}\, c_{A^-}^{m}$$

By use of the solubility product, the maximum concentration of an ion that a given solution will hold in equilibrium with the solute phase may be calculated.

Calcium Hydroxide Solution contains 1.4 g of calcium hydroxide per liter; it is 0.019 molar. The solubility product of calcium carbonate is 9 X 10^{-9}. Knowing this solubility product and the concentration of calcium ion, the maximum concentration of carbonate ion may be found.

$$S_{CaCO_3} = c_{Ca^{++}}\, c_{CO_3^{--}}$$

$$9 \times 10^{-9} = 0.019\, c_{CO_3^{--}}$$

$$c_{CO_3^{--}} = 4.7 \times 10^{-7} \text{ molar}$$

Since the molecular weight of ammonium carbonate is 96 g mole^{-1}, the weight which may be added to 1 liter is

$$4.7 \times 10^{-7} \times 96 = 4.5 \times 10^{-5} \text{ g}$$

Up to this amount of ammonium carbonate will dissolve in Lime Water to form a solution; any greater amount will remain undissolved as the solubility of calcium carbonate has been exceeded.

It is interesting to note that at times the addition of a common ion may result in the formation of a complex which is highly soluble. At first glance it might appear that the addition of a soluble iodide would, according to the solubility product, decrease the solubility of mercuric iodide; however, a more soluble complex salt is formed which dissociates

$$HgI_2 + 2I^- \longrightarrow HgI_4^{--}$$

D. Prepare 120 ml of Calcium Hydroxide Solution U. S. P. Expose 30 ml of Lime Water to the atmosphere. Observe what occurs.

Gently warm another 30 ml of Lime Water. Observe what occurs.

E. Prepare 15 ml of Strong Iodine Solution U. S. P. according to the official procedure.

Prepare 15 ml of Lugol's Solution by adding all of the water at once to dissolve the iodine and potassium iodide.

Solubility varies with temperature. Generally an increase in temperature will cause an increase in solubility, and a decrease in temperature will cause a decrease in solubility. If a solute gives off heat during the process of dissolution, its solubility is decreased by an increase in temperature.

Solutions dispensed by the pharmacist on prescriptions are not maintained by the patient at a constant temperature. If a saturated solution of a drug at 25° were dispensed, it would deposit crystals when cooled below this temperature. To avoid the deposition of crystals, some of the so-called saturated pharmaceutical solutions are not saturated at 25° in order that small temperature changes common in the home will not affect the appearance or cause crystal formation in the preparation. Similarly, mouth-washes, in which the solubility is very near saturation, are chilled during manufacture prior to filtration to prevent separation or cloudiness upon subsequent cooling of the product.

F. Prepare 15 ml of Potassium Iodide Solution U. S. P. Assume the solution will not be used in a short time and add the proper amount of sodium thiosulfate.

Prepare 15 ml of Potassium Iodide Solution, using water at room temperature. Observe the temperature change upon the addition of potassium iodide to the water. Expose half the solution to the atmosphere and observe. Bottle the remainder and compare it after several weeks to the solution containing sodium thiosulfate.

REFERENCES

American Medical Association. 1973. AMA Drug evaluations. Chapter 67. Antiseptics and disinfectants. AMA, Chicago. p. 645.

Block, J. H., E. B. Roche, T. O. Soine, and C. O. Wilson. 1974. Inorganic medicinal and pharmaceutical chemistry. Lea and Febiger, Philadelphia. pp. 83-84.

von Fenyes, C. K. 1970. Alcohols as preservatives and germicides. Am. Perfumer and Cosmetics, 85, No. 3, March.

Ito, K. and K. Sekiguchi. 1966. Studies on the molecular compounds of organic medicinals. II. Application of the solubility product principle and consideration by the phase rule to the solubility phenomena of the molecular compound of sulfanilamide and sulfathiazole. Chem. Pharm. Bull., 14:255.

Lewin, S. 1960. The solubility product principle. An introduction to its uses and limitations. Interscience Publishers, Inc. New York.

Parrott, E. L. 1970. Characteristics of solutions. Chapter 5 in Pharmaceutical technology. Fundamental pharmaceutics. Burgess Publishing Company, Minneapolis. p. 139.

Sokoloski, T. D. 1975. Solutions and phase equilibria. In Remington's Pharmaceutical sciences, Mack Publishing Company, Easton, Pa. Chapter 17, p. 229.

Saturated Solutions

Data and Conclusions

1. If Potassium Iodide Solution has a density of 1.70 g cc^{-1}, complete the following table. Show your calculations.

Solubility

Compound	Solvent	g/100 g solvent	g/100 ml solvent	g/100 g solution	g/100 ml solution
Tartaric acid	50% W/W alcohol	88.6	80.9	47.0	55.7
Potassium iodide	water	(a)_____	(b)_____	(c)_____	(d)_____

2. Record the observations made on your Peppermint Water, using various distributing agents.

Distributing Agent	pH	Clarity	Intensity of Odor	Intensity of Taste	Effect of Electrolyte
Talc					
Magnesium carbonate					
Charcoal					

3. How much silver nitrate may be added to 100 ml of a 1% aqueous solution of procaine hydrochloride before precipitation occurs?

4. What occurs when Lime Water is exposed to the air?

5. Explain your observation when Lime Water was heated.

6. What percent of iodine in what percent of ethanol is the most effective and fast-acting skin disinfectant?

7. Insoluble mercuric or mercurous halides should not be administered to a patient at the same time that soluble halides are given. Explain.

8. Is Lugol's Solution a saturated solution? Explain what occurs when preparing this solution.

9. Why is sodium thiosulfate sometimes added to Potassium Iodide Solution?

10. Drug A is expensive. It dissolves to the extent of 1 g in 0.3 ml of water. If called upon by a physician to supply 30 ml of a saturated solution of Drug A, describe the most economical method of doing so.

11. How does the U. S. P. indicate solubilities?

14. AQUEOUS SOLUTIONS

Although a saturated solution, an aromatic water contains very low concentration of the solute. Other pharmaceutical solutions may contain a very high concentration of solute and yet not form a saturated solution. Syrup contains 850 g of sucrose and 450 ml of water per liter, yet it is not saturated as 1 g of sucrose dissolves in 0.5 ml of water.

A concentrated solution is usually capable of dissolving other solutes; however, the solubility of the first solute may be increased or decreased. In many pharmaceutical solutions of nonelectrolytes, the addition of a water-soluble second solute will decrease the solubility of the first solute. When the solubility of a nonelectrolyte is decreased in this manner, the effect is referred to as salting out.

Salting out occurs because the ions of the added electrolyte combine with water to form hydrates, thus reducing the amount of water available for solution of the nonelectrolyte. The greater the degree of hydration, the greater the reduction in solubility of the nonelectrolyte.

The fact that 2 g of sugar dissolves in 1 ml of water indicates that the hydration or hydrogen bonding between sucrose and water is very strong. This strong association between the solute and solvent prevents, to any great extent, further association of the water dipoles with additional water-soluble drugs; thus, syrups have a lowered solvent power for other water-soluble drugs which may be added. This is the reason the practicing pharmacist may find it difficult to dissolve a drug in a syrup, yet the drug would readily dissolve in the same volume of water.

Dilute sucrose solutions are good media for microbial growth, and concentrated sucrose solutions retard microbial growth. If a saturated solution were employed in pharmacy, it would prevent microorganic growth, but with a change in temperature it might lead to the formation of crystals which would be difficult to redissolve. Industrially formulated syrups contain other ingredients to obtain the desired solubility for the drug as well as for improvement of taste, appearance, and stability. In developing such products it is an economic necessity to consider the additive preservative effects of ingredients such as alcohol, glycerin, sugar, propylene glycol, and dissolved solids.

Syrup U. S. P. contains 850 g of sucrose per 1000 ml of syrup or 65% sucrose by weight. The minimum amount of sucrose required to preserve a neutral syrup is about 65-68% by weight. Assuming that one wishes to formulate a syrup containing only 500 g of sucrose per 1000 ml, the amount of alcohol that must be added to preserve this product may be estimated. This requires the consideration of the U.S.P. Syrup equivalent and the free water equivalent.

If 850 g of sucrose preserves 450 ml of water in a liter of Syrup U. S. P., then 1 g of sucrose will preserve 450/850 or 0.53 ml of water. In the formulation the 500 g of sucrose will preserve 500 × 0.53 or 265 ml of water.

In Syrup U. S. P. 850 g of sucrose apparently assumes a volume of 550 ml, and 1 g of sucrose occupies a volume of 550/850 or 0.647 ml. Then, if 500 g of sucrose preserves 265 ml of water, the total volume of solution which would be equivalent to U. S. P. Syrup would be the sum of the volume occupied by the sucrose (500 × 0.647) and the volume of water preserved by this amount of sucrose (265) or 589 ml. The free-water equivalent per liter of the formulation is 1000 - 589 or 411 ml.

If this 411 ml requires 18% alcohol to preserve it, then 411 × 0.18 or 74 ml of absolute alcohol is required, and the final liter of product must contain in addition to the 500 g of sucrose, alcohol to the extent of 7.4%.

In general, when dissolved solids other than sucrose are present, the volume they assume should be subtracted from the free-water volume determined according to the previous example. If glycerin is present, the percent by volume may be doubled and this figure is also subtracted from the free-water volume. If propylene glycol is present, its preservative action is considered equivalent to alcohol.

For example, if a liter of a neutral vehicle being formulated is to contain 5% glycerin by volume, 200 g of sucrose, and 150 g of total solids (in addition to the sucrose), which occupy a volume of 60 ml, the amount of alcohol required to preserve this product can be estimated. In actual practice this calculation is followed by stability tests to determine if the formulation was correct.

The volume of Syrup U. S. P. to which this is equivalent is the sum of the volume occupied by the sucrose (200 X 0.647) and the corresponding amount of water in U. S. P. Syrup (200 X 0.53) or 235 ml. The difference between total volume (1000) and the syrup equivalent (235) is the free-water equivalent or 765 ml.

From this the volume occupied by the solids (60) and the glycerin (100) is subtracted to obtain 605 ml of free-water. It is known that 18% alcohol will prevent microbial growth; thus, 605 X 0.18 or 109 ml of alcohol is added. This 10.9% alcohol in the new vehicle in conjunction with the other ingredients will prevent microorganic growth.

The bacteriostatic effect of ethyl alcohol varies according to the pH of the medium. Acidic solutions require 15% alcohol, while neutral or slightly alkaline solutions require 17.5%.

Retardation of gastrointestinal absorption of drugs dissolved in a 50% sucrose solution has been reported. In rats it has been found that increasing the concentration of sucrose in aqueous solutions of phenobarbital sodium has lengthened the induction time.

PROCEDURE. In preparing syrups, clean equipment and careful manipulation must be used to prevent contamination. There are three methods of preparing syrup: (1) solution in boiling water, (2) agitation without heat, and (3) percolation without heat.

The hot method of preparing a syrup cannot be used to make a syrup containing a thermolabile or volatile ingredient. When using the hot method, the temperature should be carefully observed to avoid the darkening of the syrup. If a concentrated solution of sugar is heated, the sweet taste is destroyed and a dark-brown liquid is formed. This mixture of decomposition products of sugar is known as Caramel or Burnt Sugar Coloring. Excessive heating during the process of manufacture of a syrup, probably results in the breakdown of sugar, and the resulting caramel imparts a dark color to the syrup.

A. Prepare 500 ml of Syrup U.S.P. Determine and record the density of the Syrup by means of a Westphal balance.

   Fluidextracts, tinctures, and other liquids may be added to a syrup to medicate it. If not mixe in the proper sequence, a clear solution will not result, for many of the alcohol-soluble substan will precipitate in the high concentration of water in the syrup. To avoid this, the tincture or fluidextract may be mixed with water and a distributing agent and filtered. Sucrose and water are added to the filtrate to form the syrup.

B. Place 10 ml of water in a test tube. Add 0.5 ml of Tolu Balsam Tincture. Observe.

C. Prepare 200 ml of Tolu Balsam Syrup N. F. following the official procedure.

Percolation is the extraction process in which the desired constituents are removed from a granulated or powdered drug by descent of a suitable solvent through the drug at a controlled rate.

In preparing Wild Cherry Syrup, the coarse Wild Cherry is macerated and percolated with water, which in the presence of an enzyme, emulsin, forms hydrolytic products which give the flavor to Wild Cherry Syrup. Heat is not used, as the syrup contains volatile constituents and the hydrolytic enzyme is deactivated by heat.

D. Prepare 200 ml of Wild Cherry Syrup U. S. P. XVIII following the official procedure. Describe the odor of the completed syrup.

Test the Wild Cherry Syrup for the presence of tannins. Add a few drops of Ferric Chloride T. S. to 2 ml of syrup in a test tube. Observe the color. Add 5 ml of water and observe the color.

Using a solution of codeine phosphate supplied by the instructor, determine if the tannins in the syrup have any effect on the alkaloidal salt.

Test the syrup for the presence of hydrocyanic acid by using the Guignard test. Prepare a strip of filter paper by moistening with Picric Acid T. S. and after draining, immerse it in a 10% sodium carbonate solution. Suspend the wet strip in a stoppered ounce bottle approximately half filled with Wild Cherry Syrup. Observe the color change.

E. Prepare 200 ml of syrup by boiling 30 g of Wild Cherry with approximately 250 ml of water for half an hour. Complete the preparation according to the official procedure. Repeat all tests as described above in D and compare the two syrups.

REFERENCES

Bean, H. S. 1972. Preservatives for pharmaceuticals. J. Soc. Cosmet. Chem., 23:703-720.

Grote, I. W. and P. Walker. 1946. Studies in the preservation of liquid pharmaceutical preparations. I. The relationship between the preservative action of alcohol and the solid content of the preparation. J. Am. Pharm. Assoc. Sci. Ed. 35:182.

Kato, R., A. Takanaka, K. Onoda, and Y. Omori. 1969. Effect of syrup on the absorption of drugs from gastrointestinal tract. The Japanese Journal of Pharmacology, 19:331.

Malone, M.H., R. D. Gibson, and T. S. Miya. 1960. A pharmacologic study of the effects of various pharmaceutical vehicles on the action of orally administered phenobarbital. J. Pharm. Sci., 49:529.

Schumacher, G. E. 1972. Formulation of non-sterile dosage forma. In Perspectives in clinical pharmacy. D. E. Francke and H.A.K. Whitney, Jr., Eds. Drug Intelligence Publications, Hamilton, Illinois. Chapter 18, p. 368.

Sugisawa, H. 1966. The thermal degradation of sugars. II. The volatile decomposition products of glucose caramel. Journal of Food Science, 31:381.

Sugisawa, H. and H. Edo. 1964. Thermal polymerisation of glucose. Chemistry and Industry, 1964:892.

The United States Pharmacopeia, 19th rev. 1975. Storage temperature. p. 8.

Aqueous Solutions

Data and Conclusions

1. Explain what occurs when Tolu Balsam Tincture is added to water.

2. Explain the purpose of magnesium carbonate in the manufacture of Tolu Balsam Syrup.

3. Complete the following chart for Wild Cherry Syrup:

	Odor	Presence of Tannins	Effect on Alkaloidal Salts	Presence of Hydrocyanic Acid
Official Method				
As Made In Part E				

4. What is the density of the Syrup prepared in A?

5. What occurs when an aqueous solution of sucrose is heated?

6. Syrup U. S. P. contains 85% w/v sucrose and has a density of 1.313 g cc^{-1}. Show how one may calculate its concentration in terms of weight-weight percentage.

7. If 5% propylene glycol had been added to the vehicle being formulated as discussed in the introductory remarks, how much alcohol would then be needed to prevent microbial growth?

8. A pharmacist is frequently called upon to dispense a prescription which he prepares by mixing equal volumes of U. S. P. Syrup and an aqueous proprietary solution. To save time, the pharmacist decides to prepare 5 liters which will be available immediately for dispensing to the patient. To avoid microorganic growth in this stock preparation, he decides to add alcohol. Calculate what percent of alcohol should be contained in the stock solution.

9. What occurs when Syrup U. S. P. is stored in a refrigerator (between 2-8°C)?

15. NONAQUEOUS SOLUTIONS

Although from their physical properties many solvents appear to be desirable for use in pharmaceutical products, the physiological actions of the solvents greatly limit their use. With few exceptions, most organic solvents are irritating or toxic.

Aromatic hydrocarbons cause paralysis of the central nervous system and are irritating to the skin; methyl alcohol is toxic, and butyl and amyl alcohol are irritating; volatile ethers paralyze the central nervous system, and as this effect decreases with an increase in molecular weight and a decrease in volatility, irritation to mucous membrane increases; ketones are mildly irritating; and the low molecular weight esters are irritating. Thus, toxicity and irritation limit the solvents employed to a few compounds such as glycerin, alcohol, and propylene glycol for internal use. For external use saturated aliphatic hydrocarbons, ether, and glyceryl esters of aliphatic acids may be added to the list of acceptable pharmaceutical solvents.

Propylene glycol has been employed as a solvent for oral and parenteral solutions of drugs such as antihistamines, barbiturates and vitamins. Although orally administered propylene glycol has a low toxicity in animals, it may exhibit a weak central nervous system depressant activity and an antagonistic action against pentylenetetrazol. Thus, the use of propylene glycol as a physiologically inert solvent is not recommended. Infants with rickets have become stuporous for hours after treatment with 600,000 units of vitamin D administered in 60 ml of propylene glycol as single or divided doses in a 24-hour period.

Although molecules as a whole are not charged, a noncoincident negative and positive electrical center within the molecule may cause one portion of the molecule to be negatively charged relative to another portion of the molecule. Such a molecule is a dipole or a polar compound. For example, in the case of an ethanol molecule the electron pair responsible for the O-H bond is not equally shared by the two atoms. As the oxygen kernel possesses a higher central charge than the proton, the bonding electron pair tends to be displaced toward the oxygen atoms, resulting in a deficiency of electrons in the vicinity of the hydrogen atom. As the molecule is not linear, this tendency of electronic displacement toward the oxygen atom results in a deficiency of electrons at the hydrogen atom making it a more positive center than the oxygen atom, which has an excess electron density giving it a negative center:

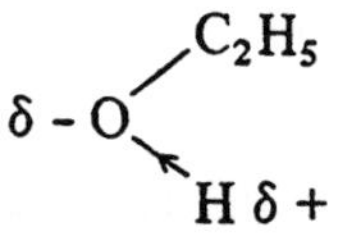

The dissymmetry in the electric charge distribution makes a dipole responsive to electric fields and to other dipoles. In a pure solvent, such as alcohol, it is the alignment and attraction between positive and negative portions of adjacent molecules which cause a weak transient bond. Although weak, this bond or dipole-dipole interaction is the force responsible for the condensed state of a substance; that is, it is the dipole-dipole interaction which maintains alcohol as a liquid at room temperature.

This type of bond is called a hydrogen bond if the association is formed through a hydrogen atom. The alcohol, phenol, amide, carboxyl, nitrile, oxime, mercaptan, thio-acid, primary amine, nitro, aldehyde, and ketone radicals tend to confer polarity on a molecule.

Solution of a solute in a solvent is due to interaction between the solute molecule and the solvent molecules. This interaction depends on the nature of the solvent and solute. A dipole such as benzoic acid dissolves in alcohol by a dipole-dipole interaction in which the oppositely charged parts of the benzoic acid and alcohol align and are attracted with sufficient force to cause the benzoic acid molecule to leave its crystal lattice and enter solution solvated by the alcohol. Other polar pharmaceutical solvents such as glycerin, propylene glycol, polyethylene glycols, and water behave in a similar fashion.

Solvents may be classified as polar and nonpolar solvents. A molecule which is electrically neutral and has symmetrical distribution of its electrons is known as a nonpolar substance. Because a nonpolar substance is symmetrical, little attraction is exerted on neighboring molecules. Actually, oscillations of the electrons within the molecule produce a very feeble, internal fleeting electronic polarization. This molecule may than induce a temporary dissymmetry of electrical centers in an adjacent molecule forming an induced dipole. This phenomenon exists in all matter and is known as van der Waals' force.

PROCEDURE. Alcohol or a binary mixture containing alcohol is the most commonly used nonaqueous solvent. In addition to the pharmaceutical classes of elixirs, spirits, tinctures, and fluidextracts, individual products such as Chloroform Liniment and Coal Tar Solution are alcoholic solutions.

Elixirs are flavored hydroalcoholic solutions to which glycerin often is added to enhance the solvent properties and as a preservative. The alcoholic content of elixirs varies widely; actually a few commercial elixirs contain no alcohol, while other elixirs may contain as much as 40% alcohol. The concentration of alcohol is determined by the amount required to maintain the drug or volatile oil in solution. The addition of aqueous solutions to elixirs may cause turbidity or separation by lessening the alcohol concentration.

A. Prepare 120 ml of Aromatic Elixir U. S. P.

B. A commercial elixir will be supplied by the instructor. Divide the elixir into 5-ml portions and place in test tubes. Add measured volumes of water to the test tubes and determine to what extent the elixir may be diluted with water and still maintain a clear solution. Observe these dilutions for one week.

C. Add 2.5 ml of Belladonna Tincture U. S. P. to 15 ml of Low Iso-Alcoholic Elixir N. F. Observe.

Calculate by alligation the amounts of Low and High Iso-Alcoholic Elixir to be used to dilute 10 ml of Belladonna Tincture to a final volume of 60 ml. Mix the elixirs and tincture according to your calculations and observe.

Spirits or essences are alcoholic solutions of volatile substances. Some spirits are used for their medicinal effect, but most spirits are a convenient means of obtaining a proper amount of a flavoring oil. All essences have a high alcohol content, and the addition of water invariably causes turbidity and separation.

Examination of unofficial liquid pharmaceutical speciality products and similar official products indicates that a minimum of 15% alcohol is required to preserve the product from microbial growth if no other preservative agents are present. Industrial pharmacists usually regard 15% alcohol as adequate for the preservation of products with a pH of 5, while 18% has been considered adequate for neutral or slightly alkaline preparations. It is obvious that products such as tinctures, spirits, and fluidextracts possess alcohol in concentrations that far exceed these values and need no further preservative.

Whisky and Brandy are prepared by distillation. Compound Orange Spirit, Camphor Spirit, and Compound Cardamon Spirit are prepared by simple solution.

D. Prepare 120 ml of Peppermint Spirit N. F.

E. Prepare 120 ml of Aromatic Ammonia Spirit N. F.

Tinctures are alcoholic solutions of nonvolatile substances which are generally extracted by maceration or percolation. Tinctures of potent drugs represent the activity of 10 g of the drug in each 100 ml of the tincture; they are 10% tinctures. With a few exceptions, nonpotent tinctures represent 20 g of the drug per 100 ml of tincture.

Tinctures are prepared chiefly by percolation and maceration. Percolation is the procedure of choice when the crude drugs are cellular in structure; plant exudates tend to become impacted in the percolator and stop the flow so that maceration is preferred in such preparations. Moderately coarse powders are preferred, because coarse powders are slowly penetrated by the menstruum and fine powders tend to clog the percolator.

Usually alcohol or a hydroalcoholic menstruum is employed. The choice of menstruum depends on the solubility, stability, and ease of removal of the desired constituent. Other inactive constituents are extracted, but if the material is not objectionable, it is allowed to remain.

In the process of percolation, the drug is dampened with the menstruum and allowed to stand for a short period before packing the percolator so that the drug may expand as the menstruum is absorbed. If the drug is packed into the percolator and moistened, the swelling would pack the drug so firmly that the percolate could not flow.

The menstruum is then added to cover the drug and the lower opening is closed when the liquid is about to drip from the percolator. This permits the air between the particles to escape as the menstruum descends. Maceration for a prescribed time permits saturation of the menstruum in contact with the drug, assuring a more nearly complete extraction.

The menstruum is then allowed to flow or percolate at a definite rate. Normally the percolate collected is assayed before final volume is reached, and then it is adjusted to the proper strength.

In the process of maceration the drug is soaked with the menstruum in a closed container. The closed container prevents the loss of volatile constituents and evaporation of the menstruum. The mixture is agitated frequently so the menstruum at the bottom of the container does not become saturated and incapable of extracting further drug. Circulatory maceration is an efficient modification which eliminates the need for agitation. When heat is employed in maceration, the process is known as digestion. The mixture is then transferred to a filter, and the residue is washed with sufficient menstruum to bring the tincture to final volume.

F. Prepare 60 ml Iodine Tincture U. S. P.

G. Prepare 50 ml of Sweet Orange Peel Tincture N. F. or Compound Benzoin Tincture U. S. P. or the tincture assigned by the instructor.

Other alcoholic solutions and solutions made with other polar solvents find use in medicine. Glycerites are solutions of drugs in glycerin. Glyceryl triacetate, a semipolar and inert solvent, is used as a solvent for chloroazodin.

Avertin with Amylene Hydrate is a solution of tribromoethanol in amylene hydrate. The uniqueness of this solution lies in the fact that not only the solute but also the solvent functions as a central nervous system depressant so that the solvent contributes somewhat to the anesthesia.

H. Prepare 60 ml of Coal Tar Solution U. S. P. Determine the extent to which 10 ml of Coal Tar Solution may be diluted with water before separation occurs.

The nonpolar solvents used in pharmacy are essentially hydrocarbons or glyceryl esters. Peanut, sesame, corn, cottonseed, and mineral oil are most frequently chosen as solvents or vehicles.

Two rather unusual solutions in nonpolar solvents are Floropryl and 622 Mixture. Ophthalmic solutions are usually aqueous so that they are physiologically similar to the lachrymal fluid. Peanut oil is used as a solvent in Isoflurophate Ophthalmic Solution. Dimethyl phthalate is an insect repellant but is most commonly used as a solvent for ethohexadiol and butopyronoxyl for enhanced effect.

REFERENCES

Block, J. H., E. R. Roche, T. O. Soine, and C. O. Wilson. 1974. Inorganic medicinal and pharmaceutical chemistry. Lea and Febiger, Philadelphia. pp. 84-96.

Martin, G. and L. Finberg. 1970. Propylene glycol: A potentially toxic vehicle in liquid dosage form. The Journal of Pediatrics, 77:877.

Martin, A. N., J. Swarbrick, and A. Cammarata. 1969. Intermolecular forces and states of matter. In Physical pharmacy 2nd ed. Lea and Febiger, Philadelphia. Chapter 4, p. 65.

Saski, W. 1955. A modified colorimetric assay for Belladonna alkaloids. Drug Standards. 23:149.

Spott, D. A. and W. B. Shelley. 1970. Exanthem due to contact allergen (benzoin) absorbed through skin. J.A.M.A., 214:1881.

Stadelmann, E. J. 1969. Permeability of plant cell. Annual Review of Plant Physiology, 20:585-606.

U.S.I. Chemicals. 1969. Ethyl alcohol handbook. Pure ethyl alcohol. Specially denatured alcohol. Completely denatured alcohol. U.S.I. Proprietary solvents. U.S.I. New York, N.Y.

Zaroslinski, J. F., R. K. Browne, and L. H. Possley. 1971. Propylene glycol as a drug solvent in pharmacologic studies. Toxicology and Applied Pharmacology, 19:573.

Nonaqueous Solutions

Data and Conclusions

1. To what extent could the commercial elixir supplied in B be diluted with water? May water be added to most elixirs without separation of precipitation occurring?

2. Is Low Iso-Alcoholic Elixir a suitable vehicle for Belladonna Tincture? Show your calculation from C. Were your calculations correct in actual practice?

3. Is microbial growth a problem in preserving elixirs?

4. Differentiate between Brandy and Whisky.

5. Why is Polysorbate 80 included in Coal Tar Solution?

6. For what type of vegetable drug is maceration preferred to percolation? Give examples.

7. What determines the fineness to which powders are ground prior to extraction?

8. Define maceration and percolation.

9. How much morphine is present in Paregoric and Brown Mixture? In your state may either of these preparations be sold without a prescription?

10. How may alkaloids be colorimetrically determined in Atropa Belladonna?

11. Name nonaqueous solvents that may be used in parenterals.

16. PARTITION COEFFICIENT

A solute dissolved in one phase in equilibrium with another immiscible phase will be distributed between the two phases so that the ratio of the concentrations in the two phases is a constant at a given temperature. This constant, K, referred to as the distribution constant or partition coefficient, is then defined as

$$K = \frac{C_U}{C_L}$$

where C_U and C_L are the concentrations in the upper and lower phase, respectively.

This equation holds in the case where the molecules in each phase are in the same state of aggregation. If the solute is dissociated or associated, more complex forms of the equation must be applied. It is also recognized that only in an ideal system is the partition coefficient independent of the total solute present; this deviation is so well known that in the literature of chemical engineering, the equation above is considered to be a limiting case. Fortunately, in most pharmaceutical extractions the solutions are dilute enough so that the above equation is valid for all practical purposes.

In most procedures of pharmacy it is desired in extraction to remove a particular solute from a heterogeneous system. At its simplest the number of extractions is governed by the partition coefficient and the relative volumes of the two phases. At equilibrium the fraction, U, of the total solute found in the upper layer may be expressed

$$U = \frac{Kr}{Kr + 1}$$

where K is the partition coefficient and r is the ratio of the volumes of the upper and lower phases, respectively.

The fraction, L, remaining in the lower phase is then

$$L = \frac{1}{Kr + 1}$$

If the lower phase is re-extracted with n successive equal volumes of the upper layer, each nth extract will contain U_n of the solute

$$U_n = \frac{Kr}{(Kr + 1)^n}$$

and the L_n fraction of the solute will remain in the lower layer

$$L_n = \frac{1}{(Kr + 1)^n}$$

A more exhaustive extraction is obtained by using a given volume in several portions than in a single extraction. If the same volume is used but in divided portions the fraction, L_n, in the lower phase at the nth extraction is

$$L_n = \frac{1}{\left(\frac{Kr}{n} + 1\right)^n}$$

where n is the number of equal portions of the extracting liquid.

A liter of an aqueous solution of a drug is to be extracted by using a liter of ether. The partition coefficient is 2. In a single extraction, two-thirds of the drug is removed by the ether phase

$$U = \frac{Kr}{Kr + 1} = \frac{2 \times 1}{(2 \times 1) + 1} = 0.667$$

If the liter of ether is divided into four 250-ml portions, a larger fraction of the drug will be extracted than by a single extraction. The fraction of the drug remaining in the lower phase after the fourth extraction is

$$L_n = \frac{1}{\left(\frac{Kr}{n} + 1\right)^n}; \quad L_{4th} = \frac{1}{\left(\frac{2 \times 1}{4} + 1\right)^4} = 0.197$$

In this case, the same volume of ether used in four portions extracts about 20% more than in a single extraction.

In extraction from solids equilibrium proceeds very slowly so extraction is not usually carried out under equilibrium conditions. When the intact plant cells of a crude drug are in contact with the extracting liquid, a partition ratio is the limiting factor in the extraction of a cellular solute. A cellular solute at equilibrium with the whole cell will be partitioned between the cellular fluid and the lipoidal cell membrane; this particular partition ratio will maintain practically all the solute in the cell fluid. The cellular solute which has partitioned into the cell membrane will, in turn, partition between the cell membrane and the extraction medium. An equilibrium will be set up between the two partitions. The partition from the cell interior into the membrane probably is the limiting coefficient as shown by the resistance normal plant cells exhibit to penetration.

Since the diffusion of a solute throughout the body of a solid or from the cell interior to the external environment is very slow, the material to be extracted should be ground finely for the most intimate contact. In grinding the drug the cell wall is weakened or ruptured, permitting the extracting menstruum to come into direct contact with the cellular fluids. If the crude drug were completely free of moisture, extraction from the ruptured cells would be a simple dissolving or leaching out of the desired cell solute. Actually, a dried plant will contain several percent of moisture. Thus, in practice, even though the plant cell is ruptured, the solute is in an aqueous phase of the residual moisture after drying the plant, and if the menstruum were a solvent not miscible with water, a partition would exist between the two phases.

Extraction is not a simple process but a complex one involving not only leaching out of cellular constituents but also partition ratios.

The use of a proper solvent and the addition of other substances to improve extraction is more important in extraction from solids than from liquids. Often it is necessary to first extract some interfering substance, such as wax or gum, by a solvent in which the desired solute is insoluble. In the extraction of plant material the addition of a small amount of acid or alkali will greatly increase the extractability of the desired solute.

Partition coefficients are of interest not only in alkaloidal separations and assay procedures but in the isolation of antibiotics from fermentation broths. The importance of the addition of a substance to control the pH to obtain the most favorable partition coefficient is shown in the butanol extraction of tetracycline from the fermentation broth. The optimum partition coefficient for this system appears to exist at pH 1 as shown in Figure 9.

Partition is significant in dosage forms. In flavoring emulsions the partition must be considered so that the flavor does not equilibrate with too low a concentration in the phase to be flavored.

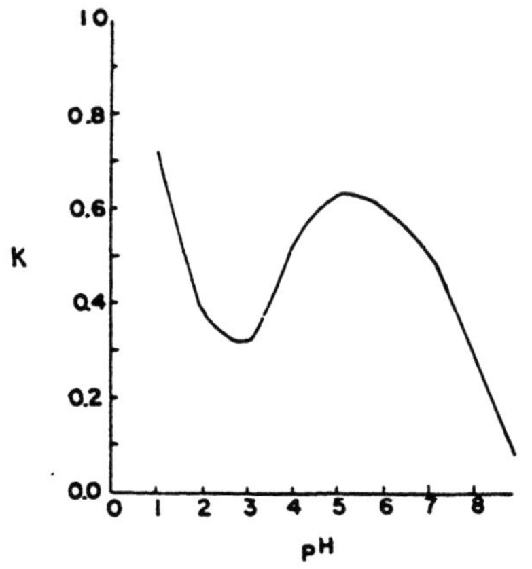

Figure 9 – Distribution of tetracycline between butanol and water.

In oily-type suppository bases which melt at body temperature, the release of the drug depends on the form of the drug and its partition coefficient. If a drug has a high partition coefficient favoring the oil phase, it will be slowly released and perhaps not rapidly enough to provide a concentration required for a therapeutic effect.

PROCEDURE. Fluidextracts are alcohol-containing solutions of the therapeutically active constituents of vegetable drugs. Each milliliter of a fluidextract represents the soluble components of 1 g of the drug. The alcoholic content of the fluidextract acts as a preservative.

All fluidextracts are prepared by percolation. The menstrua employed in making fluidextracts are chosen to obtain a complete and economical extraction of the desired solute while avoiding extraction of unwanted material. Usually the drug is allowed to macerate while in the percolator to permit equilibrium to be reached in the case of partitioning and to permit leaching out of the desired solutes.

The N. F. describes three processes used in preparing fluidextracts. The most common process, A, consists of percolating the drug with alcohol or hydroalcoholic menstruum. The first 85% of the percolate is set aside and the drug is further percolated. The weak percolate, after collection, is concentrated usually by low heat and under reduced pressure. This concentrate is then dissolved in the first percolate, and the fluidextract is adjusted to final volume using water and alcohol.

Process D utilizes boiling water as a menstruum and is limited to the extraction of water-soluble constituents. Alcohol is added to preserve the percolate.

Pressure percolation of Process E may save menstruum and eliminates the concentration of the weak percolate. Industrially, several tubes or percolators are connected by U-tubes to adjacent vertical tubes. The premoistened drug is packed into each tube and U-tube. The U-tube is then attached to the bottoms of the first and second tube, a second U-tube is attached to the top of the second and third tubes, etc. A reservoir for the menstruum is connected to the first tube and a pressure system.

The techniques of the preparation of tinctures and fluidextracts are employed in preparing extracts, resins, and oleoresins; however, with the latter the solvents are removed after extraction.

Extracts are semisolids or solids obtained by extracting desired constituents with an appropriate menstruum, evaporating the solvent, often under controlled temperature and reduced pressure, and adjusting the residue with inert substances to the prescribed standards.

Often the menstruum used in preparing an extract is more alcoholic than that used in the preparation of a tincture of fluidextract. This reduces the extraction of inert material such as sugars which would dilute the extract. The fatty material of some drugs may interfere with the extraction of the active constituents and hinder the final drying of the extract. In such cases the crude drug or the extract are defatted.

Oleoresins are liquid preparations of natural oils and resins extracted by percolation, generally using acetone or ether as a menstruum. Fundamentally oleoresins are similar to fluidextracts but differ in the lack of a uniform relationship to the drug, in the menstruum used, and in the removal of the menstruum after percolation.

Resins are solids made by percolating a drug with an alcoholic menstruum, removing the volatile portion of the menstruum from the percolate, and precipitating the resins by pouring the concentrated percolate into water. A resin consists of vegetable drug constituents which are soluble in alcohol but insoluble in water.

A. Prepare 100 ml of Aromatic Cascara Sagrada Fluidextract U. S. P. or Cascara Sagrada Fluidextract N. F.

The semipermeable membrane, which separates the lumen of the gastrointestinal tract from the blood, is a highly complex structure composed of lipids, proteins, lipoproteins and polysaccharides. The membrane is selectively permeable to the passive diffusion of lipid soluble compounds. To be readily absorbed a medicinal compound must have an appropriate lipid solubility. A crude guide to the lipid solubility of a medicinal compound is provided by its partition coefficient between a lipid-like solvent and water. In general, all other factors being equal, the percent of a medicinal compound absorbed is increased as the chloroform to water partition coefficient is increased.

Biotransformation is the conversion of a medicinal compound into a metabolite; detoxification is the conversion into a pharmacologically inactive metabolite. Drug metabolites are less lipid soluble than the parent compound and consequently have no or a decreased capacity to permeate membranes. Simultaneously drug metabolites are more polar than the parent compound and are consequently more poorly reabsorbed by the renal tubules and are more readily cleared by the kidney. Thus, biotransformation eliminates drugs from the body by metabolism of the drug to a polar compound which is excreted in the urine.

Salicylic acid may be used as a model compound to represent salicylates which are widely used as analgesics. Salicylic acid is biotransformed in the human to gentisic acid by aromatic ring hydroxylation.

B. Determine the partition coefficient of salicylic acid between water and chloroform. An aqueous solution of a known concentration of salicylic acid will be supplied by the instructor.

   Accurately pipet 25.0 ml of the aqueous solution of salicylic acid into a separatory funnel. Then pipet an equal volume of chloroform into the separatory funnel and close with a glass stopper. Shake the funnel frequently for ten minutes. Allow to sit in a ring stand until the two phases have separated. Discard the bottom layer.

   Dilute the aqueous layer by pipetting 5.0 ml of the aqueous layer into a 50-ml beaker containing 20.0 ml of distilled water measured by a pipet. By pipet remove 5.0 ml of the diluted solution and place in a cuvette containing 1.0 ml of color reagent. In each 100 ml of aqueous solution the color reagent contains 4 g of ferric nitrate [$Fe(NO_3) \cdot 9H_2O$] and 12 ml of N hydrochloric acid. The absorbance is determined using a spectrophotometer at 540 nm. A standard curve relating the absorbance to concentration of salicylic acid is provided by the instructor. Record the absorbance.

   Considering the fivefold dilution of the solution of salicylic acid, calculate and record the concentration of salicylic acid in the extracted aqueous layer. Calculate by difference the concentration of salicylic acid in the chloroform solution. Calculate the partition coefficient.

C. Determine the partition coefficient of gentisic acid between water and chloroform. An aqueous solution of a known concentration of gentisic acid will be supplied by the instructor.

Accurately pipet 25.0 ml of the aqueous solution of gentisic acid into a separatory funnel. Then pipet an equal volume of chloroform into the separatory funnel and close with a glass stopper. Shake the funnel frequently. Allow to sit in a ring stand until the two phases have separated.

Dilute the aqueous layer by pipetting 5.0 ml of the aqueous layer into a beaker containing 45.0 ml of distilled water measured by pipet. By pipet remove 5.0 ml of the diluted solution and place in a cuvette containing 1.0 ml of color reagent. Shake. The absorbance is measured exactly one minute after the two solutions are mixed at 595 nm. A standard curve relating the absorbance to concentration of gentisic acid is provided by the instructor. Record the absorbance.

Considering the tenfold dilution of the solution of gentisic acid calculate and record the concentration of gentisic acid in the extracted aqueous layer. Calculate by difference the concentration of gentisic acid in the chloroform solution. Calculate the partition coefficient.

REFERENCES

Bates, T. R. and M. Gibaldi. 1970. Gastrointestinal absorption of drugs. In Current concepts in pharmaceutical sciences: Biopharmaceutics. J. Swarbrick, Ed., Lea and Febiger, Philadelphia. Chap. 2, p. 62.

Brochman-Hanssen, E. 1954. Studies on the effect of surface-active agents on the extraction of crude drugs. J. Am. Pharm. Assoc., Sci. Ed. 43:28.

Connors, K. A. 1975. Solvent extraction. In A Textbook of pharmaceutical analysis, 2nd ed., John Wiley & Sons, Inc., New York, Chap. 16, p. 333.

Craig, L. C. and D. Craig. 1956. In A. Weissberger, Ed., Techniques of organic chemistry, 2nd ed., Vol. III. Interscience Publishers, Inc., New York, Chap. II.

Daniels, T. C. and E. C. Jorgensen. 1971. Metabolic changes of drugs and related organic compounds (detoxification). In Textbook of organic medicinal and pharmaceutical chemistry, 6th ed., C. O. Wilson, I. Gisvold, and R. F. Doerge, Eds. J. B. Lippincott Company, Philadelphia, Chap. 3, pp. 82 and 91.

Flynn, G. L. 1971. Structural approach to partitioning: Estimation of steroid partition coefficients based upon molecular constitution. J. Pharm. Sci., 60:345.

Goldsmith, R. H. 1974. Solubility relationships of drugs and their metabolites, J. Chem. Ed., 51:272.

Hansch, C. and S. M. Anderson. 1967. The effect of intramolecular hydrophobic bonding on partition coefficients. J. Org. Chem., 32:2583.

Hober, R. 1945. Physical chemistry of cells and tissues. Blakiston Co., Philadelphia. p. 229.

Mary, N., B. Christensen, and J. Beal. 1957. The effect of some selected surface-active agents on the extraction of Cape Aloe. J. Am. Pharm. Assoc., Sci. Ed. 45:370.

Schanker, L. S. 1959. Absorption of drugs from the rat colon. J. Pharmacol. Exp. Ther., 126:283.

Smith, M. J. H. and P. K. Smith. 1966. The salicylates. Interscience Publishers, London, Chap. 1.

Terada, H. 1972. Partition behavior of p-aminobenzoic acid and sulfonamides at various pH values. Chem. Pharm. Bull., 20:765.

The National Formulary 14th ed. 1975. Mack Publishing Co., Easton, Pa. p. 931.

Weddenburn, D. L. 1964. Distribution or partition of preservative between phases. In Advances in Pharmaceutical Sciences, Vol. I. H. S. Bean, A. H. Beckett, and J. E. Carless. Academic Press, London and New York. p. 218.

Partition Coefficient

Data and Conclusions

1. A kilogram of Belladonna Leaf yields 95 g of dry extract which assays 4.8% of the alkaloids. How many grams of a diluent must be added to adjust the strength of the Belladonna Extract to the required concentration? Name diluents that could be used for pillular and powdered Belladonna Extract.

2. Although the same amount of crude drug is used to prepare Aromatic Cascara Sagrada Fluidextract and Cascara Sagrada Fluidextract, the dose of the former is twice that of the Cascara Fluidextract. Explain.

3. In what galenical preparations are alkaline solvents used?

4. What is the role of glycerin in the extraction of and the stabilization of tannin-containing preparations?

5. A crude vegetable drug with thick-walled tissue contains valuable thermolabile alkaloids as a tannoid complex. Outline and justify a method for fully extracting the alkaloids and preparing a fluidextract beginning with the unground drug.

6. What effect do surface-active agents have in the extraction of crude drugs?

7. Show your calculations for determining the partition coefficient of salicylic acid in B.

8. If 100 ml of a 5% aqueous solution of salicylic acid were extracted with four 25-ml portions of chloroform, how much more would be removed from the aqueous phase than by a single extraction with 100 ml of chloroform?

9. If three successive 100-ml portions of chloroform were used to extract 100 ml of a 5% solution of salicylic acid, how much salicylic acid would remain in the water?

10. Show if it is possible or not to extract 90% of salicylic acid using an equal volume of chloroform.

11. Show your calculations for determining the partition coefficient of gentisic acid in C.

12. The *in vivo* enzymatic hydrolysis of aspirin to salicylic acid in man occurs rapidly ($t_{1/2}$ = 0.3 hr). Considering your experimentally determined partition coefficients for salicylic acid and gentisic acid, discuss the removal of salicylate from the body.

13. By means of structural formulas show the biotransformation of aspirin in man.

14. Salicylamide has a chloroform to water partition coefficient of 2.8. Would you predict a more rapid gastrointestinal absorption of a solution of salicylamide or salicylic acid? Explain.

15. How does alkalinization of the urine affect the excretion of salicylates?

17. FLAVOR AND COLOR

For patient acceptance, drug and cosmetic preparations must be aesthetically presentable. The patient assumes pharmaceuticals to be therapeutically effective and judges the product on its appearance, flavor, color, and even package design at times. Pediatric patients especially insist on a pleasant-tasting medication.

Pharmaceutical firms are greatly concerned with flavor since with the similarity and duplication of products it is often the flavor and patient acceptance which will sell a product.

Generally, a pharmaceutical manufacturer will utilize blended mixtures obtained from frutal companies rather than individual flavor constituents. Although a few very general rules are known to the product development pharmacist, the flavoring of each pharmaceutical is an individual problem solved by empirical means. This is to be expected when one considers that flavor is a subjective phenomenon. A flavor is evaluated by a taste panel, and although the taste is acceptable to the panel and most persons, it is not necessarily acceptable to each patient who will eventually take the medication.

There are four primary tastes: sweet, sour, salty, and bitter. Actually, the flavor of a substance depends not only on the primary tastes but on the composite sensation resulting from modification of the primary tastes by smell, feel, sight, and psychological associations.

Attempts have been made to correlate chemical structure with taste; however, the few correlations reported are so restricted that they are of little use.

Essentially, there are five techniques used in flavoring liquids. Addition of strong flavoring agents to overshadow or cover up an unpleasant taste is known as masking technique. Magnesium Citrate Solution illustrates the technique of carbonation; however, this is seldom applicable. More often effervescent granules are used; they react in water to form carbon dioxide effecting partial anesthesia of the sensory buds of the oral cavity, thereby covering up saline and bitter tastes. Emulsification is employed when unpalatable oils are placed in the internal phase where they are surrounded by a flavored, aqueous phase. Emulsification also eliminates the unpleasant tactual sensation which oils produce in the mouth. The colloidal technique consists of the preparation of the drug or of its derivative in a water-insoluble, colloidal state or else, if the drug is soluble, it is adsorbed on a suitable resin by bonding the taste-producing radical which, after adsorption, loses its taste-producing capacity. Thereafter, a suspension of the obtained material is made.

Microencapsulation is the process by which a liquid or a solid is encased in a thin coating forming a particle smaller than a millimeter. The complications arising with the incorporation of liquids into solid dosage forms may be alleviated by the use of powdered flavors which are available from most frutal companies. Dry flavors are microencapsulated by spray-drying liquid flavors with arabic.

PROCEDURE. Pharmaceutical flavoring is more difficult than food or beverage flavoring as most soluble drugs taste unpleasant. Although each product must be approached individually, generally in flavoring a bitter solution the first step is to add a sweetening agent such as sugar or saccharin. A small amount of citric acid, sodium glutamate, or some salt helps to cover up bitterness. If the bitterness cannot be completely masked by a flavor or a combination of flavors, then a flavor is chosen which is associated with a bitter aftertaste such as wild cherry or a citrus-vanilla combination.

Most fruit flavors can be used with sour or acid ingredients. Salty taste is often masked by the use of butterscotch in which a slightly saline taste is not unpleasant.

Some older remedies contain anise or peppermint oil to mask a foul taste; however, these essential oils are not sufficiently soluble in aqueous solutions, and the droplets of undissolved oil have an irritating effect on mucous membranes. Industrially, these older volatile oil flavors have given way to newer complex blends of chemical compounds which give better flavors and the desired solubility.

The practicing pharmacist by suitable choice of vehicles and official flavoring agents could often improve the taste of liquid prescriptions. For example, alcoholic vehicles intensify a saline taste while a syrup will decrease it. Cinnamon syrup is reputed to be a good vehicle for salty drugs. Suitable vehicles may be prepared by using Merco flavored syrup bases or similar preparations.

A. Prepare 20 ml of an aqueous solution of each of the following drugs so that each ml contains the amount of drug specified:

sodium bromide	0.6 g
sodium salicylate	0.3
chloral hydrate	0.3
penicillin G potassium	40,000 units.

B. Place 5 ml of each vehicle listed in Question 1 of the Data and Conclusions section into test tubes and add one of the solutions prepared in A, drop by drop. Taste after each addition and continue the process until the taste of the drug is just perceptible.

Taste each vehicle and indicate your personal taste preference. The mouth should be rinsed with distilled water at room temperature before and after each sample.

Color complements the flavor of a pharmaceutical, and it should be associated with the flavor. For example, mint-flavored pharmaceuticals are colored green, and cherry-flavored liquids are colored red.

A few natural coloring principles are still employed in pharmacy, but for the most part, they have been replaced by the synthetic coal tar dyes. Dyes are certified by the Food and Drug Administration and are classified into three categories: Group I, the F. D. & C. dyes may be used in foods, drugs, and cosmetics; Group II, the D. & C. dyes may be used in drugs and cosmetics; Group III, the Ext. D. & C. dyes may be used in externally applied drugs and cosmetics only.

The coal tar dyes are used in a liquid internal medication in a concentration sufficient to color the liquid but not concentrated enough to stain fabrics. Usually a solution will be adequately colored with 0.0005 to 0.001% dye. A pastel shade may be given to a white powder by incorporating 0.1% of a coal tar dye.

Many of the certified coal tar dyes are water-soluble as the sodium salt. The addition of acids to an acidic dye will precipitate the color acid. Sulfonic acid dyes are not precipitated by acidic vehicles, as the sulfonic acids are strong acids which ionize readily, carrying the large molecule into aqueous solution. F. D. & C. Red No. 3 is a cherry-red in aqueous solution, but if the solution is acidified, a yellowish-brown precipitate is formed.

Acidic or anionic dyes may be precipitated or their color lost when mixed with basic or cationic dyes or drugs. For example, F. D. & C. Yellow No. 5, when added to a 1:1000 Zephiran chloride solution, will deposit a yellow precipitate on standing.

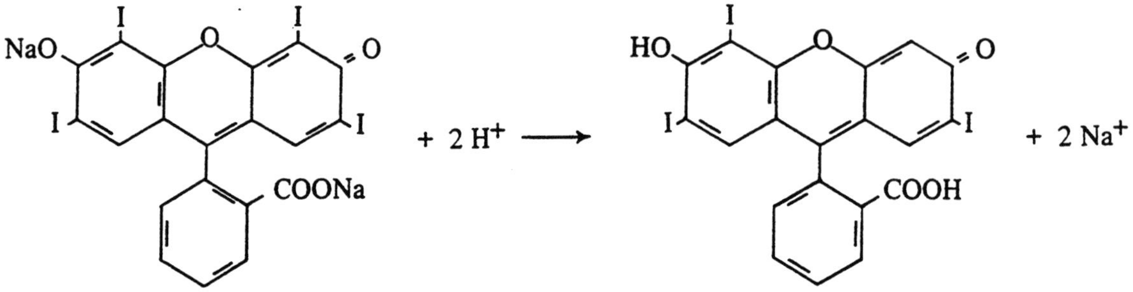

In choosing a dye to be used in a new formulation, the pharmacist must consider several physical and chemical properties of the dye. Depending on the type of preparation, a dye of appropriate solubility must be chosen.

C. Determine the solubility of the dyes listed in Question 2 of the Data and Conclusions section. To do this, place a small amount of the dye in a test tube and add 15 ml of the solvent in question. Remember that dyes are used in very low concentrations.

Stability to acids generally is tested with 10% acetic acid and glacial acetic acid, and 10% and 30% hydrochloric acid; likewise, resistance to alkali is tested with 10% and 30% sodium hydroxide solutions. In addition, resistance of the dye to light, oxidizing agents, reducing agents, and the presence of salts must be determined. In product development the complete formula is prepared and subjected to stability tests for long periods of time and at various temperatures to ensure an active medicinal product with no unwanted changes either in the drugs or the additives.

D. To determine the effect of pH on a dye, place a dilute solution of the dye in four test tubes. Reserve one as the control. Add 30% hydrochloric acid to one test tube until definitely acid; add 30% sodium hydroxide solution to another test tube until definitely alkaline. Record your observations.

   In the same manner, test the stability of the dye to metallic ions by adding an equal volume of 10% ferrous sulfate solution. Record your observations.

   Determine the effect of pH and metallic ions on the colorants in Question 3 of the Data and Conclusion section.

There are three primary colors: yellow, red, and blue. By blending two of these colors one obtains a secondary color, for example, a mixture of yellow and blue produces a green color. A tertiary color is achieved by mixing a secondary with a primary color as in the case of brown, which is a mixture of primary red with secondary green.

Delicate shades of colors are achieved by blending several colors. For illustrative purposes, green is often used to color external preparations such as after-shaving lotions, hair tonics, etc. It may be obtained by blending Tartrazine and Brilliant Blue.

E. Prepare a delicate, attractive blend of green by using Tartrazine and Brilliant Blue. Place the solution in an appropriate bottle and label with your name and amount of each dye used.

   Prepare a violet-shaded solution using Amaranth and Indigotine.

REFERENCES

Amoore, J. E. 1971. Molecular basis of odor. C. C. Thomas, Publisher, Springfield, Illinois.

Anonymous. 1976. FDA declares ban on red dye No. 2 (amaranth). APhArmacy Weekly, 15, No. 4, p.1.

Anonymous. 1974. Cyclamate data "inconclusive." FDA Drug Bulletin. September 1974. p. 4.

Anonymous. 1974. Artificial sweeteners, old and new, and new exotic natural sweeteners being studied as sugar prices climb. Worthington's World, 3, October 1974, p. 3.

Bryan, G. T and O. Yoshida. 1971. Artificial sweeteners as urinary bladder carcinogens. Arch. Environ. Health, 23:6.

Cain, W. S., Ed. 1974. Psychological and medical importance of odors. In Odors: Evaluation, utilization, and control. Annals of the New York Academy of Sciences, Vol. 237, September 27, 1974. p. 217.

Clauss, K. and H. Jensen. 1973. Oxathiazinone dioxides – A new group of sweetening agents. Angewandte Chemie. International Edition in English. 12:869.

Davies, J. T. 1970. Recent developments in the "penetration and puncturing" theory of odour. In Ciba Foundation Symposium on Taste and Smell in Vertebrates. pp. 265-291.

Faull, J. R., H. L. Meiselman, and B. P. Halpern. 1971. Tastelessness: A poorly defined concept – The example of quinine ethylcarbonate. The Psychological Record, 21:219-228.

Fennelly, D., C. Perry, J. Nelson, M. Madeiros, T. MacLeod, W. Taylor, M. DeCenzo, and S. Bartucca. 1972. A method to improve patient acceptance and administration of liquid psychoactive drugs. Am. J. Pharm., 144:88.

Forss, D. A. 1969. Role of lipids in flavors. Agricultural and Food Chemistry, 17:681.

Furia, T. E. 1971. Fenaroli's Handbook of flavor ingredients. CRC Press, Inc., Cleveland, Ohio.

Gangolli, S. D., P. Grasso, L. Golberg, and Jean Hooson. 1972. Protein binding by food colouring in relation to the production of subcutaneous sarcoma. Fd Cosmet. Toxicol., 10:449.

Ghadimi, H. and S. Kumar. 1972. Current status of monosodium glutamate. The American Journal of Chemical Nutrition, 25:643.

Green, M. 1974. Sublingual provocative testing for foods and FD & C dyes. Annals of Allergy, 33:274.

Heller, W. M. 1972. USAN 10 and the USP dictionary of drug names. Aspartame. Page 11.

Kare, M. R. 1969. Some functions of the sense of taste. Agricultural and Food Chemistry, 17:677.

Kier, L. B. 1972. A molecular theory of sweet taste. J. Pharm. Sci., 61:1394.

Kuehner, R. L., Ed. 1964. Recent advances in odor: Theory, measurement, and control. Annals of the New York Academy of Sciences, 116:357-746.

McBurney, D. H. 1974. Are there primary tastes for man? Chemical Senses and Flavor, 1:17-28.

McConnell, R. J., C. E. Menendez, F. R. Smith, R. I. Henkin, and R. S. Rivlin. 1975. Defects of taste and smell in patients with hypothyroidism. The Am. J. of Medicine, 59:354-364.

Moncrieff, R. 1967. The chemical senses, 3rd ed. Leonard Hill Ltd., London.

Moulton, D. G. and L. M. Beidler. 1967. Drugs and injected odorants. In Structure and function in the peripheral olfactory system. Physiological Reviews, 47:33.

Ohloff, G. and A. F. Thomas. 1971. Gustation and olfaction. An International symposium, Geneva, June 1970. American Press, New York.

Peacock, W. H. No date. The application properties of the certified "coal tar" colorants. Calco Technical Bulletin No. 715. American Cyanamid Co., Bound Brook, N.J.

Peacock, W. H. 1952. The coloring of pharmaceutical preparation. Calco Technical Bulletin No. 730. American Cyanamid Co., Bound Brook, N.J.

Price, S. 1969. Chemoreceptor proteins from taste buds. Agricultural and Food Chemistry, 17:709.

Shallenberger, R. S. and T. E. Acree. 1969. Molecular structure and sweet taste. Agriculture and Food Chemistry, 17:686.

Stone, H. and S. M. Oliver. 1969. Measurement of relative sweetness of selected sweeteners and sweetener mixtures. J. of Food Science, 34:215.

Swartz, C. J. and J. Cooper. 1962. Colorants for pharmaceuticals. J. Pharm. Sci. 51:89.

Taylor, J. D., R. K. Richards, R. G. Wiegand, and M. S. Weinberg. 1968. Toxicological studies with sodium cyclamate and saccharin. Fd Cosmet. Toxicol., 6:1.

Teranishi, R., I. Hornstein, P. Issenberg, and E. L. Wick. 1971. Flavor research: Principles and techniques. Food Science Series, Volume 1, Marcel Dekker, Inc., New York.

Wolfe, S. M. and R. I. Herkin. 1970. Absence of taste in type II familial dysautonomia: Unresponsiveness to methacholine despite the presence of taste buds. The J. of Pediatrics, 77:103.

Wurster, D. E. 1970. Dyes. In Prescription pharmacy, J. B. Sprowls, Ed. 2nd ed. J. B. Lippincott Co., Philadelphia, p. 395.

Yamaguchi, S., T. Yoshikawa, S. Ikeda, and T. Ninomiya. 1970. Studies on the taste of some sweet substances. Part I. Measurement of the relative sweetness. Part II. Interrelationships among them. Agricultural and Biological Chemistry, 34:181, and 34:187.

Zanda, G., P. Franciosi, G. Tognoni, M. Rizzo, S. M. Standen, P. L. Morselli, and S. Garratini. 1973. A double blind study on the effects of monosodium glutamate in man. Biomedicine, 19:202.

Flavor and Color

Data and Conclusions

1. Complete the following chart using the following symbols to express taste preference:

4 very good
3 good
2 fair
1 poor
0 very poor

Drug	Vehicle	Taste Preference	Drops Added	Amount of Drug Masked by 5 ml
Sodium bromide	Cherry Syrup Glycyrrhiza Syrup Aromatic Elixir Lactated Pepsin Elixir Peppermint Water			
Sodium salicylate	Cherry Syrup Cinnamon Syrup Cinnamon Water Citric Acid Syrup Tolu Balsam Syrup			
Chloral hydrate	Glycyrrhiza Syrup Eriodictyon Syrup Aromatic Elixir Acacia Syrup Raspberry Syrup Cinnamon Syrup			
Penicillin	Raspberry Syrup Tolu Balsam Syrup Citric Acid Syrup Anise Water Eriodictyon Syrup			

2. Complete the following table:

Dye	Common Name	Water Soluble	Oil Soluble
F. D. & C. Blue No. 1			
F. D. & C. Blue No. 2			
F. D. & C. Green No. 3			
F. D. & C. Red No. 32			
F. D. & C. Red No. 3			
F. D. & C. Violet No. 1			
F. D. & C. Yellow No. 5			

3. Complete the following table:

Colorant Solution	Effect of		
	Acid	Alkali	10% Ferrous Sulfate
Caramel			
Methylene blue			
Brilliant Blue			
Erythrosine			
Fast Green			
Indigotine			
Tartrazine			

4. List the official flavoring agents. Whenever possible in the case of crude drugs and volatile oils, name the active flavor constituent. When the flavoring agent is a liquid, state if it is acid, neutral, or alkaline.

5. What are the dangers, if any, of the condition known as hypogeusia if it should remain untreated?

6. List the official coloring agents.

7. What is meant by the term "chromophore"? Briefly, what is necessary in the structure to produce a colored compound?

8. What does the term pigment mean to a phytochemist? What does pigment mean to a dye chemist?

9. List the official medicinal dyes. Give the use and dose of each when applicable.

18. COLLIGATIVE PROPERTIES OF SOLUTIONS

According to the kinetic theory, matter is in a state of constant motion, with the molecules at the surface of a liquid or solid tending to leave the surface. If a liquid is confined to an evacuated vessel, the molecules at the surface escape and pass into the vapor phase. Eventually, a state of equilibrium will be reached between the liquid and its vapor, when the rate of escape is equal to the rate of condensation of the vapor. The pressure exerted by the vapor when it is in equilibrium with its liquid is known as vapor pressure. Vapor pressure of a liquid is a constant at a given temperature, and it increases with an increase in temperature.

The addition of a solute to a liquid decreases the concentration of the solvent and the tendency of the molecules to escape into the gas phase; that is, the vapor pressure of the solvent is lowered. In an ideal or very dilute solution, the partial vapor pressure of one component, p_1, is directly proportional to the fraction of the molecules of that component in the mixture

$$p_1 = N_1 p_1^0$$

where N_1 is the mole fraction and p_1^0 is the vapor pressure of the pure substance.

If the solution contains a nonvolatile solute, the total pressure of the system is the partial pressure of the volatile solvent. As the solute molecules reduce the effective concentration of the solvent, the solvent molecules have less chance to escape and the vapor pressure is lowered. The lowering of vapor pressure, $p^0 - p$, may be expressed

$$p^0 - p = N_2 p^0$$

where p^0 is the vapor pressure of the pure solvent, p is the partial pressure of the solvent in the solution, and N_2 is the mole fraction of the solute.

Since the vapor pressure of a solvent is lowered by the addition of a nonvolatile solute, the solution must be heated to a higher temperature than the pure solvent if both are to have the same vapor pressure; thus, the boiling point of a solvent is elevated by the addition of a nonvolatile solute.

The freezing point of a liquid is lowered by the addition of a solute. At the freezing point the solid and liquid are in equilibrium and most have the same vapor pressure. If a solute is added and the temperature is held constant, the solid phase will disappear; however, a state of equilibrium between the solid and the liquid phase may be maintained by lowering the temperature.

The vapor pressure-temperature curve of a solid is steeper than that of the corresponding liquid because the heat of sublimation of the solid is greater than the heat of vaporization of the liquid. At the intersection of the two curves, the solid and liquid are in equilibrium, and the corresponding temperature is the freezing point.

With an increase in concentration of the solution, the lowered vapor pressure curve intersects the vapor pressure curve of the solid at a lower freezing-point temperature. This is shown for an ice-water system in Figure 10.

The relationship between the concentration of the solution and the freezing-point depression, ΔT_f, is

$$\Delta T_f = \frac{RT_0^2 m}{\Delta H_{fusion} \dfrac{1000}{M_1}} = K_f m$$

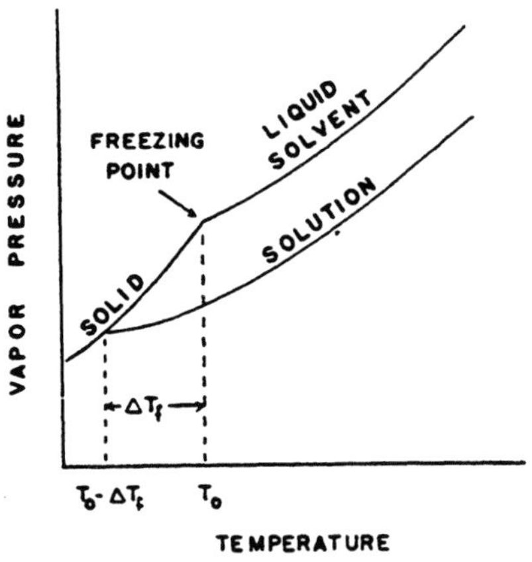

Figure 10 — Lowering of the freezing point.

where R is the gas constant (1.987 cal deg^{-1} $mole^{-1}$), T_0 is freezing point of the pure solvent, ΔH_{fusion} is the molar heat of fusion, M_1 is the molecular weight of the solvent, K_f is the molal freezing-point depression constant, and m is the molality of the solution. For water K_f has the value 1.86°, provided the solute is undissociated.

Osmosis is the diffusion of a solvent through a membrane from a dilute solution to a more concentrated one. The solvent moves from a region where its escape tendency or vapor pressure is great to where it is small. The presence of dissolved material lowers the vapor pressure and increases osmotic pressure.

Osmosis is independent of the membrane although the rate at which equilibrium is reached may depend on the membrane. The pressure exerted by the process of osmosis for dilute solutions of low molecular weight solutes may be calculated.

$$\pi = \frac{gRT}{Mv}$$

where π is the osmotic pressure, g is the weight of the solute of molecular weight M, T is the absolute temperature (C + 273), v is the volume of solvent, and R is the gas constant (0.08205 liter-atm deg^{-1} $mole^{-1}$).

To illustrate the above relationships, consider an aqueous solution of a nonvolatile solute. Twenty grams of a nonelectrolyte with a molecular weight of 350 g $mole^{-1}$ is dissolved in 1000 g of water at 37°. The vapor pressure of water at 37°C is 47.067 mm of mercury. The partial pressure of the solution may be calculated

$$p_1 = N_1 p_1^0 = \frac{\dfrac{1000}{18}}{\dfrac{1000}{18} + \dfrac{20}{350}} \times 47.067 = 47.02$$

The vapor pressure lowering may be expressed

$$p^0 - p = N_2 p^0 = \frac{\dfrac{20}{350}}{\dfrac{1000}{18} + \dfrac{20}{350}} \times 47.067 = 0.048$$

Since the molal freezing-point depression constant of water is 1.86°, the freezing-point depression of this solution is

$$\Delta T_f = K_f m = 1.86 \times \frac{20}{350} = 0.106°$$

In examining the handbooks of chemistry and physics, one finds that a kilogram of water at 37°

occupies a volume of 1006.7 ml. The osmotic pressure of the solution can be found

$$\pi = \frac{gRT}{Mv} = \frac{20 \times 0.08205 \times 310}{350 \times 1.0067} = 1.44 \text{ atm}$$

Since the colligative properties discussed depend on the number of particles in solution, all solutes which ionize will have an increased effect on the colligative properties. An equal molal solution of a nonelectrolyte and an electrolyte, which completely ionizes into two ions, will not produce the same freezing-point depression. The electrolyte will cause twice as great a depression of the freezing point of the solvent as there are twice as many particles.

In very dilute solutions the freezing-point depression of a solvent is a multiple of the number of ions into which the electrolyte dissociates. For example, in very dilute solutions potassium sulfate completely dissociates into three ions, and the freezing-point depression is three times as great as an equal molal nonelectrolyte ($3 \times 1.86° = 5.58°$). In very dilute solution the ions are so far apart that they exert no attraction on each other so ionization is complete.

As the concentration increases, the ions are closer together and exert a strong attraction for each other, suppressing dissociation. With a suppression of dissociation, there are fewer particles per unit weight of electrolyte available to lower the freezing point of the solvent. For example, in the range of 0.05 molal solutions, potassium sulfate is only 80% ionized. Thus 100 molecules of potassium sulfate would yield 160 K^+ and 80 SO_4^{--} plus 20 undissociated molecules of K_2SO_4 or a total of 260 particles. As there are 2.6 times as many particles as when no dissociation occurred, the freezing-point depression is 2.6 times as great as an 0.05 molal nonelectrolyte solution ($2.6 \times 1.86 = 4.84°$).

Fortunately the molal freezing-point depression lowering has been determined experimentally in the concentration ranges employed in pharmacy. The ionization and ionic interactions have been combined into a single experimentally determined constant, L, which may be substituted for K_f

$$\Delta T_f = Lm$$

Tables of L values have been compiled (see Appendix: Molal Freezing-Point Depression Constants, page 320).

Solutions which have the same osmotic pressure are said to be isotonic solutions. A more concentrated solution is a hypertonic solution; a more dilute solution is a hypotonic solution. Blood serum and tear fluids, which have a freezing point of -0.52°C, are isotonic with 0.9% sodium chloride solution. Isotonic solutions have identical values of their colligative properties.

When a red blood cell is placed in water, the water diffuses through the cell membrane into the cell, and if sufficient pressure is exerted to rupture the cell wall, hemolysis results. Conversely, if a red blood cell is placed in a hypertonic solution, the water will diffuse out of the cell and the cell shrinks; this is known as crenation.

To prevent hemolysis of the red blood cells, solutions of drugs to be given intravenously are made isotonic with blood serum by the addition of a physiologically inert additive such as sodium chloride.

The same consideration applies to all living cells whether found in the muscle, blood, eye, or elsewhere. For example, if a hypotonic solution is dropped into the eye, water diffuses into the cells of the eye. In most cases the cell is not ruptured but the distention causes a sensation of stinging pain. Similarly, a hypertonic solution will cause cellular crenation, which probably does no permanent damage but does elicit a sensation of pain. The comfort of the patient may be increased with the elimination of this unnecessary pain by adjusting the ophthalmic solution until it is isotonic with the lachrymal secretion.

The measurement of osmolality by the freezing point depression has become a readily available clinical laboratory determination. An osmol, Osm, is related to the gram molecular weight of the molecules or ions in solution. For example, one mole or 180 g of glucose dissolved in 1 kg of water has an osmolality of 1 Osm or 1000 mOsm per kilogram of water, while 58.5 g of sodium chloride dissolved in 1 kg of water has an osmolality of slightly less than 2000 mOsm per kilogram of water, because the high dissociation of sodium chloride results in almost two particles per molecule.

The measurement of plasma and urine osmolality is useful in diagnosis. Serum hyperosmolality may be indicative of chronic renal disease, diabetes mellitus and acute brain trauma. Hypoosmolality is observed in Addison's disease and in diseases with inappropriate secretion of antidiuretic hormone. Osmolality reflects the pathophysiological state more accurately than the volume of urine because of variation in emptying of the bladder.

PROCEDURE. The temperature at which the solid and liquid phases are in equilibrium is the freezing point of the solvent. To aid in the experimental determination of the freezing point a cooling curve is plotted. As the solvent is cooled, temperatures are recorded at various time intervals. The plateau or stationary temperature is taken as the freezing point.

A. Using a Beckmann molecular weight apparatus, determine the freezing point of a solvent assigned by the instructor.

   The inner tube contains the solvent in which a Beckmann thermometer is immersed. The stirring rod should be bent so it does not touch or damage the thermometer. An air jacket around the tube minimizes the rate of cooling after the apparatus is set in the cooling bath.

   With a pipet introduce about 20.0 ml or enough solvent to cover the bulb of the thermometer. Cool quickly to approximately the freezing point of the solvent, then immerse it in the freezing mixture. To prevent supercooling, operate the stirrer until the freezing point has been found. Tap the thermometer gently before a reading is taken.

B. A solution using the solvent for which you have determined the freezing point will be supplied by the instructor. Determine the freezing point of this solution from a cooling curve. Measure and record the temperature at 15- or 30-second intervals. Plot the temperature on the ordinate against time. The stationary temperature is taken as the freezing point.

If two solutions have the same freezing point, all their colligative properties are of the same magnitude. If a drug with a molecular weight of 200 g $mole^{-1}$ has a molal freezing point lowering constant of 3.4, calculate how much sodium chloride must be added to 60 ml of a 1% solution of the drug to make it isotonic with body fluids.

The depression of freezing point caused by the drug is

$$\Delta T_f = Lm = 3.4 \frac{10}{200} = 0.17^\circ$$

To lower the freezing point to that of blood serum, sufficient sodium chloride must be added to further depress the freezing point 0.52 - 0.17° or 0.35°,

$$\frac{\Delta T_f}{L} = \frac{0.35}{3.44} = m = 0.102$$

Converting this into weighable terms, 0.102 X 58.5 or 5.96 g of sodium chloride are required per liter. As only 60 ml are to be prepared, 0.102 X 58.5 X 0.06 or 0.358 g of sodium chloride and 0.6 g of drug will be used in making 60 ml of isotonic solution containing 1% of the drug.

Several methods have been advanced to facilitate the calculations involved in preparing isotonic solutions; however, all methods are based on the fundamental relation just expressed. To illustrate, let us consider the sodium chloride equivalent method.

The sodium chloride equivalent is the weight of sodium chloride that will produce the same osmotic or freezing depression effect as one unit of a drug. Antistine hydrochloride has a sodium chloride equivalent, E, of 0.19, that is, 0.19 unit weight of sodium chloride and 1 unit weight of antistine hydrochloride have identical colligative properties.

Using the basic relationship, the sodium chloride equivalent may be calculated. For the drug

$$\Delta T_f = L_d m_d$$

and for sodium chloride

$$\Delta T_f = L_{NaCL} m_{NaCl}$$

By definition the freezing-point depression for 1 g of drug is equal to that of E g of sodium chloride so

$$\Delta T_f = L_d m_d = L_{NaCl} m_{NaCL} = \frac{3.44\ E}{58.5}$$

and since E is being calculated in relation to 1 g of drug

$$\frac{L_d \times 1}{M_d} = \frac{3.44\ E}{58.5}$$

Thus, the sodium chloride equivalent, E, is expressed in terms of molecular weight of drug, M, and molal freezing-point depression constant of the drug, L_d,

$$E = 17 \frac{L_d}{M_d}$$

To illustrate the application of the sodium chloride equivalent method, consider 30 ml of solution containing 1.5% of Drug A with an E of 0.19 and 0.5% of Drug B with an E of 0.16. The weight of each drug to be used is determined and multiplied by the E

$$\begin{aligned} 0.45 \times 0.19 &= 0.0855 \\ 0.15 \times 0.16 &= \underline{0.0240} \\ & 0.11 \end{aligned}$$

The 0.45 g of Drug A and the 0.15 g of Drug B are osmotically equal to 0.11 g of sodium chloride.

Recall that a 0.9% saline solution is isotonic with body fluids; therefore, a solution containing 30 X 0.009 or 0.27 g of sodium chloride in 30 ml of solution is isotonic with body fluids. The difference between the amount of sodium chloride required to make 30 ml of isotonic saline solution and the amount of sodium chloride osmotically equal to the two drugs is the amount of sodium chloride yet to be added to adjust the solution to isotonicity

$$0.27 - 0.11 = 0.16 \text{ g of sodium chloride}$$

If a substance other than sodium chloride were being used to make an isotonic solution, the amount of sodium chloride required would be divided by the E of the additive to give the amount of the additive to be added to adjust to isotonicity.

C. Prepare 30 ml of an ophthalmic solution containing 60 mg of zinc sulfate in sterile distilled water. Place 1 or 2 drops in one of your eyes and record your observations.

Prepare 30 ml of an ophthalmic solution containing 60 mg of zinc sulfate in 2.5% saline solution. Place 1 or 2 drops in one of your eyes and record your observations. Allow 15 minutes to elapse between administration of each solution.

Prepare 30 ml of an ophthalmic solution containing 60 mg of zinc sulfate and, using sodium chloride, adjust until isotonic with body fluids. Place 1 or 2 drops in one of your eyes and record your observations.

REFERENCES

Bordalen, B. E., H. Wang, and H. Holtermann. 1970. Osmotic properties of some contrast media. Investigative Radiology, 5:559.

Daniels, F., J. W. Williams, P. Bender, R. A. Alberty, and C. D. Cornwell. 1962. Experimental physical chemistry. 6th ed. McGraw-Hill Book Company, New York. p. 78.

Deardorff, D. L. 1975. Isotonic solutions. In Remington's Pharmaceutical sciences. 15th ed. Mack Publishing Co., Easton, Pa. Chapter 79, p. 1405.

Hendry, E. B. 1961. Osmolarity of human serum and of chemical solutions of biologic importance. Clinical Chemistry, 7:156.

Moses, A. M. and M. Miller. 1972. Urine and plasma osmolality in differentiation of polyuric states. Postgraduate Medicine, 52:187.

Riegelman, S. and D. Sorby. 1971. EENT medications. In Dispensing of medication. E. W. Martin, Ed. Mack Publishing Co. Easton, Pa. Chapter 24, p. 880.

Robinson, A. G. and J. N. Loeb. 1971. Ethanol ingestion – Commonest cause of elevated plasma osmolality? New England Journal of Medicine, 284:1253.

Wallach, J. 1970. Interpretation of diagnostic tests. A handbook synopsis of laboratory medicine. Little, Brown and Company, Boston. pp. 33 and 61.

Wolf, A. V. and P. G. Prentiss. 1968. Osmotic concentrations: Comparison of vapor pressure and freezing point methods. The Journal of Laboratory and Clinical Medicine, 72:688.

Colligative Properties of Solutions

Data and Conclusions

1. Enter the data obtained in B. Plot a cooling curve using this data. Explain the form of the cooling curve.

2. What is the depression of freezing point in the solution given to you in B? Knowing the molecular weight and the amount of solute added, how would you calculate the molal freezing-point depression constant for this substance?

3. Compare your observations in C. What concentration range of sodium chloride is tolerated in the eye without a sensation of irritation?

4. Forty-six grams of a solute with a molecular weight of 46 g $mole^{-1}$ is dissolved in 1000 g of water at 25°C forming a solution with a density of 0.992 g cc^{-1}. Express the concentration of the solution in terms of molality, molarity, mole fractions, and weight-weight percent.

5. A new volatile saturated anesthetic is to be used as a mixture with ethyl ether, which has a molecular weight of 74 g $mole^{-1}$ and vapor pressure of 545 mm Hg at 25°C. The new anesthetic has a molecular weight of 100 g $mole^{-1}$ and a vapor pressure of 180 mm of mercury at 25°C. Calculate the partial and total vapor pressures of the following mixtures:

   a. 10 g of new anesthetic and 90 g of ether.

   b. 50 g of new anesthetic and 50 g of ether.

   c. 90 g of new anesthetic and 10 g of ether.

6. How much will 5% cocaine hydrochloride (MW = 340 g $mole^{-1}$) lower the vapor pressure when dissolved in water at 25°?

7. Syrup contains 65% W/W sugar. Calculate the freezing and boiling point.

8. Calculate the osmotic pressure of a 1% solution of dextrose, expressing the answer in terms of mm of mercury.

9. Calculate the osmotic pressure of Syrup U. S. P.

10. Calculate the sodium chloride equivalent of Dextrose U. S. P., Zinc Sulfate U. S. P., and Morphine Sulfate U. S. P.

11. Using the sodium chloride equivalent method, calculate the amount of substance to be added to make the following solutions isotonic with the blood:

a. 100 ml of a 1% cocaine hydrochloride solution, using sodium chloride to make the solution isotonic.

b. Repeat (a) using dextrose rather than sodium chloride.

c. 1% ephedrine sulfate and 0.5% chlorobutanol to be made isotonic by the addition of sodium chloride.

d. 0.25% zinc sulfate and 2% boric acid solution to be made isotonic by the addition of sodium chloride.

12. Clinical pharmacists may use the term "osmolar" or "osmolal" in discussing tissue fluids and solutions to be used in tissue baths. What is meant by the terms?

13. Preservatives are added at times to ophthalmic and parenteral solutions, which the physician may desire to be isotonic with body fluids. Calculate the depression of freezing point caused by the following preservatives:

Benzalkonium chloride 0.01%

Benzyl alcohol 0.5%

Chlorobutanol 0.5%

Methylparaben 0.02% and propylparaben 0.01%

Phenol 0.5%

19. HYDROGEN ION CONCENTRATION

Hydrogen ion concentrations are determined to very small values, and to avoid the nuisance of writing many zeros to describe the concentrations, an exponential notation has been adopted. The term, pH, is defined as the negative exponent of 10 which gives the hydrogen ion concentration.

Thus,

$$10^{-pH} = C_{H^+}$$

or

$$pH = -\log C_{H^+} = \log \frac{1}{C_{H^+}}$$

For example, the hydrogen ion concentration in a solution with a pH of 5 is

$$C_{H^+} = 10^{-pH} = 10^{-5} = 0.00001 \text{ moles liter}^{-1}$$

The pH of blood in the healthy individual is 7.4. The hydrogen ion concentration of blood is calculated as follows:

$$pH = -\log C_{H^+} = 7.4$$

$$\log C_{H^+} = -7.4$$

$$-7.4 = (-8 + 0.6) = \bar{8}.6$$

$$\text{antilogarithm of } 0.6 = 3.98$$
$$\text{antilogarithm of } -8 = 10^{-8}$$

$$C_{H^+} = 3.98 \times 10^{-8} \text{ moles liter}^{-1}$$

In treating achlorhydria a solution of hydrochloric acid with a hydrogen ion concentration of 0.05 moles liter^{-1} was used; the solution had

$$pH = \log \frac{1}{0.05} = \log 20 = 1.3$$

Color is due to resonance or the motion of electrons in a suitable structure. The vibration period of electrons in an acid in the ionized form is different than that of the acid in the undissociated form, thus the color is different. Phenolphthalein, for example, is a weak colorless acid which reacts with a base to form a salt which dissociates to give a red colored anion.

Use is made of certain weak acids and bases which change color in definite pH ranges to measure hydrogen ion concentration. In titrating a strong acid or base using phenolphthalein as an indicator, the weak indicator acid competes with the strong acid for the base, and only after the strong acid is neutralized is it successful. The end point is reached when the acid is equivalent to the amount of base present. If the salt formed is hydrolyzed, an indicator is required which does not change its color at exact neutrality but at the pH which is produced by the addition of the salt to the water.

An acid indicator reacts

$$\underset{\text{color I}}{HIn} \rightleftharpoons H^+ + \underset{\text{color II}}{In^-}$$

The pH range in which these indicators change color depends on their ionization constant. Phenolphthalein is used in the pH range of 8.3-10.

Buffer solutions are used as standards in determining the pH of a solution by comparing the color of the solution with an indicator and the color of a series of buffer solutions and the indicator. The pH of the solution is the same as that of the particular buffer whose color matches that of the solution.

Mixed indicators are used to estimate the pH of solutions, as a wide range of pH may be covered with a single solution of mixed indicators. Test strips may be prepared by placing these solutions on filter paper and allowing them to dry. As an initial screening technique such paper is useful in selecting the final method by which the exact pH will be determined.

The electrometric method of determining pH is more exact than the colorimetric method. The electrometric method is based on the fact that when two electrodes of the same material are immersed in solutions of their ions at different concentrations, the cell will exhibit a definite electromotive force which depends on the ratio of the concentrations of the ions in the two solutions.

At equilibrium for positive ions the potential, E, may be expressed

$$E = -\frac{RT}{nF} \ln \frac{c_1}{c_2}$$

where R is the gas constant (8.314 joules deg^{-1} $mole^{-1}$), T is the absolute temperature, n is the valence change, F is the faraday, and c_1 and c_2 are concentration of the ions.

The determination of hydrogen ion concentration was first made utilizing a hydrogen electrode, which is the standard of reference for all electrodes. One of the two hydrogen electrodes is held in a standard state of 1 atm of pressure and in a solution having a hydrogen ion concentration of unity. The potential as measured is then related to the concentration of hydrogen ion

$$E = -\frac{RT}{nF} \ln C_{H^+}$$

Thus, at 25° the potential of the cell is related to the hydrogen ion concentration

$$E = -0.0591 \log C_{H^+}$$

or

$$pH = \frac{E}{0.0591}$$

In actual practice other more convenient electrodes such as the calomel and glass electrode are used; however, all electrode potentials are based on the standard hydrogen electrode.

It should be realized that the actual measurement of pH involves the activity of the hydrogen ion rather than its concentration. Since the activity of the hydrogen ion or any other single ion is not directly measurable, pH measurements are experimental measurements of the difference of hydrogen ion activity between unknown solutions and standard buffers with assigned pH values.

The pH is an index of the chemical potential of the protons including dissociable protons incorporated in proton-donor molecules as well as free or hydrated protons. The hydrogen ion differs from a stable ion (sodium ion) in that the average life of a hydrogen ion is approximately 10^{-6} seconds. There is a dynamic release and combination of protons with acceptor molecules.

The hydrogen ion concentration of solutions is of paramount importance to pharmacy. The stability of a drug in solution often depends on the pH. Hydrolysis of ester-containing drugs is suppressed at a low pH. With such drugs as ascorbic acid, epinephrine, eserine, and thiamine, oxidative degradation is promoted by a high pH; therefore, such drugs are dispensed in acid solution. Antioxidants are sometimes incorporated. Certain antibiotics, such as oxytetracycline and chloramphenicol, are rapidly destroyed in neutral or alkaline solutions.

It is believed that most amine and alkaloid type drugs are absorbed as the free base which is unstable and insoluble in water. Although a drug such as atropine may be most stable at pH 4, a compromise between drug stability and therapeutic effectiveness is reached by dispensing the drug at a pH 6.8. At this pH and at room temperature the atropine will be stable for approximately a month, yet it is readily converted to the base form by the body buffers enhancing absorption.

Benzoic acid shows its greatest effectiveness as a preservative in acid solutions where it is commonly employed in 0.2% concentration. In neutral or alkaline solutions benzoic acid is used as an inhibitor of microbial growth, but it is not bacteriostatic even at 3% concentration. Similarly, hexylresorcinol is most effective in an acid medium. Thimerosal is unsatisfactory in acid medium and shows its greatest preservative action in alkaline solutions.

Control of pH in ointments not only prevents irritation and promotes stability of the drugs, but it may enhance the activity of the drug. Ammoniated mercury and mercurous iodide ointments have greater antiseptic value as the pH decreases.

In manufacturing processes, control of pH is important. In extracting crude drugs, the hydrogen ion concentration is adjusted not only to facilitate extraction but at times to prevent degradation of the extracted drug. The preparation of various insulins is an excellent example to illustrate the importance of pH in drug extraction and preparation.

The semipermeable membrane of the gastrointestinal tract permits the passive diffusion of lipid soluble drugs. Many drugs are weak acids or weak bases, which exist in solution in partly ionized and partly un-ionized form. Only the un-ionized form is lipid soluble and can be absorbed. If the pH is altered so that a greater fraction of the drug molecules exist in the un-ionized form, the concentration gradient of the un-ionized form is greater, and the absorption rate is increased.

The pH-partition theory also applies to the elimination of a drug from the body. Phenobarbital is a weak acid with a pK_a of 7.41. The percent of ionized phenobarbital may be calculated by

$$\text{Percent of weak acid ionized} = \frac{100}{1 + \text{antilog}\,(pK_a - pH)}$$

In cases of poisoning with phenobarbital, the percent of phenobarbital ionized in the blood plasma (pH 7.4) is 49.4% and in the cerebrospinal fluid (pH 7.3) is 43.7%. If an intraveneous injection of sodium bicarbonate solution is given until the blood plasma has a pH 8, 79.55% of the phenobarbital is ionized in the blood plasma. With this change in pH the distribution between the cerebrospinal fluid and the blood plasma will be such that the concentration in the cerebrospinal fluid will decrease, and the alkaline urine produced will result in less tubular reabsorption and greater excretion of phenobarbital in the urine.

For a weak base, the percent ionized may be calculated by

$$\text{Percent of weak base ionized} = \frac{100}{1 + \text{antilog}\,(pH - pK_a)}$$

PROCEDURE. To the pharmacist the most obvious effect of pH is on solubility. In addition to stability, local anesthetics and alkaloidal-type compounds are usually dispensed as the salt of an acid to increase their water solubility, as the free base usually is only slightly water-soluble. In compounding presciptions the pharmacist may encounter incompatibilities in which the salt of an alkaline water-insoluble drug is to be dispensed in an alkaline vehicle. Such an acid-base incompatibility is the most common incompatibility met at the prescription counter today. With the increased use of admixtures for intravenous administration, it is imperative that the pharmacist recognize and avoid the mixing and injection of incompatible solutions into hospitalized patients.

A. Using pH indicator paper, determine the pH of the following vehicles: Cherry Syrup N. F., artificial cherry syrup, Aromatic Eriodictyon Syrup N. F., glycyrrhiza syrup, Orange Syrup N. F., Cocoa Syrup U. S. P., Tolu Balsam Syrup N. F., wild cherry syrup, Aromatic Elixir U. S. P.; lactated pepsin elixir, citric acid syrup. Record the pH of each.

B. Prepare 50 ml of a 1.5% phenobarbital sodium solution. When 4 ml of this solution is mixed with 4 ml of a vehicle, the resulting mixture contains a usual dose of phenobarbital sodium in each 4 ml.

Mix 4 ml of the phenobarbital sodium solution with 4 ml of each of the vehicles listed in A. Observe and record the results.

C. Prepare 50 ml of 0.5% amphetamine sulfate solution. To obtain a concentration which gives a usual dose in 4 ml, mix equal volumes of the amphetamine sulfate solution and the vehicles listed in A. Observe and record the results.

REFERENCES

Astrup, P., K. Engel, K. Jorgensen, and O. Siggaard-Andersen. 1966..Definitions and terminology in blood acid-base chemistry. Annals of The New York Academy of Sciences, 133, Art. 1, p. 59.

Austin, W. H. 1965. Acid-base balance. A review of current approaches and techniques. Am. Heart J., 5:691.

Bates, R. G. 1964. Determination of pH: Theory and practice. Wiley, New York.

Bates, R. G. 1966. Acids, bases and buffers. Annals of the New York Academy of Sciences, 133, Art. 1, p. 25.

Bates, R. G. and M. Paabo. 1970. Measurement of pH. In Handbook of biochemistry. Selected data for molecular biology. 2nd ed. H. A. Sober, Ed. The Chemical Rubber Company, Cleveland, Ohio. p. J-227.

Butler, T. C. 1973. pH: Another view. Science, 179:854.

Carter, N.W. 1972. Intracellular pH. Kidney International, 1:341.

Christensen, H. N. 1963. pH and Dissociation. A learning program for students of the biological and medical sciences. W. B. Saunders Company, Philadelphia.

Dale, J. K. 1971. Drug interactions and incompatibilities. In Dispensing of medication, 7th ed., E. W. Martin, Ed., Mack Publishing Co., Easton, Pa., Chap. 4, p. 113.

Feldman, I. 1956. Use and abuse of pH measurements. Analytical Chemistry, 28:1859.

Hopgood, M. F. 1970. Nomogram for calculating percentage ionization of acids and bases. J. Chromatog., 47:45.

Klahr, S., S. Wessler, and L. V. Avioli. 1972. Acid-base disorders in health and disease. J.A.M.A., 222:567.

Kramer, W. R., A. S. Inglott, and R. J. Cluxton, Jr. 1972. Incompatibilities of drugs for intravenous administration. In Perspectives in clinical pharmacy. D. E. Francke and H. A. K. Whitney, Jr., Eds. Drug Intelligence Publications, Hamilton, Illinois. Chap. 21, p. 438.

Morgan, H. G. 1969. Acid-base balance in blood. Brit. J. Anaesth., 41:196.

Niebergall, P. J. 1969. Ionic equilibria. In Physical pharmacy, 2nd ed. A. N. Martin, J. Swarbrick, and A. Cammarata. Lea and Febiger, Philadelphia. Chapter 9, p. 189.

Seeman, P. 1972. The pH concept. Science, 177:835.

Siegel, P. D. 1973. The physiologic approach to acid-base balance. Medical Clinics of North America, 57:863.

Siggaard-Andersen, O. 1966. Titratable acid or base of body fluids. Annals of The New York Academy of Sciences, 133, Art. 1, p.41.

Tannen, R. L. 1969. The relationship between urine pH and acid excretion – The influence of urine flow rate. The Journal of Laboratory and Clinical Medicine, 74:757.

Van Slyke, D. D. 1966. Some points of acid-base history in physiology and medicine. Annals of the New York Academy of Sciences, 133, Art. 1, p. 5.

Webb, J. W. 1969. A pH pattern for I. V. additives. Am. J. Hospital Pharm., 26:31.

Weisberg, H. F. 1959. A better understanding of anion-cation ("acid-base") balance. The Surgical Clinics of North America, 39:1.

Whipple, H., Ed. 1966. Current concepts of acid-base measurement. Annals of The New York Academy of Sciences, 133, Art. 1, pp. 1-274.

Wurster, D. E. 1970. In J. B. Sprowls, Prescription pharmacy. 2nd ed. J. B. Lippincott Co., Philadelphia. Chap. 10, pp. 373-395.

Hydrogen Ion Concentration

Data and Conclusions

1. Complete the following chart using the following symbols:

N C	no change
Op	opalescence
Ppt. Sl.	slight precipitate
Ppt. Mod.	moderate precipitate
Ppt. Hvy.	heavy precipitate

Vehicle	pH	Phenobarbital Sodium			Amphetamine Sulfate		
		Immediate	1 hour	1 week	Immediate	1 hour	1 week
Cherry Syrup N. F.							
Cherry Syrup, Artificial							
Aromatic Eriodictyon Syrup N. F.							
Glycyrrhiza Syrup							
Orange Syrup N. F.							
Cocoa Syrup U. S. P.							
Syrup U. S. P.							
Tolu Balsam Syrup N. F.							
Wild Cherry Syrup							
Aromatic Elixir U. S. P.							
Lactated Pepsin Elixir							
Citric Acid Syrup							

What generalization can one arrive at based on these data?

2. The urinary antiseptic effect of methenamine depends on the liberation of formaldehyde in the presence of acids. To be effective, the urine must have a pH no greater than 5.2. Calcium mandelate is an effective urinary antiseptic at a pH of 5.5 or less. Calculate the hydrogen ion concentration required for each of these drugs to be effective.

3. Three commonly used hydrogen ion concentrations in collyria are 1.6×10^{-7}, 2.5×10^{-9}, and 10^{-5}. Calculate the corresponding pH's.

4. Define the term "activity of a solute" in an aqueous solution.

5. The germicidal effect of benzoic acid resides mainly in the un-ionized molecule. At pH 3.5 a 1:800 benzoic acid solution will kill colon bacillus and the staphylococcus in an hour; at a pH of 5 it is not too effective in a 1:20 dilution. To what magnitude of hydrogen ion concentration do these 1.5 units of pH change correspond?

6. A physician would like to administer intravenously solutions of the following pairs of drugs. Discuss what would occur and what you would observe on mixing the solutions of the drugs.

   a. ampicillin and oxytetracycline

   b. kanamycin and heparin

   c. dilantin and promazine

   d. warfarin and vitamin B complex with C

20. BUFFER SOLUTIONS

The salt of a strong acid and a strong base dissociates completely when dissolved, giving rise to positive and negative ions with no change in hydrogen of hydroxyl ions. However, in a salt made by neutralization of a weak acid with a strong base, the negative ions of the salt will react with the hydrogen ions of the water to form the weak acid, thus upsetting the equality of hydrogen and hydroxyl ions. Sodium acetate hydrolyzes to give an alkaline reaction

$$CH_3COONa \rightleftharpoons Na+ + CH_3COO^-$$

$$HOH \rightleftharpoons OH^- + H^+$$

$$\upharpoonleft\downharpoonright \quad \upharpoonleft\downharpoonright$$

$$NaOH \quad CH_3COOH$$

The sodium ion and the hydroxyl ion attract each other, but as sodium hydroxide is strongly dissociated, there is no change in concentration of hydrogen ion. The acetate ion and the hydrogen ion react to give undissociated molecules of acetic acid. More and more water dissociates to produce hydrogen ions for the formation of acetic acid. Finally, at equilibrium, there is an excess of hydroxyl ions over hydrogen ions yielding an alkaline solution

$$CH_3COO^- + H_2O \rightleftharpoons CH_3COOH + OH^-$$

Buffer solutions are solutions which tend to resist changes in pH when acids or bases are added. Buffer solutions usually contain a salt of a weak acid or base and the corresponding weak acid or base. If a base is added to a buffer solution containing a weak acid, HA, and one of its salts, MA, the alkali is neutralized by the acid

$$OH^- + HA \longrightarrow H_2O + A^-$$

If an acid is added, the hydrogen ions of the acid react with the anions of the salt forming the undissociated weak acid, thus resisting a change in pH

$$H^+ + A^- \longrightarrow HA$$

The ionization constant, K_a, of an acid is given by the expression

$$K_a = \frac{(H^+)(A^-)}{(HA)}$$

where concentrations are expressed in moles per liter.

Knowing the ionization constant of acetic acid to be 1.8×10^{-5}, one may calculate the hydrogen ion concentration of a solution containing 0.140 mole per liter of acetic acid. Let x equal the number of moles of acetic acid ionized per liter, then 0.140 - x is the number of moles of undissociated acid at equilibrium, and x is the number of moles of hydrogen and acetate ions. Substituting these values one has

$$K_a = 1.8 \times 10^{-5} = \frac{(H^+)(A^-)}{(HA)} = \frac{x^2}{0.140 - x}$$

$$x = 0.158 \times 10^{-3}$$

Calculations may be simplified by assuming that since the acid is only very slightly ionized, there is no practical difference between the total or original concentration of the acid and the concentration of the acid after ionization occurs. Such an assumption introduces less than one percent error,

$$K_a = 1.8 \times 10^{-5} = \frac{(H^+)(A^-)}{(HA)} = \frac{x^2}{0.140}$$

$$x = 0.159 \times 10^{-2}$$

Henderson and Hasselbalch derived an equation by which the pH of a buffer solution consisting of a weak acid, HA, and its salt, MA, may be calculated.

The equation defining ionization constant may be transposed

$$(H^+) = K_a \frac{(HA)}{(A^-)}$$

A weak acid is only slightly dissociated and the addition of a salt with a common ion will further decrease dissociation. Thus, if the salt of a weak acid is added to a weak acid, the anions for all practical purposes come from the highly dissociated salt. The concentration of anion, A^-, is equal to the concentration of the salt, MA. As shown in the previous calculation, ignoring the dissociation of a weak acid will produce an error of less than one percent. The hydrogen ion concentration of the buffer solution is then equal to the product of the ionization constant and the ratio of the concentrations of the acid and the salt

$$(H^+) = K_a \frac{(HA)}{(MA)}$$

If the negative logarithm of this equation is taken, pH may be calculated directly

$$pH = -\log(H^+) = -\log K_a - \log \frac{(HA)}{(MA)}$$

Since $pK_a = -\log K_a$ and $-\log \frac{(HA)}{(MA)} = \log \frac{(MA)}{(HA)}$ the relationship may be written

$$pH = pK_a + \log \frac{(MA)}{(HA)}.$$

In examining the handbooks of chemistry and physics, one finds the pK_a of acetic acid at 25° is 4.73. The pH of a buffer solution consisting of equal volumes of 0.1 N acetic acid and 0.1 N sodium acetate may be calculated. As equal volumes are mixed, the final concentrations of acetic acid and sodium acetate are 0.05 N. Substitution produces

$$pH = pK_a + \log \frac{(MA)}{(HA)} = 4.73 + \log \frac{0.05}{0.05} = 4.73$$

In other words, the pH is numerically equal to the pK_a of the acid in a buffer solution which contains equal moles of a weak acid and its salt. This offers one method of determining pK_a. A solution of equal concentration of the weak acid and its salt are made up and the pH is determined.

The Henderson-Hasselbalch equation has certain limitations. It does not apply when the proportion of the weak acid in the form of its salt is less than about 10% of the total buffer concentration, or when the hydrogen ion concentration is great enough to constitute a significant part of the total ions present. These limitations do not detract from its use in the cases commonly encountered in pharmacy.

Comparable relationships may be derived for buffers composed of weak bases and the corresponding salt of a strong acid

$$pH = pK_w - pK_b + \log \frac{(Base)}{(Salt)}$$

Atropine has a pK_b of 4.35. Generally, it is recommended that atropine be dispensed at a pH 6.8. Calculate the percent of the total atropine in a 1% solution which exists in the base form.

$$pH = 6.8 = pK_w - pK_b + \log \frac{(Base)}{(Salt)} = 14 - 4.35 + \log \frac{(Base)}{(Salt)}$$

$$-2.85 = \log \frac{(Base)}{(Salt)} = 7.15 - 10.00$$

Antilogarithm of 7.15 - 10.00 = 0.0014

$$\frac{(Base)}{(Salt)} = \frac{0.0014}{1}$$

Thus, approximately 0.14% of the atropine exists in the base form at pH 6.8.

Buffer capacity is the ability of a buffer solution to resist pH change. The smaller the pH change caused by the addition of a given amount of acid or alkali, the greater the buffer capacity of the solution. When equimolar amounts of the buffer acid and buffer salt are used, the buffer capacity is greatest.

If 1 ml of 0.1 N HC1 is added to 99 ml of pure water at pH 7, the hydrogen concentration of the solution will be approximately 10^{-3}. The pH of the water has been changed 4 units by the addition of the acid. If 1 ml of 0.1 N HC1 is added to 99 ml of a buffer solution containing 0.1 N acetic acid and 0.1 N sodium acetate, the pH changes 0.01 units. The buffer solution has a much greater buffer capacity than pure water.

The buffer capacity is determined by the actual concentration of the salt and acid present as well as by their ratio. At the same pH, twice as much buffer has twice the buffer reserve.

The pH of blood and most body fluids is 7.4 and although a change in pH of 0.4 units may be fatal, all solutions used in the body do not have to be adjusted to pH 7.4. The natural body buffers assimilate and bring medicinal solutions to the pH of body fluids. For this reason pharmaceutical buffers for medicinal solutions for injection or placement in the eye should have a low buffer capacity. If buffers with high buffer capacity were used, they would resist change and interfere with the normal pH and buffer mechanisms of the body.

Boric acid, for example, has a pH of 5, but it may safely be used in the eye as it has a low buffer capacity and is rapidly adjusted to the physiological pH of the lachrymal fluid. Pyridoxine hydrochloride solutions are acid in reaction with a pH of approximately 3, yet when a small dose is given intravenously, it is rapidly diluted and buffered by the blood. It is somewhat irritating when administered subcutaneously or intramuscularly, but even in such cases, it is buffered by the blood as it is absorbed.

The buffer capacity at any hydrogen ion concentration may be calculated by means of the Van Slyke equation

$$\beta = 2.3\,C \frac{K_a[H^+]}{(K_a + [H^+])^2}$$

where β is the buffer capacity or the number of gram equivalents of an acid or base that changes the pH of a liter of buffer solution one unit, and C is the total buffer concentration or the sum of the molar concentrations of the acid and the salt.

The amounts of buffer components and sodium chloride required to prepare one liter of an isotonic 0.5% solution of tetracaine hydrochloride buffered at pH 5 with a buffer capacity of 0.05 may be calculated. The selected buffer components are propionic acid, which has a molecular weight of 74.08 g $mole^{-1}$, a sodium chloride equivalent of 0.46, and a K_a of 1.34×10^{-5} moles $liter^{-1}$, and sodium propionate, which has a molecular weight of 96.07 g $mole^{-1}$ and a sodium chloride equivalent of 0.61.

For a buffer composed of propionic acid and sodium propionate,

$$pH = pK_a + \log \frac{(MA)}{(HA)}$$

$$5.0 = 4.87 + \log \frac{(MA)}{(HA)}$$

$$0.13 = \log \frac{(MA)}{(HA)}$$

and

$$\frac{(MA)}{(HA)} = \text{antilog } 0.13 = \frac{1.35}{1}$$

The total buffer concentration may be calculated by use of the equation

$$\beta = 2.3\,C \frac{K_a\,[H^+]}{(K_a + [H^+])^2}$$

$$0.05 = 2.3\,C \frac{(1.34 \times 10^{-5})\,(10^{-5})}{[(1.34 \times 10^{-5}) + (10^{-5})]^2}$$

$$C = \frac{0.05}{2.3} \frac{[(1.34 \times 10^{-5}) + (10^{-5})]^2}{(1.34 \times 10^{-5})\,(10^{-5})}$$

$$C = 0.088 \text{ moles liter}^{-1}$$

Since (MA)/(HA) is 1.35, (MA) = 1.35 (HA). As the total buffer capacity is the sum of the acid and salt components,

$$C = (HA) + 1.35\,(HA) = 0.088 \text{ moles liter}^{-1}$$

$$(HA) = 0.037 \text{ moles liter}^{-1} \text{ of propionic acid}$$

and

$$(MA) = C - 0.037 = 0.053 \text{ moles liter}^{-1}$$

Converting to units of weight, the amount of propionic acid is

$$74.08 \times 0.037 = 2.741 \text{ g liter}^{-1}$$

and the amount of sodium propionate is

$$96.07 \times 0.053 = 5.092 \text{ g liter}^{-1}$$

The amount of sodium chloride necessary to adjust the solution to isotonicity with body fluids may be calculated by the sodium chloride equivalent method in which the summation of the products of the quantity and the sodium chloride equivalent of each solute is subtracted from the quantity of sodium chloride required to prepare normal saline.

Tetracaine hydrochloride	5.0	X 0.15	=	0.75
Propionic acid	2.741	X 0.46	=	1.261
Sodium propionate	5.092	X 0.61	=	3.105
				5.116

$$9.00 - 5.116 = 3.88 \text{ g of sodium chloride per liter}$$

Thus, the formulation is

Tetracaine hydrochloride	5.000 g
Propionic acid	2.741 g
Sodium propionate	5.092 g
Sodium chloride	3.88 g
Purified water q.s.	1 L

The use of buffer solutions to adjust pH may be employed to increase the solubility of drugs. Many organic acids are water-insoluble, but they dissolve readily in alkaline solution. Enhanced solubility is due to salt formation. The undissolved phase in equilibrium with the saturated solution is composed of unreacted acid and the increase in solubility is not influenced by the solubility of the salts formed.

The dissolution of a relatively insoluble organic acid occurs in two consecutive steps

$$HA_{(\text{solid phase})} \rightleftharpoons HA_{(\text{solution phase})}$$

$$HA_{(\text{solution phase})} \rightleftharpoons H^+ + A^-$$

The equilibrium constant, K_s, for the first reaction corresponds to the concentration of undissociated acid in equilibrium with the solid phase or the solubility of the acid in pure water.

The equilibrium constant for the second reaction is the ionization constant, K_a. The total amount, S_a, of the compound in solution is the sum of the ionized, A^-, and nonionized, HA, forms,

$$S_a = (HA) + (A^-) = (HA) + K_a \frac{(HA)}{(H^+)}$$

and as $K_s = (HA)$

$$S_a = K_s + K_s \frac{K_a}{(H^+)} = K_s \left[1 + \frac{K_a}{(H^+)} \right]$$

Thus, the total solubility of an acid is related to the hydrogen ion concentration of the solution.

In cases where the hydrogen ion concentration is appreciably less than the ionization constant, $K_a/(H^+)$ becomes the dominant term and 1 is of little significance. The equation then becomes approximately

$$S_a = \frac{K_a K_s}{(H^+)}$$

In logarithmic form it may be expressed

$$\log S_a = \log K_a + \log K_s - \log (H^+)$$

but since $-\log (H^+) = pH$ and $-\log K_a = pK_a$,

$$\log S_a = \log K_s + pH - pK_a$$

Benzoic acid is soluble in water to the extent of 0.028 mole liter^{-1} and has an ionization constant of 6.8×10^{-5}. The total amount of acid that would dissolve in a solution with a pH of 5 may be calculated

$$S_a = \frac{K_a K_s}{(H^+)} = \frac{6.8 \times 10^{-5} \times 0.028}{10^{-5}} = 0.19$$

Corresponding relationships exist for the dissolution of a slightly soluble nitrogenous base which dissolves in two steps

$$R_3N_{\text{(solid phase)}} \rightleftharpoons R_3NH_2O_{\text{(solution phase)}}$$

$$R_3NH_2O_{\text{(solution phase)}} \rightleftharpoons R_3NH^+ + OH^-$$

The ionization constant for the basic compound is

$$K_b = \frac{(R_3NH^+)(OH^-)}{(R_3NH_2O)}$$

The total solubility, S_b, is the sum of the undissociated and the ionized form

$$S_b = K_s + \frac{K_b K_s}{(OH^-)} = K_s \left[1 + \frac{K_b}{(OH^-)}\right]$$

Since the dissociation constant of water, K_w, at 25° is

$$K_w = (OH^-)(H^+) = 10^{-14}$$

the hydroxyl ion concentration may be expressed in terms of the more commonly used hydrogen ion concentration

$$S_b = K_s \left[1 + \frac{K_b}{\frac{K_w}{(H^+)}}\right] = K_s \left[1 + \frac{K_b (H^+)}{K_w}\right]$$

If hydroxyl ion concentration or $K_w/(H^+)$ is much less than the dissociation constant, the total solubility is approximately

$$S_b = \frac{K_s K_b}{K_w}(H^+)$$

or in logarithmic form

$$\log S_b = pK_w - pH - pK_b + \log K_s.$$

If a pharmacist were called upon to prepare a 1% apomorphine solution maintaining as high a pH as possible, he could calculate the required pH. The molecular weight of apomorphine is 267 g mole^{-1}, its pK_b is 7, and it is soluble to the extent of 4×10^{-4} mole liter^{-1}.

$$\log S_b = \log \frac{10}{267} = pK_w - pH - pK_b + \log K_s = 14 - pH - 7 + \log 0.0004$$

$$\log 0.0376 = 7 - pH + \log 0.0004$$

$$-1.427 = 7 - pH + (-3.398)$$

$$pH = 5$$

PROCEDURE. Various buffer systems have been suggested for different pharmaceutical solutions. Probably no one system will be suitable in all preparations; however, Sørensen phosphate buffer and its modifications have been widely adopted. The phosphate buffer system consists of two stock solutions, M/15 sodium acid phosphate and M/15 disodium phosphate, which are mixed in various volumes to obtain a desired pH.

If an alkali is added to the phosphate buffer, the hydroxyl ions are removed by reacting with the monobasic sodium phosphate

$$H_2PO_4^- + OH^- \longrightarrow H_2O + HPO_4^{--}$$

and if an acid is added, the hydrogen ions are removed by reacting with the dibasic sodium phosphate,

$$HPO_4^{--} + H^+ \longrightarrow H_2PO_4^-$$

A. Prepare 350 ml of each of aqueous M/15 sodium acid phosphate and M/15 disodium phosphate.

   Using a pH meter, determine the pH of each solution. Record.

   Mix 75, 50, 25, and 10 ml of M/15 sodium acid phosphate with 25, 50, 75, and 90 ml of M/15 disodium phosphate, respectively. Measure and record the pH of the four solutions after mixing well.

B. A drug will be assigned to each student by the instructor. Prepare 30 ml of an aqueous 0.2% solution of the drug buffered at an appropriate pH or with another buffer system satisfactory for the drug. Make this solution isotonic by the addition of sodium chloride.

C. Prepare 90 ml of a 5% aqueous solution of sodium sulfathiazole. Determine the pH. Expose 15 ml to the atmosphere for twenty-four hours. Record your observations.

   To 75 ml of the sodium sulfathiazole solution gradually add, while agitating, 0.1 N hydrochloric acid until sulfathiazole precipitates. Determine the pH at which precipitation begins.

   A borate buffer with a pH of 9 has been recommended as a vehicle for sulfathiazole sodium. Prepare the following solution and store under the same conditions as the 5% aqueous solution and compare the two solutions after a week.

Sulfathiazole sodium		1.5
Boric acid		0.013
Sodium borate		0.126
Sodium sulfite		0.30
Purified water	q. s.	30

D. Prepare 100 ml of an aqueous buffered solution containing 100 mg per ml of quinidine. Calculate the pH required to dissolve the quinidine. Measure the pH of your solution.

REFERENCES

Boylan, J. C. 1976. Liquids. In The theory and practice of industrial pharmacy, 2nd ed. L. Lachman, H. A. Lieberman, and J. L. Kanig, Eds. Lea and Febiger, Philadelphia. Chapter 19, p. 541.

Deardorff, D. L. 1975. Ophthalmic preparations. In Remington's Pharmaceutical sciences, 15th ed. Mack Publishing Company, Easton, Pa. Chapter 85, p. 1488.
Martin, A. N., J. Swarbrick, and A. Cammarata. 1969. Buffers and buffered isotonic systems. In Physical pharmacy, 2nd ed. Lea and Febiger, Philadelphia. Chapter 10, p. 236.
Niebergall, P. J. 1975. Buffers. In Remington's Pharmaceutical sciences, 15th ed. Mack Publishing Company, Easton, Pa. Chap. 18, p. 268.
Riegelman, S. and D. L. Sorby. 1971. EENT Medications. In Dispensing of medication, 7th ed. E. W. Martin, Ed. Mack Publishing Company, Easton, Pa. Chap. 24, p. 880.
Ritschel, W. A. 1972. pKa values and some clinical applications. In Perspectives in clinical pharmacy. D. E. Francke and H. A. K. Whitney, Jr., Eds. Drug Intelligence Publications, Hamilton, Illinois. Chap. 17, p. 325.
The United States Pharmacopeia, 19th rev. 1975. pH, pp. 653-654. Buffer solutions, pp. 761-762. Buffering ophthalmic solutions, pp. 702-703.

Buffer Solutions

Data and Conclusions

1. Complete the following chart and show a sample calculation:

pH	Volume of M/15 Sodium Acid Phosphate Solution	Volume of M/15 Disodium Phosphate Solution	Grams of Sodium Chloride to Make 100 ml Isotonic
	100 ml	0 ml	
	75	25	
	50	50	
	25	75	
	10	90	
	0	100	

2. Show calculations and final formula used to prepare 30 ml of the 0.2% isotonic and buffered solution in B.

3. What occurs and what is observed when a 5% aqueous solution of sodium sulfathiazole is exposed to the air? How may a stable solution be prepared?

4. At what pH does sulfathiazole begin to precipitate?

5. What is meant by the general term, pK? What is meant by the specific term, pK_w?

6. Calculate the total solubility of benzoic acid in a buffer containing 0.15 M sodium acetate and 0.1 M acetic acid.

7. In product research and development it is desired to formulate a morphine solution containing 15 mg per teaspoonful (5 ml). Other medicinal drugs in the product give rise to a pH of 7.5. Can the desired concentration of morphine be obtained in this preparation, and if not, what pH would be required? The pK_b of morphine is 6.13 and it is soluble 1 g in 5000 ml of water.

8. The ionization constant of acetic acid is 1.8×10^{-5}. Calculate and tabulate the hydrogen ion concentration and pH of the following mixtures of acetic acid and sodium acetate.

Parts of Undissociated Acetic Acid	Parts of Anions or Salt	Hydrogen Ion Concentration	pH
99	1		
95	5		
90	10		
85	15		
80	20		
75	25		
70	30		
65	35		
60	40		
55	45		
50	50		
45	55		
40	60		
35	65		
30	70		
20	80		
10	90		
5	95		
1	99		

Plot the pH of each solution as an abscissa and [acid] or [salt] as an ordinate. Based on this curve, what is the zone of greatest buffer capacity? Give a sample of the calculations used to complete the table.

9. What is the relationship between pK_a and pK_b?

10. For D show your calculations for the pH required to dissolve the quinidine.

11. For D give your formulation and observations. How does the calculated pH compare to the measured pH of your solution?

21. PARENTERAL SOLUTIONS

Parenteral solutions are sterile solutions to be administered by intravenous, subcutaneous, intramuscular, or intraspinal injection. An ampul is a hermetically sealed container, usually of glass, which maintains in a sterile condition a single dose of medicament that may be in the form of a solution, dry powder, or a suspension. A vial is a stoppered glass container which preserves, in a sterile condition, multiple doses of a medicament.

Rubber closures may reduce the concentration of preservatives in solutions packaged in multidose vials. Solutions containing chlorobutanol, methyl paraben, p-chloro-β-phenylethyl alcohol, phenylethyl alcohol and benzyl alcohol in multi-dose vials stoppered with natural and synthetic rubber closures exhibit a greater loss of preservative than those solutions packaged in ampuls. Vials stored in an inverted position showed a greater loss of preservative than those stored upright. Natural rubber stoppers exert a less deleterious effect than butyl rubber closures.

Accelerators (diphenyl guanidine, zinc diethyl dithiocarbate) are employed in vulcanization of rubber for increasing the rate of the process and reducing the amount of sulfur. Fillers (carbon black, talc, zinc oxide) softeners (petroleum), antioxidants and pigments (iron oxide) are used in processing rubber. Any of these substances or the reaction products of the vulcanization process may be leached from the closure by solutions and may be potentially toxic or promote degradation of the medicinal compound in the parenteral solution.

The method used to sterilize a parenteral preparation depends primarily on the thermostability of the drug. The fundamental techniques of sterilization involve the use of heat, gas, radiation, and bacterial filtration.

Substances which are decomposed by moisture or are not readily permeated by steam are sterilized by dry heat. Dry-heat sterilization kills microorganisms by oxidation, while moist-heat sterilization destroys microorganisms by coagulation of the cellular protein. Although the dry-heat method is limited in use, it is the usual procedure for sterilizing glassware, porcelain, and metallic containers, and instruments. Containers should be clean and free of organic matter. To ensure sterility the container should be exposed to a temperature not less than 170° for a period of 1-2 hours. To avoid cracking the glassware, heating and cooling should be gradually accomplished. Equipment to be used sometime after sterilization should be wrapped in strong paper, and nonabsorbent cotton plugs may be used to stopper flasks. Cotton and paper brown at 190°.

Arrangement of the materials to be sterilized by dry heat is important. Glassware should not be tightly packed in a hot-air oven but should be loosely arranged so that air currents may readily diffuse. Care should be taken that substances, such as glycerin, propylene glycol, liquid petrolatum and fixed oils, are heated so that the entire content of each container is maintained at 170° for the designated time. Powdered drugs usually are spread in a 1/4-inch layer to facilitate the uniform distribution of heat.

To autoclave or to use steam under pressure is generally the most satisfactory method of sterilization. At 121° saturated steam will kill in 2 minutes not only the microorganisms but also bacterial spores. Steam at atmospheric pressure, 14.7 lb in $^{-2}$, cannot exceed a temperature of 100°; however, if the steam is confined and the pressure is increased, the temperature of the steam is elevated. Air should be excluded from the autoclave prior to the sterilization period, as only the pressure exerted by the steam is effective in elevating the temperature of the steam. For example, at 20 and 40 lb in $^{-2}$ the temperature of steam is 109° and 130°, respectively.

Water possesses a rather large latent heat, which is available upon the condensation of the steam. The temperature of the steam is maintained by the condensed water, and the condensed water supplies the hydrating and coagulating factors essential to the destruction of spores.

The total time required in the sterilization process is the sum of the time needed to heat the solution to the temperature at which it is to be sterilized and the exposure time. A temperature of 121° at a pressure of 15 lb in $^{-2}$ for an exposure time of 20 minutes is the usual sterilization time; however, time must be allowed for the solution to attain this temperature and added to the 20 minutes for actual sterilization time. For example, it requires 35-40 minutes to bring a gallon of water to 115° but only 6 minutes to bring 50 ml to the same temperature. The total time to process a gallon is then approximately twice that of the smaller 50 ml in a small container.

Sterile solutions of a thermolabile drug are generally prepared by passing the solution through a bacteria-retaining filter under aseptic technique. With a few exceptions, a bacteriostatic agent is added to the parenteral solutions prepared in this manner. Liquid petrolatum and oily vehicles are commonly thought to increase the permeability of a bacterial filter and cannot be sterilized by this method. By controlling pore size and the thickness of the filter plate, a filter, which is effective and has a rapid filtration rate, can be produced. For example, a Selas 02 porosity porcelain filter has an average pore radius of 0.42 μ and approximately 8×10^8 capillaries in $^{-2}$ of filter plate.

The mechanism of bacteriological filtration is complicated by the fact that with the great surfaces involved, adsorption of the bacteria and the drug may occur. The pH of the solution may affect the form of the drug or the charge on the protein of the bacteria and introduce more variables in the mechanism of filtration. Since these effects occur, industrially each parenteral solution is developed after experiments have shown the effectiveness of a particular type of filter for a given solution.

Gaseous sterilization has become industrially popular since the advent of antibiotics. A chemical in the gaseous or vapor state can be used to sterilize solid drugs which are thermolabile or decomposed by moisture. Ethylene oxide by virtue of its ability to diffuse and penetrate through dry materials is the chemical of choice for gas sterilization. Pure ethylene oxide is flammable and when mixed with from 3-80% air, forms an explosive mixture. To reduce fire hazards, ethylene oxide is used as a mixture with carbon dioxide. Carboxide, which is used in the pharmaceutical industry, is a mixture of 10% ethylene oxide and 90% carbon dioxide. Ethylene oxide may be used to sterilize packaged products. Small surgical dressings, hermetically sealed in cellophane envelopes, packaged in small cartons and placed in large fiberboard sealed shipping containers, are placed in an air-evacuated chamber. Upon exposure to a concentration of 450 mg liter^{-1} of ethylene oxide, the dressings are sterilized in 4-6 hours exposure at 45°. Since ethylene oxide readily diffuses, it is rapidly dissipated from materials after sterilization has been completed.

Ultraviolet radiation is used commercially to protect workers, to sterilize, and to maintain sterile areas. Ultraviolet radiation of 2500 Å is lethal to bacteria, mold spores, and other microorganisms in the air or on exposed surfaces; however, it will not penetrate most substances and is useless in the sterilization of drugs, foods, and fabrics. Investigation of radiation technique is required to utilize it successfully. For example, ultraviolet radiation of 2500 Å is lethal to microorganisms and destroys vitamin D, while ultraviolet radiation of 2900 Å builds vitamin D and has little effect on bacteria.

Higher energy radiations with greater penetrating ability are being investigated as a means of sterilizing packaged materials. Beta rays, gamma rays, x-rays, and accelerated electron beams produce ionization that is lethal to bacteria. It should be noted that identical radiations may be described by different terms. This arises from the conventional practice of naming radiations according to the mode by which they are produced. The number of surviving bacteria exposed to such radiations decreases logarithmically with the time of exposure. Rarely will a microorganism survive an exposure of 2×10^6 rad. The rad, radiation absorbed dose, is a measure of the energy absorbed from any radiation by any material. One rad represents an energy absorption of 100 ergs g^{-1}.

The effectiveness of these radiations varies with the ionization produced and their penetrating ability. Beta particles and x-rays probably can be discounted for most industrial applications. The beta particle has limited penetrating ability and is limited to surface sterilization. The higher energy x-rays are penetrating but their production is inefficient and more costly than the production of accelerated electrons.

Gamma radiation and highly accelerated electrons appear to present the most promise for sterilizing packaged goods. By means of a linear accelerator, electrons may acquire the energy of several million electron volts, MeV. The charge on an electron somewhat limits its penetration. Eight MeV electrons will penetrate water only to a depth of 4 cm. By irradiation from opposite sides, an effective, uniform dose of radiation could be delivered through a material with unit density only to a thickness approximately 7 cm. This would barely be adequate for most packaged products. Greater penetration could be achieved by increasing the energy of the electrons; however, the risk of residual radioactivity following absorption of the incident energy by atomic nuclei then becomes a significant factor.

Gamma radiation is available from Cs^{137}. This isotope has a half-life of twenty-seven years. The energy of the gamma ray is 0.66 MeV so there is no danger of residual radioactivity in the irradiated material. Gamma rays are very penetrating; they will sterilize material with unit density, when exposed on opposite sides, to a thickness of 25 cm.

Whatever method is used, adequate shielding must be provided to protect the operator from radiation.

Radiation may be used with thermolabile drugs, since the heat released when 2×10^6 rad is absorbed is approximately two calories. Penicillin G potassium, streptomycin-potassium chloride complex, chlortetracycline, chloramphenicol, and oxytetracycline have been treated in the dry state with 2×10^6 rad. All samples were sterile after irradiation and maintained their antibiotic potency and normal solubility, although some of the powders became slightly discolored. Before radiation can be used commercially, each product must be examined for alteration in the color, stability of the product toward and after irradiation, formation of toxic by-products, and the possible pyrogenic activity of the irradiated bacteria. For example, plasma can be sterilized by gamma radiation, but whole blood cannot be, as hemolysis occurs. Irradiation of liquid dosage forms may not only affect the active ingredient but may also degrade carbohydrates used as suspending and emulsifying agents with changes in the physical stability of the suspension or emulsion.

Attention should be given briefly to several methods of sterilization of limited or questionable value. Boiling water is a household means of sterilizing instruments and rubber goods. The item to be sterilized is completely immersed in water and boiled for at least 15 minutes. As an emergency measure, solutions sealed in an ampul may be sterilized in a similar manner; these solutions should be boiled for 30-60 minutes on three consecutive days. If therapeutically suitable, the addition of a bactericide such as 0.2% chlorocresol or 0.002% phenylmercuric nitrate may be added to facilitate sterilization of the solution.

In industry, free-flowing steam is passed through pipes, vats, and containers to sterilize them. The Arnold sterilizer utilizes free-flowing steam in tyndallization; the material is exposed to the free-flowing steam at 100° for 30-60 minutes on three consecutive days. Materials that are damaged by temperatures of 100° may be sterilized by inspissation. This is a fractional heating in which the material is exposed to a temperature of 60-80° for 4-7 days. A bacteriostatic agent should be used in such instances; however, this is not a safe method of sterilization.

If a physician prescribes intravenous infusions to be used to correct electrolyte imbalance in terms of milliequivalents, mEq, the pharmacist must be able to convert into terms of weight of salts required. An equivalent weight expresses the combining power or chemical reactivity; it is the number of grams of a substance that can react with or replace one gram of hydrogen. One equivalent weight is equal to 1000 milliequivalents. The number of grams of a salt corresponding to a given number of milliequivalents may be dissolved in as little water as necessary. In practice the contents are then transferred to a large volume intravenous infusion bottle, and the concentration of electrolyte ultimately in the bottle is expressed in milliequivalents per liter. With Potassium Chloride Injection, if there are 1.5 g of potassium chloride in solution, the number of milliequivalents of K^+ and Cl^- is always 20 mEq for each regardless of the volume of solution. The number of milliequivalents may be calculated by means of the relation

$$\text{mEq} = \frac{(\text{grams of salt})\ (\text{valence of a given ion})\ (\text{number of ions})\ 1000}{\text{molecular weight}}$$

For example, in 0.143 g of magnesium chloride, the milliequivalents are

$$\frac{(0.143)\ (2)\ (1)\ 1000}{95.3} = 3\ \text{mEq of}\ Mg^{++}$$

and

$$\frac{(0.143)\ (1)\ (2)\ \ 1000}{95.3} = 3\ \text{mEq. of}\ Cl^-$$

PROCEDURE. As the majority of parenteral solutions are aqueous, the characteristics of water for injection are important. To be used for injection, water must be distilled and must be pyrogen-free, colorless, odorless, clean, and tasteless. In solutions of a volume exceeding 100 ml, 2 mg of solid residue is generally permissible upon evaporation of 100 ml of solution. The solids in water are usually expressed in terms of parts per million, ppm. Two milligrams of residue per 100 ml of water is equal to 20 ppm. Water packaged in a volume of 30 ml or less may be acceptable if it contains no more than 40 ppm.

In industry, distilled water assays are made with a Barnstead or Solu-Bridge purity meter. A purity meter is a small Wheatstone bridge equipped with a conductivity cell to be immersed in the water to be tested. The Wheatstone bridge is balanced by turning a dial calibrated in parts per million or grains of sodium chloride per gallon.

The specific resistance of an electrolyte is the resistance in ohms of a column of solution 1 cm long and 1 cm^2 in cross section. The specific conductance, L, is the reciprocal of the specific resistance and has the units of $ohm^{-1}\,cm^{-1}$.

Equivalent conductance, Λ, is obtained by multiplying the specific conductance by the volume in ml which contains 1 g equivalent of the solute, that is, 1000/c where c is the number of gram equivalents per liter

$$\Lambda = VL = \frac{1000\ L}{c}$$

To illustrate the use of these conductance terms, consider a 0.0200 M potassium chloride standard. At 18° potassium chloride has a specific conductance of 0.002394 $ohm^{-1}\,cm^{-1}$. If r is measured resistance of the conductivity cell being used, 1/r is the conductance, and the specific conductance is k (1/r) where k is a constant for a given cell. When our cell is filled with 0.0200 M potassium chloride at 18°

$$k = 0.002394\ r$$

After determining the cell constant,

$$L = \frac{k}{r}$$

When a given cell at 18° is filled with 0.0200 M potassium chloride, it has a resistance of 80 ohms as measured by a Wheatstone bridge, and when filled with 0.005 N solution of an electrolyte, it has a measured resistance of 320 ohms. The cell constant is

$$k = 0.002394 \times 80 = 0.1915$$

The specific conductance of the solution being tested is

$$L = k/r = 0.19152/320 = 0.000598 \text{ ohm}^{-1} \text{ cm}^{-1}$$

The equivalent conductance of the 0.005 N solution is

$$\Lambda = \frac{1000\ L}{c} = \frac{1000 \times 0.000598}{0.005} = 110.6 \text{ cm}^2 \text{equiv}^{-1} \text{ohm}^{-1}$$

Water that has been distilled several times and is suitable for conductivity measurements is referred to as conductivity water. Conductivity water has a specific conductance of 10^{-6} ohms^{-1} cm^{-1}.

If a purity meter is calibrated to read in terms of grains of sodium chloride per gallon, a scale reading of 0.1 grains may be converted into ppm. One-tenth grain equals 6.5 mg of sodium chloride per one gallon or 3785 ml; thus,

$$\frac{0.0065}{3785} = \frac{x}{1{,}000{,}000}$$

$$x = 1.7 \text{ g or } 1.7 \text{ ppm}$$

When there is more than 2 ppm, it indicates contamination, and the still must be examined. Since pyrogens and bacteria may be carried over with the electrolytes, it is assumed that the water is unsafe for parenteral use. Although conductivity tests are valuable, the finished parenteral solution must be subjected to a pyrogen test. Nonelectrolytes may be pyrogenic but do not conduct current in solution, and they would not be detected by a conductivity cell.

A. By means of a Barnstead purity meter, analyze a sample of water supplied by the instructor.

B. Prepare six 250-ml bottles of a 5% Dextrose Injection U. S. P. Filter the solution through a medium porosity sintered-glass filter, using an aspirator or vacuum pump to reduce pressure and hasten filtration. A Seitz filter or a Millipore filter and pressure may also be used. Seal the containers and sterilize by autoclaving at 15 psi for 20 minutes. The proper operation of an autoclave will be demonstrated by the instructor. Examine the finished solution for discoloration.

An inexpensive but efficient apparatus for washing a small number of ampuls is shown in Figure 11. A medium bore needle (A) at least 10 cm in length is mounted on one end of the axis of a glass T-tube (B) by a short length of rubber pressure tubing (C). The needle is inserted through one wall of a length of tubing (D) of approximately 6 mm so that its length lies within the lumen of the tubing and its tip projects approximately 2 cm beyond the end of the tubing. The sharp point of the needle is removed and the tip is smoothed. The opposite end of the axis of the T-tube is connected to a piece of glass delivery tubing (E) of the same bore by a rubber stopper (F) fitted into a one-liter filtration flask (G). The flask is filled with freshly distilled water. The ampul is in-

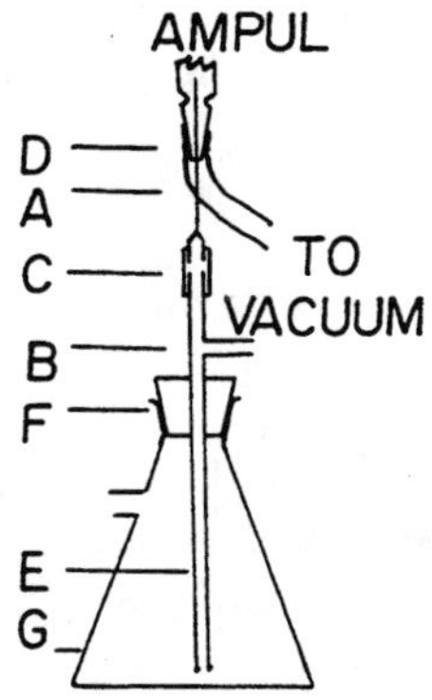

Figure 11 – Ampul cleaning device.

serted into tube D so that the tip of the needle lies within its body. Upon aspiration at the other end of tube D with the closing of the side-arm T-tube with the fingers, a jet of water issues from A and rinses the ampul. When the finger is removed from the side-arm of B, the residual water is removed from the ampul. The ampuls can be used without further treatment. If sterile ampuls are required they may be heated in a hot air oven at 150° for one hour.

C. Prepare Sodium Chloride Injection U. S. P. or Ringer's Injection U. S. P. The preparation and size of ampul to be filled will be assigned by the instructor. Sterilize by means of an autoclave. Examine the ampuls for leakage.

In addition to the usual procedures in preparing parenteral solutions, problems arise because of the structure of a drug. As an example, ascorbic acid is stable in the dry state, and its solutions are susceptible to oxidation and discoloration which are catalyzed by trace metals.

Ascorbic acid in the presence of air is oxidized to dehydro-ascorbic acid. Although dehydroascorbic acid shows the same activity as ascorbic acid, it is rapidly degraded into biologically inactive products. An increase in pH of a solution accelerates oxidation; a solution with pH 3 is stable but painful if injected in large volumes. Oxidation is minimized by bubbling carbon dioxide through the water for ten minutes prior to adding the ascorbic acid. This removes any dissolved air and saturates the solution with carbon dioxide. During compounding, bottling and sealing, air should be displaced by carbon dioxide.

Sunlight decomposes ascorbic acid in solution. Indirect or subdued light, which contains little ultraviolet light, has no effect. Bottles of bulk solutions of ascorbic acid may be wrapped in black opaque cloth or paper, and finished ampuls should be packaged in light-resistant containers.

At concentrations exceeding 10%, solutions will occasionally liberate carbon dioxide. At high concentrations the liberation of gas occurs to such an extent that dangerous pressures may result during storage. Ampuls containing 25% ascorbic acid solutions have been known to explode.

Ascorbic acid may be sterilized by autoclave at 15 psi at 120°. As ascorbic acid solutions tend to darken at elevated temperatures, bacteriological filtration is often used industrially. Phenol or the methyl and propyl esters of p-hydroxybenzoic acid may be used as bacteriostatic preservatives. Chlorobutanol is of questionable value.

Ampuls to be used for ascorbic acid solutions should meet all the requirements for Type I glass. Multiple-dose vials with rubber closures are permissible, but the stability of the solution is limited by the permeability of the rubber by oxygen. Any ascorbic acid remaining on the neck of an ampul will char upon being sealed. To eliminate this problem, a technique involving washing the neck of the ampul has been developed. Allowance is made for the dilution of the solution.

Discoloration may arise from local alkalinization during adjustment of pH. This is readily avoided by slowly adding a concentrated solution of sodium bicarbonate while the solution is being vigorously agitated by a stream of carbon dioxide.

D. Develop a method and prepare the ascorbic acid solution assigned by the instructor.

E. A parenteral solution to be packaged in multidose vials will be assigned by the instructor.

Laminar flow, a recent technique for controlling airborne contamination, has been widely used in aerospace, electronics, and other industries. Laminar air-flow lends itself very well to pharmaceutical procedures which require aseptic operation. It is being successfully used in the preparation of ophthalmic and parenteral products and in sterility testing procedures.

Laminar air-flow is defined by Federal Standard 209A as "Air flow in which the entire body of air within a confined area moves with uniform velocity along parallel flow lines." The standard states further that the velocity of the air shall be 90 feet per minute with a uniformity of ±20 feet per minute. Whenever the use of laminar flow devices is contemplated, the containment of the air flow and the uniformity of velocity must be considered.

To maintain high levels of particulate cleanliness, it is necessary to have in the air stream a filter which will effectively filter minute particulate matter. The filter which is used to provide these high levels of cleanliness is a High Efficiency Particulate Air (HEPA) filter, which with a minimum efficiency will remove 99.97% of all particles 0.3 microns and larger. Laminar flow *per se* is formed downstream of this filter.

Laminar flow may be horizontal or vertical. It may be used in an entire clean room or in a smaller work station. A work station may be preferred to a clean room, as a work station is more economical and it is easier to maintain as an ultraclean and sterile work area.

F. Using a laminar flow hood, conduct one of the sterility tests described in the U. S. P.

REFERENCES

APhA Annual Meeting Industrial Pharmaceutical Technology Section, May 5-10, 1968, Miami Beach, Florida. Symposium: Environmental control in the manufacture of pharmaceuticals.

Application Report AR-11. 1976. Low volume sterilizing filtration. Millipore Corporation, Bedford, Massachusetts.

Artz, W. J., W. T. Gloor, and D. R. Reese. 1961. Study of various methods for detecting leaks in hermetically sealed ampuls. J. Pharm. Sci., 50:258.

Autian, J. 1971. Plastics and medication. In Dispensing of medication, 7th ed. E. W. Martin, Ed. Mack Publishing Company, Easton, Pa. Chap. 15, p. 652.

Avis, K. E. 1975. Parenteral preparations. In Remington's Pharmaceutical sciences, 15th ed. Mack Publishing Co., Easton, Pa. Chap. 84, p. 1461.

Avis, K. E. 1976. Sterilization. In The theory and practice of industrial pharmacy, 2nd ed. L. Lachman, H. A. Lieberman, and J. L. Kanig, Eds. Lea and Febiger, Philadelphia. Chap. 20, p. 567.

Avis, K. E. 1976. Sterile products. In The theory and practice of industrial pharmacy, 2nd ed. L. Lachman, H. A. Lieberman, and J. L. Kanig, Eds. Lea and Febiger, Philadelphia. Chap. 21, p. 586.

Avis, K. E., H. S. Carlin, and H. L. Flack. 1961. Preparation of injectables. Philosophy and master procedures. Am. J. Hospital Pharmacy, 18:223.

Ballard, B. E. 1968. Biopharmaceutical considerations in subcutaneous and intramuscular drug administration. J. Pharm. Sci., 57:357.

Boucher, R. M. G. 1972. Advances in sterilization techniques. State of the art and recent breakthroughs. Am. J. Hospital Pharmacy, 29:660-672.

Bowman, F. W. 1969. The sterility testing of pharmaceuticals. J. Pharm. Sci., 58:1301.

Brewer, J. H. and C. B. McLaughlin. 1961. Dehydrated sterilizer controls containing bacterial spores and culture media. J. Pharm. Sci., 50:171.

Bruch, C. W. and M. K. Bruch. 1971. Sterilization. In Dispensing of medication. E. W. Martin, Ed. Mack Publishing Company, Easton, Pa. Chap. 13, p. 592.

Calhoun, M. P., M. White, and F. W. Bowman. 1970. Sterility testing of insulin by membrane filtration. J. Pharm. Sci., 59:1022.

Carleton, F. J. 1967. Aqueous and non-aqueous solvents in parenteral preparations. Bulletin of the Parenteral Drug Association, 21:142.

DeLuca, P. P. and R. J. Kowalsky. 1972. Problems arising from the transfer of sodium bicarbonate injection from ampuls to plastic disposable syringes. Am. J. Hospital Pharmacy, 29:217.

Dirksen, J. W. and R. V. Larsen. 1975. Filling vials aseptically while monitoring for bacterial contamination. Am. J. Hospital Pharmacy, 32:1031.

Food and Drug Administration, U. S. Department of Health, Education, and Welfare. July 28-29, 1966. Safety of large volume parenteral solutions. National Symposium Proceedings. Washington, D. C.

Francke, D. E., Ed. 1972. Handbook of I. V. additive reviews. Drug Intelligence and Clinical Pharmacy Publications, Hamilton Press, Hamilton, Illinois.

Groves, M. J. 1969. The size distribution of particles contaminating parenteral solutions. Analyst, 94:992.

Hem, S. L., D. R. Bright, G. S. Banker, and J. P. Pogue. 1974-1975. Tissue irritation evaluation of potential parenteral vehicles. Drug Development Communications, 1(5):471.

Hopkins, G. H. 1965. Elastomeric closures for pharmaceutical packaging. J. Pharm. Sci., 54:138.

Lachman, L., S. Weinstein, G. Hopkins, S. Slack, P. Eisman, and J. Cooper. 1962. Stability of antibacterial preservatives in parenteral solutions I. Factors influencing the loss of antimicrobial agents from solutions in rubber-stoppered containers. J. Pharm. Sci., 51:224.

Lachman, L., T. Urbanyi, and S. Weinstein. 1963. Stability of antibacterial preservatives in parenteral solutions IV. Contribution of rubber closure composition on preservative loss. J. Pharm. Sci., 52:244.

Laskaris, T. and A. L. Chaney. 1969. Reliability of biologic autoclave sterilization indicators. The American Journal of Clinical Pathology, 52:495.

Lazarus, J., P. C. Eisman, and D. Jaconia. 1963. Liquid ethylene oxide sterilization and other pharmaceutical aspects of a novel dosage form. The Bulletin of the Parenteral Drug Association, 17, No. 3, p. 1.
Lebowitz, M. H., J. Y. Masuda, and J. H. Beckerman. 1971. The pH and acidity of intravenous infusion solutions. J.A.M.A., 215:1937.
Lee, H. A., Ed. 1974. Parenteral nutrition in acute metabolic illness. Academic Press, London and New York.
Ley, F. J. 1971. Gamma radiation for product sterilization. J. Soc. Cosmetic Chemists, 22:711-723.
McDade, J. J., G. B. Phillips, H. D. Sivinski, and W. J. Whitfield. 1969. Principles and applications of laminar-flow devices. In J. R. Norris and D. W. Ribbons, Methods in microbiology, Vol. I. Academic Press, London and New York.
Morton, M., Ed. 1959. Introduction to rubber technology. Reinhold Publishing Co. New York.
Palmer, C. H. R. 1971. Pharmaceutical aspects of pyrogens in hospital and industry. In Ciba Foundation Symposium on pyrogens and fever. G. E. W. Wolstenholme and J. Birch, Eds. J. & A. Churchill, 104 Gloucester Place, London. pp. 193-205.
Parrott, E. L. 1965. Formulation of parenterals. Drug & Cosmetic Ind. 96:320.
Perkins, J. J. 1969. Principles and methods of sterilization in health sciences, 2nd ed. C. C. Thomas Co., Springfield, Illinois.
Phillips, G. B. and W. S. Miller. 1975. Sterilization. In Remington's Pharmaceutical sciences, 15th ed. Mack Publishing Co., Easton, Pa. Chap. 78, p. 1389.
Roseman, T. J., J. A. Brown, and W. W. Scothorn. 1976. Glass for parenteral products: A surface view using the scanning electron microscope. J. Pharm. Sci., 65:22.
Rosenzweig, A. L. 1964. Potential health hazards in the multiple-dose vial. Hospitals, Journal of the American Hospital Association, 38:71.
Rowe, T. W. G. 1971. Machinery and methods in freeze-drying. Cryobiology, 8:153-172.
Saski, W. 1963. Adsorption of sorbic acid by plastic cellulose acetates, J. Pharm. Sci. 52:264.
Schulman, S. G. 1973. Fundamentals of interaction of ionizing radiation with chemical, biochemical, and pharmaceutical systems. J. Pharm. Sci., 62:1745-1757.
Seligmann, E. B., Jr. and J. F. Farber. 1971. Freeze drying and residual moisture. Cryobiology, 8:138-144.
Simonelli, A. P. and D. S. Dresback. 1972. Principles of formulation of parenteral dosage forms. In Perspectives in clinical pharmacy. D. E. Francke and H. A. K. Whitney, Jr., Eds. Drug Intelligence Publications, Hamilton, Illinois. Chap. 19, p. 390.
Spiegel, A. J. and M. M. Noseworthy. 1963. Use of nonaqueous solvents in parenteral products. J. Pharm. Sci., 52:917.
Svensson, H. 1956. A discussion on the meaning of equivalent weights and transport (transference) numbers for amphoteric electrolytes, especially protolytes. Science Tools. The LKB Instrument Journal, 3:29.
Sykes, G. 1965. Disinfection and sterilization, 2nd ed. J. B. Lippincott Co., Philadelphia.
The United States Pharmacopeia, 19th rev. 1975. Sterilization, P. 709. Containers, p. 642. Injections, p. 582. Sterility tests, p. 592.
Turco, S. and R. E. King. 1974. Sterile dosage forms. Their preparation and clinical application. Lea and Febiger, Philadelphia.
Van Ooteghem, M. and H. Herbots. 1969. The adsorption of preservatives on membrane filters. Pharm. Acta Helv. 44:602.
Vidt, D. G. 1975. Use and abuse of intravenous solutions. J.A.M.A., 232:533.
White, P. L. and M. E. Nagy, Eds. 1974. Total parenteral nutrition. Proceedings of the Symposium on Total Parenteral Nutrition sponsored by the Food Science Committee, Council on Foods and Nutrition of the American Medical Association held in Nashville, Tennessee in 1972. Publishing Sciences Group, Inc., Acton, Massachusetts.
Wilkinson, G. R. and L. C. Baker. 1964. Contemporary trends in heat sterilization. In Advances in pharmaceutical sciences. Volume 1. H. S. Bean, A. H. Beckett, and J. E. Carless. Academic Press, London and New York. p. 269.
Wilson, D. A. 1971. Sterility testing procedures in a pharmaceutical factory. Medical Laboratory Technology, 28:351.
Wood, D. G. 1952. A simple ampule-washing device. The Pharmaceutical Journal, March 8, p. 159.
Wurdack, P. J. and J. L. Colaizzi. 1970. Electrolyte solution calculations. J. Am. Pharm. Assoc., NS 10:412.

Parenteral Solutions

Data and Conclusions

1. What is the purity of the sample of water tested by the Barnstead purity meter?

2. Give your formulation and method of preparation of the assigned ascorbic acid injection.

3. Give your formulation and method of preparation of the assigned multidose preparation.

4. What is the common practice regarding the buffering of parenteral solutions?

5. List the solvents which can be used parenterally.

6. What are pyrogens? Briefly, describe the pyrogen test. Some pyrogenic injections lose the pyrogenic activity upon storage. How might this occur?

7. What are the sources of pyrogen and how may they be removed from equipment, water, solutions, and drugs?

8. What antibacterial preservatives can be used in parenteral solutions, and in what concentration? When should a preservative be avoided?

9. How many grams of sodium bicarbonate are required to provide 40 mEq of bicarbonate ion?

10. Why is air excluded from the autoclave before sterilization begins?

11. Define latent heat. Saturated steam at 100° occupies 1.674 m^3kg^{-1}. An autoclave with a capacity of 0.2 m^3 is filled with steam at 100°. If all the steam condenses without a change in temperature, how much heat will be liberated?

12. Complete the following chart of bacteria-retaining filters:

Filter	Composition	Disadvantages
Berkefeld		
Millipore		
Seitz		
Selas		
Sintered-glass		

13. Calculate the mEq of each of the five ions present in Lactated Ringer's Solution.

14. Complete the following table of radiation:

Radiation	Origin	Consists of	Charge	Penetrating Ability
alpha				
beta				
gamma				
x-ray				
accelerated electron				

15. Define lyophilization utilizing a diagram of pressure against temperature. What applications of freeze-drying are made in manufacturing parenteral products?

16. What extractives from rubber may occur in solutions sterilized and preserved in multiple dose vials? What preservatives are known to have been extracted by rubber caps from solutions in multiple dose vials?

17. Describe the sterility test you performed in F.

22. KINETICS OF AN AQUEOUS SOLUTION

The shelf life or stability of all pharmaceuticals is of great practical importance. The stability of pharmaceutical preparations is often stated in ambiguous terms such as relatively stable or stable for a month. The industrial pharmacist aims by chemical kinetics to predict the rate and course of drug deterioration. The hospital pharmacist is concerned with the compatibility and stability. An understanding of kinetics is essential to adequately practice product development and to clinically select a dosage regimen.

Recent kinetic studies have involved the hydrolysis of esters, such as procaine and amyl nitrate, and amides such as procainamide and chloramphenicol. The degradation of penicillin and oxytetracycline, the oxidation of ascorbic acid, the fading of coal tar dyes, and the loss of biological activity of 1-epinephrine by racemization have lent themselves to the application of kinetics. After experimentally evaluating the velocity constant of a particular reaction, the pharmacist can predict the amount of active drug present at any time.

A reaction in which the rate of reaction is directly proportional to the concentration of the reacting substance is a first-order reaction. The amount of drug which reacts depends on the amount that is present and may be expressed mathematically

$$-\frac{dc}{dt} = kc$$

where c is the concentration of the reacting drug, k is a proportionality factor, t is the time, and -dc/dt is the rate at which the concentration is decreased.

If this equation is integrated between the limits, concentration c_1 at times t_1, and c_2 at a later time t_2, it takes the form

$$k = \frac{2.303}{t_2 - t_1} \log \frac{c_1}{c_2}$$

The constant, k, is the specific reaction-rate constant or the velocity constant. For a first-order reaction it is a number per unit time. For example, if k is 0.002 hr^{-1}, 0.2% of the drug is decomposed every hour.

This equation may also be expressed in an exponential form

$$c = c_O e^{-kt}$$

where c_O is the initial concentration, and c is the concentration at time t.

Radioactive decay, the inversion of sucrose and the acid hydrolysis of procaine are first-order reactions. The reaction rate may be described in terms of half-life as well as a velocity constant. The half-life, $t_1/_2$, is the time necessary for half of a given quantity of drug to decompose. For first-order reactions

$$k = \frac{2.303}{t_{1/2}} \log \frac{1}{1/2} = \frac{0.693}{t_{1/2}}$$

A second-order reaction is one in which the rate of the reaction is proportional to the concentration of two reacting substances. If two drugs react, A + B $\longrightarrow$ AB, then the rate at which the concentrations decrease is

$$-\frac{dc_A}{dt} = -\frac{dc_B}{dt} = kc_Ac_B$$

The value of k depends on the units in which concentration is expressed. If by convention the concentration is expressed in moles liter^{-1}, then k has the dimension of liter mole^{-1} unit time^{-1}.

Some reactions are independent of concentration (which is mathematically equivalent to the concentration to the zero power) and are known as zero order reactions. The degradation of suspensions and the degradation due to the absorption of light are zero order reactions. In suspensions only the drug in solution undergoes degradation. The degradation rate is

$$-\frac{dc}{dt} = k$$

The kinetics of photochemical degradation is complex due to many variables (wave length and intensity of light, size and shape of container). A photochemical reaction may produce a catalyst, which causes a thermal reaction that proceeds at a measurable rate and may continue after the illumination has ceased.

Although many reactions are complicated, they are usually not of an order greater than the third-order; they are often a combination of several subsequent or simultaneous first- and second-order reactions. Interpretation of the stability of some pharmaceutical products is difficult because of the complexity of the formulation and the interactions of various components in the formulation; however, kinetic data are of great value to the pharmaceutical formulator in developing a new product and of great aid in establishing a stability pattern for the finished product.

As many pharmaceuticals are stored in a refrigerator, it is well recognized that an increase in temperature will hasten degradation of a drug. In considering the stability of a given product the integrated form of the Arrhenius equation is important

$$\log\frac{k_2}{k_1} = \frac{E_a\,(T_2 - T_1)}{2.303\;RT_2\,T_1}$$

in which k_2 and k_1 are the velocity constants at the absolute temperatures T_2 and T_1, respectively, R is the gas constant (1.987 cal deg^{-1} mole^{-1}), and E_a is the energy of activation. The energy of activation is the amount of energy required to put an initial reactant molecule into an activated state from which it may react to yield the product of the reaction. The energy required for the activated state is the main factor in determining the speed of the reaction. The greater the energy of activation, the fewer the molecules possessing this energy, thus, the slower the reaction at a given temperature.

When a new product is being developed, it would not be expedient or economical to determine the stability of the product by setting up samples at room temperature for months or years, but rather, based on a consideration of Arrhenius equation, accelerated tests are carried on at 37°, 50°, and at times, 100°. The results of these accelerated stability tests are projected to room temperature, and if favorable, production is initiated with further and more elaborated stability tests at elevated as well as at room temperature for prolonged periods.

For example, a new drug received by a product research and development department was given preliminary stability tests and found to follow a first-order degradation at 100° and 110°. After 20 minutes at 110°, the drug was found to be 76.3% active; after 1 hour at 100°, the drug was found to be 70% active. Based on these data the time required for a 10% loss of potency at room temperature may be calculated:

The velocity constant at 110° and 100° may be calculated

$$k_{110^\circ} = \frac{2.303}{t_2 - t_1} \log \frac{c_1}{c_2} = \frac{2.303}{20} \log \frac{100}{76.3} = 0.0135 \text{ min}^{-1}$$

$$k_{100^\circ} = \frac{2.303}{60} \log \frac{100}{70} = 0.006 \text{ min}^{-1}$$

Knowing the velocity constants at two temperatures, the energy of activation for the drug may be determined

$$\log \frac{k_2}{k_1} = \frac{E_a (T_2 - T_1)}{2.303\, R\, T_2\, T_1} = \log \frac{0.0135}{0.006} = \frac{E_a (383 - 373)}{2.303 \times 1.987 \times 383 \times 373}$$

$$E_a = 23{,}000 \text{ cal mole}^{-1}$$

The velocity constant at 25° is found:

$$\log \frac{0.0135}{k_{25^\circ}} = \frac{23{,}000\,(383 - 298)}{2.303 \times 1.987 \times 383 \times 298} = 3.7482$$

$$k_{25^\circ} = \frac{0.0135}{5{,}600} = 2.4 \times 10^{-6} \text{ min}^{-1}$$

Having evaluated k_{25°, the length of time necessary for 10% loss at room temperature is calculated

$$t = \frac{2.303}{k} \log \frac{c_1}{c_2} = \frac{2.303}{2.4 \times 10^{-6}} \log \frac{100}{90}$$

$$t = 4.32 \times 10^4 \text{ min or 30 days}$$

Although the integrated form of the Arrhenius equation is generally used in drug and chemical studies, the exponential form is conventionally employed in radio-technology

$$A = A_o e^{-0.693\, t/t_{1/2}}$$

where A_o is the initial radio-activity, A is the activity after t, time interval, and e is the base of the natural logarithms or 2.718. In logarithmic form the equation is

$$\log A = \log A_o - 0.301\, t/t_{1/2}$$

For example, a hospital pharmacist receives a shipment of sodium iodide ^{131}I solution with the following data on the label:

Date of Assay:	Tuesday, March 19, 8:00 AM
Assay:	14.66 ±10% millicuries (mc)
Volume:	2.1 ml

It is known that the half-life of ^{131}I is 8.1 days.

A physician wishes to administer an activity of 0.5 mc on Friday at 2:00 p.m. The volume of solution to be administered with the desired radioactivity may be calculated. The activity of 1 ml of solution on Friday at 2:00 p.m. is

$$\log A = \log \frac{14.66}{2.1} - 0.301 \quad (3.25/8.1)$$

$$= 0.7247$$

$$A = \text{antilog } 0.7247 = 5.30 \text{ mc per ml after } 3.25 \text{ days}$$

and as the physician wishes to give 0.5 mc of activity the volume to be injected is

$$\frac{5.30}{1.0} = \frac{0.5}{x}$$

$$x = 0.094 \text{ ml}$$

PROCEDURE. Esters, amides, and lactams are readily hydrolyzed in water in the presence of hydrogen and hydroxyl ions. Catalysis by hydrogen and hydroxyl ions is known as specific acid-base catalysis. A pH-rate profile is a curve obtained by plotting pH against rate constant.

Many reactions follow the first-order equation although two molecules are involved in the reaction. In the acid hydrolysis of an ester two molecules are involved

$$R{-}COOR' + H_2O \xrightarrow{H^+} R{-}COOH + R'OH$$

however, the water is present in great excess and only the ester appears to change in concentration. The large excess of water also forces the equilibrium to the right so for all practical purposes the reaction goes to completion.

For a first-order reaction a plot of the logarithm of concentration of the drug against time is a straight line with the equation

$$\log c = -\frac{kt}{2.303} + \text{a constant}$$

From this equation of a straight line, k, may be evaluated by multiplying the slope of the line by 2.303.

A. The hydrolysis of aspirin in buffered solution is followed by measuring with a Spectronic 20 or another suitable spectrophotometer the concentration of salicylic acid as a function of time. A color reagent is used to produce a color with salicylic acid. The color reagent contains in each 100 ml of aqueous solution 4 g of ferric nitrate [$Fe(NO_3)_3 \cdot 9\,H_2O$], 4 g of mercuric chloride, and 12 ml of 1.0 N hydrochloric acid.

   Accurately weigh on an analytical balance 0.100 g of aspirin and quantitatively transfer it to a 100-ml volumetric flask. The pH at which you are to conduct your hydrolysis will be assigned by the instructor. Place your buffer solution in the constant temperature bath at 50°. When the buffer solution has reached 50°, add sufficient buffer solution to the 0.100 g of aspirin to make 100 ml of solution.

   Place the volumetric flask in the constant temperature bath. Immediately withdraw by pipet a 1.0 ml sample, representing the zero time sample, and add to 5.0 ml of color reagent solution. Using a spectrophotometer, measure and record the absorbance of the solution at 540 nm using a blank of 1.0 ml of buffer solution and 5.0 ml of color reagent solution for each measurement. The absorbance is converted to concentration of salicylic acid by means of the standard curve supplied by the instructor.

   Upon hydrolysis each mole of aspirin yields one mole of salicylic acid; therefore, each milligram of salicylic acid represents the hydrolysis of 1.304 mg of aspirin. Calculate and record the concentration of aspirin remaining in solution. A correction should be made for any salicylic acid present in the zero time sample.

Samples are removed at 30-minute intervals and analyzed. The time and the absorbance are tabulated. Calculate the concentration of aspirin remaining at each time a sample is withdrawn.

Draw a graph in which the concentration of aspirin is plotted as the ordinate against time.

Draw another graph in which the logarithms of concentrations of aspirin are plotted on the ordinate against times. Connect the points by the best straight line. Find the specific rate constant, k, from the slope of the line.

B. Repeat A at 60°.

REFERENCES

Abbott Laboratories. 1962. Radioisotopes in medicine. A general guide for physicians and hospital personnel. North Chicago and Oak Ridge, Tennessee.

Autian, J. 1971. Plastics and medication. In Dispensing medication, 7th ed. E. W. Martin, Ed. Mack Publishing Company, Easton, Pa. Chap. 15, p. 652.

Beal, H. M., R. J. Dicenzo, P. J. Jannke, H. A. Palmer, J. Pinsky, M. Salame, and T. J. Speaker. 1967. Pharmaceuticals stored in plastic containers. J. Pharm. Sci. 56:1310-1322.

Carless, J. E. 1970. Accelerated tests for physical stability of pharmaceutical products. Pestic. Sci., 1:270.

Carstensen, J. T. 1974. Stability of solids and solid dosage forms. J. Pharm. Sci., 63:1-14.

Chase, G. D. 1975. Fundamentals of radioisotopes & medical applications of radioisotopes. In Remington's Pharmaceutical sciences, 15th ed. Mack Publishing Company, Easton, Pa. Chap. 30, p. 473 & Chap. 31, p. 492.

Chin, T. F., P. H. Chung, and J. L. Lach. 1968. Influence of cyclodextrins on ester hydrolysis. J. Pharm. Sci., 57:44.

Christensen, H. N. and G. A. Palmer. 1974. Enzyme kinetics. A learning program for students of the biological and medical sciences. 2nd ed. W. B. Saunders Company, Philadelphia.

Colwell, J. A., A. Kravitz, J. Homi, N. Levin, R. H. Parker, and S. Poticha. 1969. The acidity of intravenous dextrose solutions. A contributing factor to thrombophlebitis? Hospital Formulary Management, 4, Number 4, p. 24.

Copelan, H. W. 1972. Burning sensation and potency of nitroglycerin sublingually. J.A.M.A., 219:176.

Dorsch, B. and R. Shangraw. 1975. Stability of stabilized nitroglycerin tablets in typical distribution and administration systems. A. J. Hosp. Pharm., 32:795 - 808.

Eriksson, S. O. 1969. Hydrolysis and aminolysis of anilides and hydrolysis of barbituric acids. Acta Pharmaceutica Suecica, 6:139-162.

Gallelli, J. F., J. D. MacLowry, and M. W. Skolaut. 1969. Stability of antibiotics in parenteral solutions. Am. J. Hospit. Pharm., 26:630.

Garrett, E. R. 1962. Prediction of stability of drugs and pharmaceutical preparations. J. Pharm. Sci., 51:811-833.

Garrett, E. R. 1967. Kinetics and mechanisms in stability of drugs. In Advances in pharmaceutical sciences. Volume 2. H. S. Bean, A. H. Beckett, and J. E. Carless. Academic Press, London and New York. p. 1.

Garrett, E. R., J. T. Bojarski, and G. J. Yakatan. 1971. Kinetics of hydrolysis of barbituric acid derivatives. J. Pharm. Sci., 60:1145.

Hamid, I. A. and E. L. Parrott. 1971. Effect of temperature on solubilization and hydrolytic degradation of solubilized benzocaine and homatropine. J. Pharm. Sci., 60:901.

Hanna, J. G. and S. Siggia. 1966. Kinetic methods of analysis. J. Pharm. Sci., 55:541-549.

Heimlich, K. R. and A. N. Martin. 1960. A kinetic study of glucose degradation in acid solution. J. Am. Pharm. Assoc., Sci. Ed., 49:592.

Hicks, C. I., J. P. B. Gallardo, and J. K. Guillory. 1972. Stability of sodium bicarbonate injection stored in polypropylene syringes. Am. J. Hospital Pharm., 29:210.

Higuchi, T. and L. W. Busse. 1950. Heat sterilization of thermally labile solutions. J. Am. Pharm. Assoc., Sci. Ed., 39:411.

Higuchi, T., A. Havinga, and L. W. Busse. 1950. The kinetics of the hydrolysis of procaine. J. Am. Pharm. Assoc., Sci. Ed. 39:405.

Ho, N. 1972. Predicting drug stability of parenteral admixtures. In Perspectives in clinical pharmacy. D. E. Francke and H. A. K. Whitney, Jr., Eds. Drug Intelligence Publications, Hamilton, Illinois. Chap. 20, p. 421.

Hou, J. P. and J. W. Poole. 1969. Kinetics and mechanism of degradation of ampicillin in solution. J. Pharm. Sci., 58:447.

Kassem, M. A., A. A. Kassem, and H. O. Ammar. 1969. Studies on the stability of injectable L-ascorbic acid solutions I. Effect of pH, solvent, light and container, and II. Effect of metal ions and oxygen content of solvent water. Pharm. Acta Helv. 44:611-623 and 667-675.

Kitler, M. E. and P. P. Lamy. 1971. Kinetics of drug absorption. Pharm. Acta. Helv., 46:193-209.

Kostenbauder, H. B. 1975. Reaction kinetics. In Remington's Pharmaceutical sciences, 15th ed. Mack Publishing Co., Easton, Pa. Chap. 19, p. 275.

Kramer, W. R., A. S. Inglott, and R. J. Cluxton, Jr. 1972. Incompatibilities of drugs for intravenous administration. In Perspectives in clinical pharmacy. D. E. Francke and H. A. K. Whitney, Jr., Eds. Drug Intelligence Publications, Hamilton, Illinois. Chap. 21, p. 438.

Lachman, L. and P. DeLuca. 1976. Kinetic principles and stability testing. In The theory and practice of industrial pharmacy, 2nd ed. L. Lachman, H. A. Lieberman, and J. L. Kanig, Eds. Lea and Febiger, Philadelphia. Chap. 2, p. 32.

Levy, G. and N. J. Angelino. 1968. Hydrolysis of aspirin by rat small intestine. J. Pharm. Sci., 57:1449.

Lordi, N. G. and M. W. Scott. 1965. Stability charts. Design and application to accelerated stability testing of pharmaceuticals. J. Pharm. Sci., 54:531.

Martin, A. N., J. Swarbrick, and A. Cammarata. 1969. Kinetics and biopharmaceutics. In Physical pharmacy, 2nd ed. Lea and Febiger, Philadelphia. Chap. 14, p. 352.

Meakin, B. J., I. P. Tansey, and D. J. G. Davies. 1971. The effect of heat, pH and some buffer materials on the hydrolytic degradation of sulphacetamide in aqueous solution. J. Pharm. Pharmacol., 23:253.

Nair, D. and J. L. Lach. 1959. The kinetics of degradation of chlorobutanol. J. Am. Pharm. Assoc., Sci. Ed, 48:390.

Nogami, H., J. Hagesawa, and M. Iwatsuru. 1970. The stabilization mechanism of acylcholinesters in aqueous solution by sodium lauryl sulfate. Chem. Pharm. Bull., 18:2297.

Parke, R. F. and G. L. Sperandio. 1959. The effect of selected additives on the stability of glucose solutions. The Bulletin of the Parenteral Drug Association, 13, Number 2, pp. 17-23.

Parrott, E. L. 1962. Hydrolytic stability of calcium acetylsalicylate carbamide in the presence of high concentrations of additives. J. Pharm. Sci. 51:897.

Parrott, E. L. 1966. Stability of pharmaceuticals. J. Am. Pharm. Assoc., NS6:73.

Parrott, E. L. 1967. Student experiments in pharmaceutical technology. V. Kinetics of aspirin hydrolysis. Am. J. Pharm. Ed. 31:4.

Pawelczyk, E., R. Wachowiak, and I. Pluta. 1970. Kinetics of drug decomposition. Part X. Decomposition of quinidine sulfate in aqueous solutions. Dissert. Pharm. Pharmacol., 22:165.

Rogers, A. R. 1963. An accelerated storage test with programmed temperature rise. J. Pharm. Pharmacol., 15:101 T.

Schwartz, M. A. 1971. Stabilization. In Dispensing of medication, 7th ed. E. W. Martin, Ed. Mack Publishing Company, Easton, Pa. Chap. 14, p. 624.

Sherwin, E. R. 1967. Methods for stability and antioxidant measurement. J. Am. Oil Chamists' Soc., 45:634 A.

Smith, G. 1965. Stability of medicinal preparations. The Pharmaceutical Journal, 6 March, pp. 219-223.

Tatum, J. H., P. E. Shaw, and R. E. Berry. 1969. Degradation products from ascorbic acid. J. Agr. Food Chem., 17:38.

The Food and Drug Administration and the School of Pharmacy University of Connecticut. 1967. Drug stability as affected by environment and containers. Seminar summary. Washington, D.C.

The United States Pharmacopeia, 19th rev. 1975. Stability considerations in dispensing practice. pp. 707-709.

Varsano, J. and S. Gilbert. 1969. Pharmaceuticals in plastic packaging. Drug and Cosmetic Industry, January, February & March.

Webb, N. E., Jr., G. J. Sperandio, and A. N. Martin. 1958. A study of the decomposition of glucose solutions. J. Am. Pharm. Assoc., Sci. Ed. 47:101.

Wing, W. T. 1960. An examination of the decomposition of dextrose solution during sterilization. J. Pharm. Pharmacol. 12:191 T.

Kinetics of an Aqueous Solution

Data and Conclusions

1. Complete the following table:

Time	Absorbance	C_{sal}	C_{asa}	log C_{asa}	k_{calc}
At __°C	and pH __				
At __°C	and pH __				

2. Calculate the value of k between successive samples and tabulate in Question 1. How do the calculated k values compare with the k value determined from the slope of the graph?

3. What is the half-life of aspirin at 50° at the pH used in A?

4. What is the half-life of aspirin at 60° at the pH used in B?

5. Calculate the energy of activation of aspirin from your experimental data.

6. Calculate $k_{25°}$, using your experimental data.

7. Knowing the above constants, how long will it require at 25° for 10% of the aspirin in solution at the pH of your exercise to be hydrolyzed?

8. At what pH is a solution of aspirin most stable? Sketch a pH-rate profile for a solution of aspirin.

9. Based on your experiment, what predictions can you make concerning the stability of aspirin in the presence of moisture?

10. A buffered solution of Terramycin at pH 7 has a half-life of 9.5 days at room temperature. When placed in a refrigerator at 5°, the same solution has a half-life of 93 days. Assuming that the solution is therapeutically effective with a loss of 20% potency, how much longer would the solution be effective if refrigerated rather than stored at room temperature? Loss of potency follows a first-order equation.

11. A hospital pharmacist received a solution of sodium radio-iodide which at the time of packaging had 1000 microcuries of ^{131}I per 40 ml. Three days after the date of packaging a physician requested that the hospital pharmacist prepare an injection of 25 microcuries for a diagnostic study of thyroid uptake and excretion. What volume of solution would the pharmacist prepare for the injection?

12. Give the pathway(s) for degradation of dextrose solution upon autoclaving. In the process of manufacturing intravenous solutions of dextrose, what can be done to prevent or minimize degradation of the dextrose?

POLYPHASIC SYSTEMS

23. CHARACTERISTICS OF COLLOIDAL DISPERSIONS

Colloids, emulsions, and suspensions are polyphasic systems in which the dispersed phase is found in discrete particles many times the size of most molecules and ions. The degree of subdivision and the forces associated with the large surface distinguish the colloid from a crystalloid. The characteristics of a colloid are a result of its enormous surface per unit weight or specific surface.

Colloids may be classified as lyophobic or lyophilic colloidal dispersions. Lyophobic colloids have no affinity for the dispersing medium and are not solvated. They are stabilized by a charge acquired by preferential adsorption of ions. If water is the dispersing medium, they are known as hydrophobic colloids.

Lyophilic colloids are highly solvated as well as charged. The charge usually is a result of ionization. If water is the dispersing phase, they are called hydrophilic colloids. Hydrophobic colloids will precipitate if their electrical charge is removed; however, hydrophilic colloids, although their electrical charge is neutralized, often remain dispersed as they are hydrated. Fortunately, most of the pharmaceutical colloids are of the hydrophilic type and are stabilized by a dual mechanism.

The large surface of a lyophobic colloid preferentially adsorbs ions. Trace ions will induce an opposite charge in a neighboring molecule and will then be held to the surface of the colloid by an ion-induced dipole attraction. It is the adsorption of trace ions which gives a lyophobic colloid its charge; the charged particles repel each other and prevent aggregation and precipitation of the colloidal substance.

The adsorbed ions on the surface of the colloidal particle tend to attract oppositely charged ions, and two layers of oppositely charged electricity result. The thickness of this double layer is small compared to the diameter of the colloidal particle, and the repulsive force of the charged colloid does not extend beyond the thickness of the double layer.

The double layer consists of two shells of ions of opposite charge. The inner shell is narrow and compact, adhering tightly to the colloidal particle whenever it moves. The outer shell is wide and diffused, with a high concentration of ions near the inner shell and a progressively lower concentration of ions as the distance from the surface of the particle to the bulk of the dispersing medium (where the positive and negative ions are present in equal numbers) is increased. The outer shell is easily removed as the colloidal particle moves.

Between the surface of the colloidal particle and the main body of the solution there exists a potential. This total potential, E, may be divided into two parts. The first is the potential between the inner shell and the surface of the colloid. The second is the zeta or electrokinetic potential and is the potential difference through the outer shell extending from the outer edge of the inner shell to the body of the solution.

Let us represent trace ions in water in terms of sodium and chloride ions. Due to a dipole-ion interaction between the molecules making up the colloidal particle and the anion, the chloride ions are held tightly to the surface of the colloid, conferring a negative charge upon it. The inner shell which remains with the particle has a negative potential.

The counter ions, cations in this case, in the outer diffuse shell cause a positive potential, and since the diffused shell does not migrate with the colloidal particle as does the inner shell, there exists a permanent difference in potential. The total potential is measured from the surface of the particle to the bulk of the solution where there is equal distribution of anions and cations.

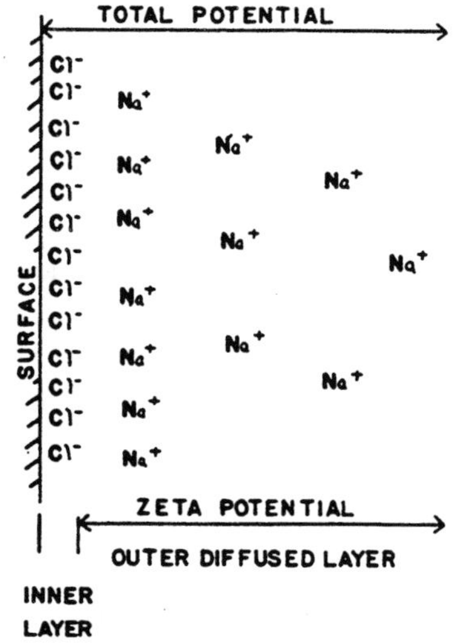

Figure 12 — Schematical drawing of the double layer of ions around a colloidal particle.

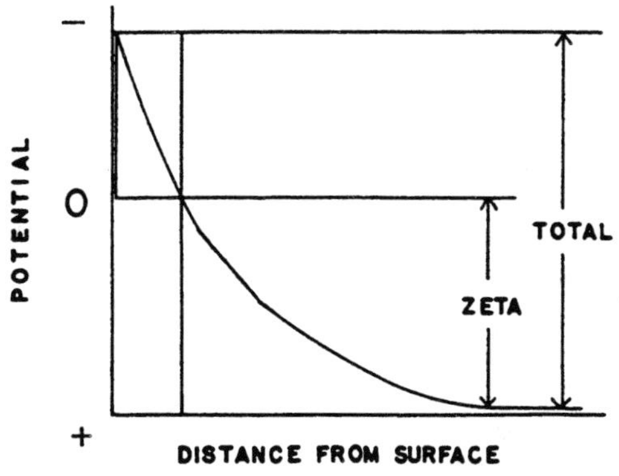

Figure 13 — Diagram defining zeta potential of a suspensoid.

The potential that exists from the outer edge of the inner layer of adsorbed chloride ions extending to the bulk of the solution is the zeta potential. The greater the zeta potential of a lyophobic colloid, the greater its stability.

When an external voltage is applied to a colloidal dispersion, the charged colloidal particles migrate to the oppositely charged electrode. This is known as electrophoresis. Electrophoretic experiments have shown that most colloids are negatively charged, such as gold, silver, sulfur, arsenic trisulfide, bacteria and virus, as well as many colloidal dispersions which acquire a negative charge by ionization, such as acacia, Pharmagel B, and algin.

Although colloidal particles are much larger than individual ions, the rate of movement toward an electrode is greater than expected. Colloids have approximately one-tenth the mobility of ions. The National Institutes of Health have set up electrophoretic mobility specifications for testing Poliomyelitis Immune Globulin (Human).

The factors governing the selective adsorption of ions are not completely known. For example, if dilute solutions of silver nitrate and sodium iodide are mixed, the colloidal silver iodide may be positively or negatively charged. It appears that the sign on the colloidal silver iodide depends on the ions in excess. If the iodide ion is in excess the colloid will be negatively charged; if the silver ion is in excess the colloid will be positively charged. The sodium and nitrate ions are not adsorbed. Fajans and Paneth concluded that ions which form slightly soluble compounds with the adsorbent will be adsorbed rather than those that form more soluble compounds.

Hydrophilic colloids acquire a charge by ionization. Acacia is a high molecular weight substance containing d-galactopyranose, d-glycuronic acid, 1-rhamnopyranose and 1-arabofuranose; it is acidic due to the ionization of the glycuronic portion of its structure. Most of the plant gums utilized in pharmacy are negatively charged emulsoids by virtue of a carboxylic or sulfuric acid radical within their structures.

Due to the zwitter ion or amphoteric nature of proteins the charge on a protein is dependent on the pH of the dispersing medium. Gelatin, obtained by the partial hydrolysis of collagen, consists of polypeptide chains of various lengths. Gelatin may have a positive or a negative charge, depending on the pH at which hydrolysis occurred.

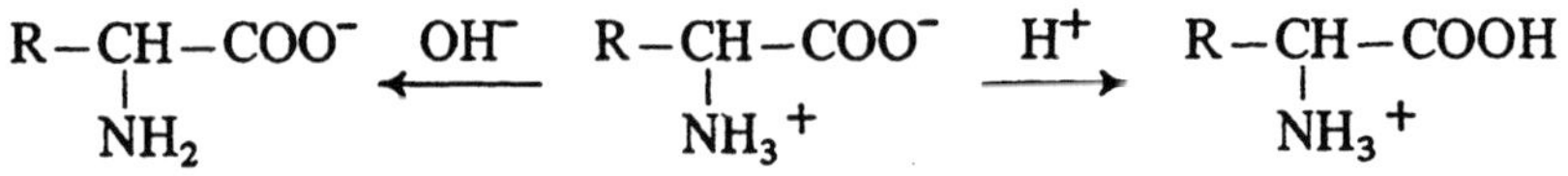

$$\underset{\text{Pharmagel B}}{\text{R}-\text{CH}-\text{COO}^- \atop \text{NH}_2} \xleftarrow{\text{OH}^-} \underset{\text{zwitter ion}}{\text{R}-\text{CH}-\text{COO}^- \atop \text{NH}_3^+} \xrightarrow{\text{H}^+} \underset{\text{Pharmagel A}}{\text{R}-\text{CH}-\text{COOH} \atop \text{NH}_3^+}$$

The isoelectric point of a substance is the pH at which it has no net charge but exists as a zwitter ion. At the isoelectric point the zeta potential is zero, and the colloid has its minimum stability, viscosity, and electrical conductance.

Gelatin derived from an acid treated precursor exhibits an isoelectric point between pH 7-9; it is highly hydrated and positively charged at pH 4-4.5. Gelatin derived from an alkaline treated precursor exhibits an isoelectric point between pH 4.7-5.0; it is negatively charged and highly hydrated at pH 8.

Hydrophobic colloids are precipitated by small concentrations of electrolytes or oppositely charged colloids. Emulsoids are much more stable than hydrophobic colloids due to a high degree of hydration. In fact, when a hydrophilic colloid is added to a hydrophobic colloid, the suspensoid particles become coated with the emulsoid and acquire some of the properties of the emulsoid. The hydrophilic substance acts as a protective colloid as it protects the suspensoid from being precipitated by electrolytes.

In pharmacy, colloidal silver iodide, colloidal silver chloride, mild silver protein, and strong silver protein owe their stability to a protective colloid. In addition to stabilizing the colloid, a protective colloid permits a colloidal system to be dried to a solid state, which upon the addition of a dispersing phase will readily form a sol. Colloidal silver iodide, for example, if dried will not be redispersed upon the addition of water; however, colloidal silver iodide rendered colloidal in the presence of gelatin becomes a reversible colloid, which may be dried and will redisperse in a colloidal form upon the addition of water.

When surface-active agents at very low concentrations are dispersed in water, they tend to become adsorbed as a closely packed monolayer at the air-water interface. If additional surface-active molecules are added, they cannot be accommodated at the air-water interface, and they agglomerate in the bulk of the solution-forming aggregates called micelles. Micelles of a given surface-active agent at a given concentration and temperature contain the same number of molecules (25 to 100). The diameters of micelles range from 30 to 80 Å. Because of their ability to form aggregates of colloidal size, surface-active agents are called association colloids. In a hydrophilic sol, the nonpolar portions of the surface-active molecules are oriented toward the center of the micelle shielding themselves from the polar environment. In a hydrophobic sol, the orientation of the surface-active molecules is reversed. Micelles of association colloids are in dynamic equilibrium with their monomeric constituents, so that each molecule alternates between the single and aggregate state. The lowest concentration at which micelles form is known as the critical micelle concentration (CMC). Micelles have the ability to increase the solubility of liquid or solid compounds that are only slightly soluble or insoluble in the solvent used. Solubilization has been defined by McBain as the spontaneous passage of solute molecules of a substance insoluble in water into an aqueous solution of a surface-active agent in which a thermodynamically stable solution is formed.

PROCEDURE. Hydrophilic colloids are commonly used in pharmaceuticals. Many have been suggested as protective colloids for hydrophobic colloidal particles. Gelatin, acacia, agar, and sodium carboxymethylcellulose have been used in this capacity.

A. Prepare 60 ml of Acacia Mucilage N. F. XII. Use powdered acacia in making this preparation.

B. Acacia Mucilage may be used as a protective colloid. Dissolve 0.66 g of potassium iodide and 0.66 g of silver nitrate in two separate 10-ml portions of water. Add 15 ml of Acacia Mucilage to the potassium iodide solution. To this mixture with constant agitation add in a thin stream the solution of silver nitrate. Evaporate the preparation to dryness on a water bath.

C. Prepare a 5% dispersion of colloidal silver iodide prepared and dried in B. Compare the solubility of silver iodide with the apparent solubility of your preparation.

One common method of obtaining a colloidal dispersion is by causing aggregation of a dissolved substance by decreasing its solubility. The resulting dispersion may be either reversible or irreversible.

D. Pour about 1 ml of benzoin tincture into 25 ml of water in a beaker. Observe.

Evaporate to dryness on a water bath. Add water to the residue and determine if the colloid is reversible.

E. To 10 ml of a 2% sodium carboxymethylcellulose solution add, dropwise, 2.5 ml of benzoin tin tincture. Observe.

Evaporate on a water bath. Add water to the residue and determine if the colloid is reversible.

Capillarity may be used to determine the electrical charge on a colloidal particle. If one end of a filter-paper strip is dipped into a colored hydrosol, the ascent of the color will depend on the charge of the colloid. If the colloid has a positive charge, a distinct separation between the dispersed phase and the dispersing medium occurs in the ascending portion of the sol. Such a separation does not occur if a negatively charged colored sol is used.

This phenomenon is probably due to wetted filter paper acquiring a negative charge. The negatively charged capillary will allow negatively charged colloids to rise, but it will attract and hold positively charged colloids and clog the capillary preventing the ascent of a positive hydrosol.

F. Prepare a 1% aqueous solution of amaranth and a 1% aqueous solution of methylene blue. Into each solution place the end of a strip of filter paper and observe what occurs.

Solubilization refers to the dispersion of a water-insoluble substance by means of a surface-active agent, in so fine a particle size that the preparation appears to be a true solution. Many imitation flavors are solubilized oils which may be diluted with water to the required strength and remain sparkingly clear. Water-insoluble antiseptics such as hexachlorophene may be incorporated into aqueous vehicles by solubilization.

Oil-soluble vitamins, estrogens, steroids, griseofulvin, and other drugs for systemic administration have been solubilized. Several studies have been made to elucidate the effect of solubilization on the availability of the drug in the body. The biological and medicinal activity and stability of the drug is greatly affected by the interaction of the surface-active agent and drug. The effects differ with the characteristics of the drug, the surface-active agent, and their relative concentrations. This particular area of research and study provides a better understanding of the effects of formulation of pharmaceutical products on therapeutic activity of drugs.

In the development of solubilized pharmaceutical products, ternary phase diagrams may be used. In an equilateral triangle, the sum of the perpendiculars from a given point to the three sides is a constant. The perpendicular distance from each apex, representing a pure compound, to the opposite side is divided into 100 equal parts corresponding to percent. The variable is labeled on the side to the right of the perpendicular. A point situated on one of the sides of the triangle indicates that only two components are present with the percentage composition indicated. The composition corresponding to any point within the triangle is obtained by measuring on these coordinates the distances toward apex A, B, and C. The total of these three distances is 100%.

G. Prepare a three-component phase diagram for a benzyl benzoate-water-polyoxyethylene sorbitan monolaurate system, or a peppermint oil-water-polysorbate 80 system as assigned by the instructor.

Prepare several samples by pipetting a definite volume of the organic substance to be solubilized into a 125-ml flask with a definite volume of the solubilizing agent. Mix gently. Titrate with purified water until the cloud point, i.e., point where system is turbid, remains for one minute when observed in a beam of light passing through the system perpendicular to the line of vision. The cloud point is utilized as a reproducible point, but it does not represent the equilibrium value. Record the volumes of each.

Using the specific gravities of the liquids, convert the volumes to weights. Record and plot the weights on a triangular coordinate paper. Identify the homogeneous phases.

Hydrophobic colloids are sensitive to electrolytes. A negatively charged colloid is coagulated by the cation of an electrolyte. The greater the valence of the coagulating ion, the more effective an electrolyte will be in precipitating a colloid. In precipitating a negative suspensoid, aluminum chloride is more effective than barium chloride, which is more effective than sodium chloride.

H. Prepare 10 ml of a 10% ferric chloride solution. Prepare a hydrophobic sol by pouring 10 ml of the ferric chloride solution into 500 ml of boiling purified water.

To 50 ml of the sol add 2.0 ml of 0.8 M potassium sulfate solution. Observe.

REFERENCES

Braun, R. J. and E. L. Parrott. 1972. Influence of viscosity and solubilization on dissolution rate. J. Pharm. Sci. 61:175.

Carey, M. C. and D. M. Small. 1972. Micelle formation by bile salts. Physical-chemical and thermodynamic considerations. Arch. Intern. Med. 130:506.

Elworthy, P. H., A. T. Florence, and C. B. MacFarlane. 1968. Solubilization by surface-active agents and its application in chemistry and biological sciences. Chapman and Hall Ltd., London.

Martin, A. N., J. Swarbrick, and A. Cammarata. 1969. Physical pharmacy, 2nd ed. Lea and Febiger, Philadelphia. Chap. 16.

Mitchell, A. G. and J. F. Broadhead. 1967. Hydrolysis of solubilized aspirin. J. Pharm. Sci. 56:1261.

Mulley, B. A. 1964. Solubility in systems containing surface-active agents. In Advances in pharmaceutical sciences, Vol. 1. H. S. Bean,, A. H. Beckett, and J. E. Carless, Eds. Academic Press, New York, p. 86.

Nakagawa, T. 1967. Solubilization. In M. J. Schick, Ed., Nonionic surfactants, Marcel Dekker, Inc., New York, Chap. 17.

Parrott, E. L. and R. J. Braun. 1973. Determination of micelle size by the Stokes-Einstein equation. Chem. Pharm. Bull. 21:1042.

Parrott, E. L. and V. K. Sharma. 1967. Dissolution kinetics of benzoic acid in high concentrations of surface active agents. J. Pharm. Sci. 56:1341.

Prince, L. M. 1975. Microemulsions versus micelles. J. Colloid and Interface Sci. 52:182.

Reber, L. A. and H. Schott. 1975. Colloidal dispersions. In Remington's Pharmaceutical sciences. 15th ed. Mack Publishing Co., Easton, Pa. Chap. 21, p. 299.

Riddick, T. M. 1968. Control of colloid stability through zeta potential with a closing chapter on its relationship to cardiovascular disease, Vol. 1. Livingston Publishing Company, Wynnewood, Pennsylvania.

Riegelman, S. 1960. The effect of surfactants on drug stability. J. Pharm. Sci. 49:339.

Saski, W. 1968. Effect of a nonionic surface-active polymer on passage of hydrocortisone across rat intestine *in vitro*. J. Pharm. Sci. 57:836.

Saski, W. and S. G. Shah. 1965. Availability of drugs in the presence of surface-active agents I. Critical micelle concentrations of some oxyethylene oxypropylene polymers. J. Pharm. Sci. 54:71

Saski W. and S. G. Shah. 1965. Availability of drugs in the presence of surface-active agents II. Effects of some oxyethylene oxypropylene polymers on the biological activity of hexetidine. J. Pharm. Sci. 54:277.

Schott, H. and A. N. Martin. 1974. Colloidal and surface-chemical aspects of dosage forms. In Sprowls' American pharmacy, L. W. Dittert, Ed., 7th ed. J. B. Lippincott Co., Philadelphia. p. 103.
Sheth, P. B. and E. L. Parrott. 1967. Hydrolysis of solubilized esters. J. Pharm. Sci. 56:983.
Swarbrick, J. 1965. Solubilized systems in pharmacy. J. Pharm. Sci. 54:1229.
Vervey, E. J. W. and J. T. G. Overbeek. 1948. Theory of the stability of lyophobic colloids. The interaction of sol particles having an electric double layer. Elsevier Publishing Company, Inc., New York.
Weiser, H. B. 1949. A Textbook of colloid chemistry, 2nd ed., John Wiley & Sons, New York, pp. 266-268.

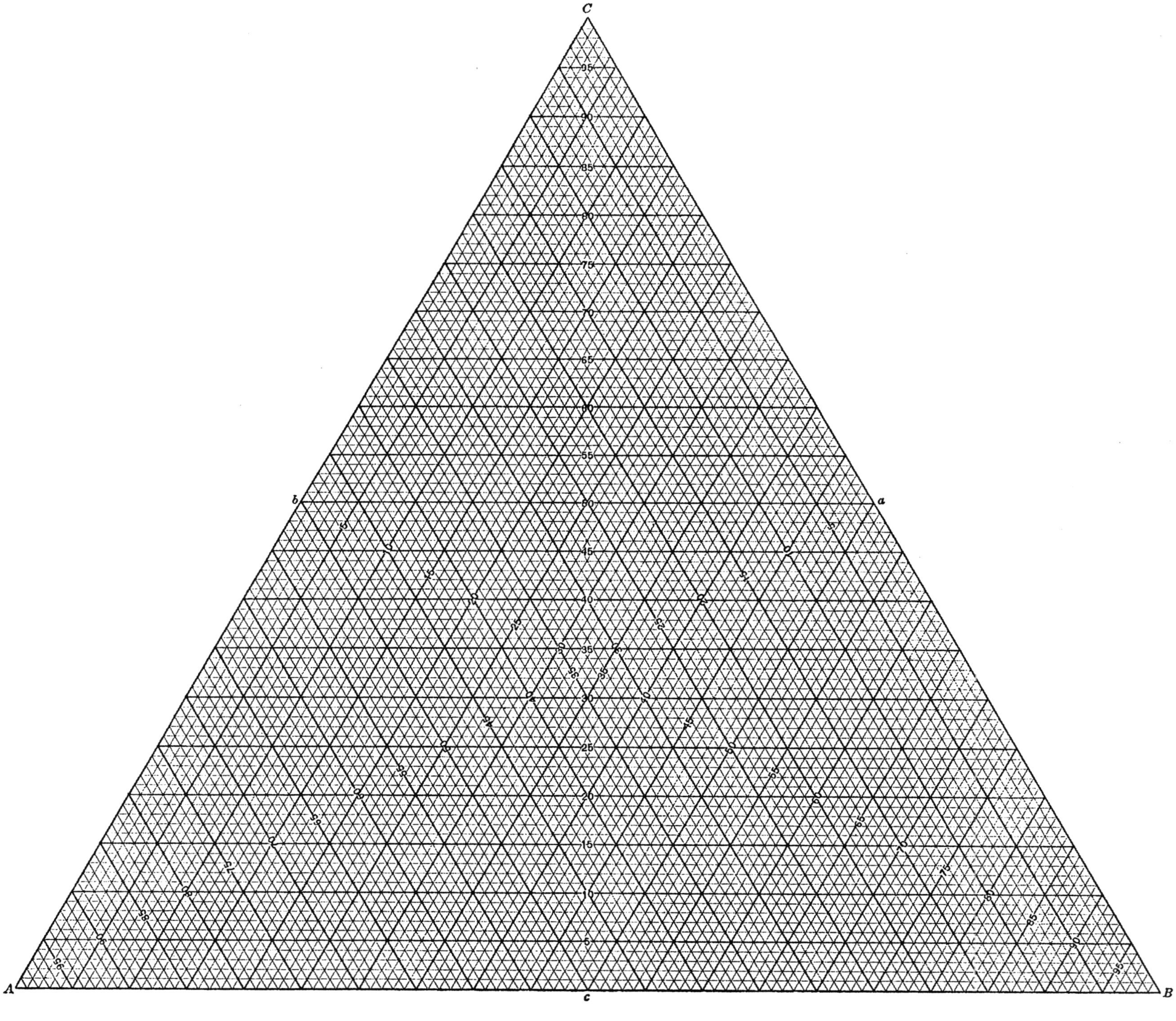
C
b
a
A
c
B

Characteristics of Colloidal Dispersions

Data and Conclusions

1. Complete the following chart:

Property	Characteristics	
	Lyophobic Sol	Lyophilic Sol
Reversibility		
Effect of Electrolytes		
Viscosity of Sol		
Surface Tension of Sol		
Tyndall Effect		
Electrophoretic Migration		

2. In B stoichiometric amounts of potassium iodide and silver nitrate are used in preparing colloidal silver iodide. If an excess of silver nitrate is used, the colloid becomes gray or black upon evaporation. Explain.

3. Name a commercial product which resembles the protected colloid prepared in B.

4. Which of the colloidal dispersions in D and E are reversible?

5. What is the charge on amaranth and methylene blue? Give the structural formula of each.

6. What is a micelle?

7. Complete the following table for G showing a sample calculation:

Organic Substance		Solubilizing Agent		Water	
Volume	Percent	Volume	Percent	Weight	Percent

8. What is a Hofmeister series?

9. Explain the mechanism by which the organic substance in G was dispersed in water.

10. How do colloids become charged?

11. What is zeta potential?

12. Cite an example of a surface-active agent enhancing the absorption of an orally administered medicinal compound.

13. What influence may solubilization have on the stability of a slightly water-soluble ester in a liquid pharmaceutical? Explain.

14. What is the approximate range of size of colloidal particles? How does this compare with the wave length of visible light?

15. Plasma albumin has a molecular weight of approximately 70,000 g $mole^{-1}$. If albumin is present in blood to the extent of 4 g per 100 ml, how much does it contribute to lowering the freezing point of blood below that of water?

16. Draw a diagrammatic sketch illustrating the electrostatic fields about a particle in the red sol of hydrated ferric oxide formed in H. How did the addition of potassium sulfate affect the system?

24. RHEOLOGY

Rheology is the study of the flow of fluids and the deformation of solids. Resistance is offered when one part of a liquid is moved past another. The force required to slip one layer of a liquid past another with a given velocity depends directly on the viscosity of the liquid and on the areas exposed to each other, and inversely on the distances separating the two surfaces. The coefficient of absolute viscosity of a liquid, η, can be defined as the force per unit area necessary to maintain a unit velocity gradient between two parallel planes separated by a unit distance. Mathematically this may be expressed

$$\eta = \frac{\frac{F}{A}}{\frac{dv}{dx}}$$

where F/A is the force per unit area acting parallel to the planes in dynes cm^{-2}, and dv/dx is the velocity gradient perpendicular to the planes per second. Although the dimension of absolute viscosity is g cm^{-1} sec^{-1}, this unit is designated as a poise. A liquid has a viscosity of one poise when the force required to maintain a relative velocity of 1 cm sec^{-1} between two parallel planes 1 cm apart is 1 dyne cm^{-2}.

As most liquids used in pharmacy have a viscosity of less than one poise, the centipoise, equal to 0.01 poise, is commonly used to express viscosity.

Pure liquid compounds (acetone, alcohol, glycerin, water) and true solutions have a constant viscosity at a given temperature and pressure. Thus, when the liquid is placed in a rotational viscometer and subjected to a given rate of shear, the observed stress becomes constant and is directly proportional to the rate of shear. Such fluids are known as Newtonian fluids. Flow curves are obtained by plotting the rate of shear (r.p.m.) against the shear stress (divisions of rotational viscometer). Newtonian fluids produce a straight line which passes through the origin as shown in Figure 14. Viscosity is the reciprocal of the slope of the flow curve. Curve A represents a less viscous fluid than Curve B. A given stress causes a lower shear rate for fluid B than for A.

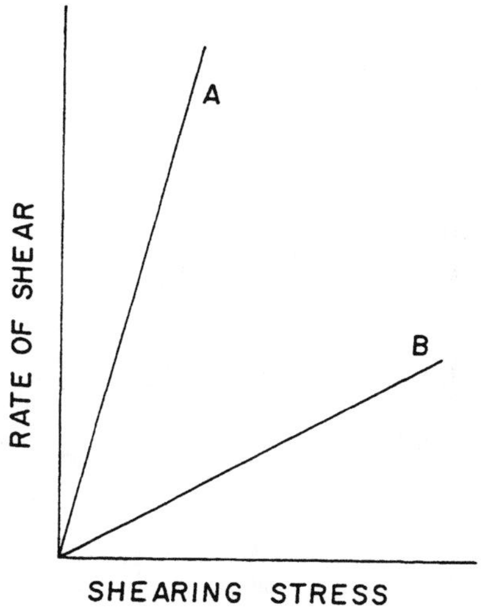

Figure 14 — Flow curve or rheogram for a Newtonian system.

The viscosity of most liquids decreases with an increase in temperature. This suggests the existence of molecular clustering or association in liquids. An increase in temperature or kinetic energy disrupts these associations wiht a resulting decrease in viscosity. Solutions of liquids which associate to a great degree or which are strong dipoles may vary greatly in viscosity. Such solutions may exhibit a maximum in their viscosity-composition curve which is greater than the viscosity of either pure liquid. The maximum represents the greatest degree of association or hydrogen bonding between the components of the solution, and this large association complex increases the resistance to movement within the solution which is apparent as an increase in viscosity.

In the case of an ideal solution in which no interactions occure, viscosity is additive. Mathematically this may be expressed

$$\frac{1}{\eta} = \frac{1}{\eta_1} V_1 + \frac{1}{\eta_2} V_2$$

where η is the viscosity of the solution composed of volume fractions, V_1 and V_2, of pure liquids 1 and 2 with viscosities of η_1 and η_2, respectively.

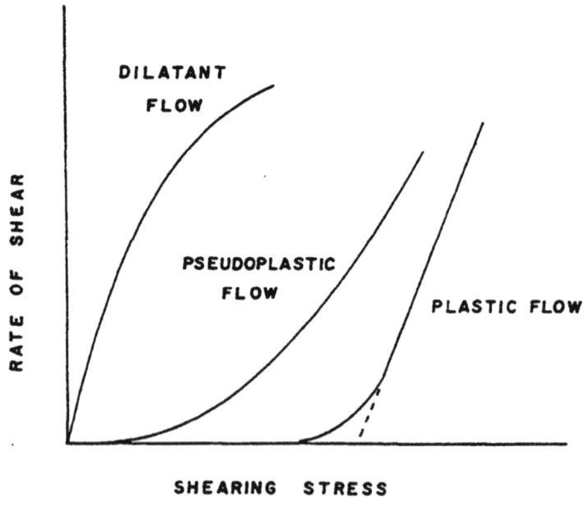

Figure 15 — Flow curves for non-Newtonian systems.

In liquid polyphasic pharmaceuticals (dispersions of tragacanth, algin, methylcellulose) the rate of shear is not directly proportional to the shearing stress, and the viscosity changes as the rate of shear is changed. Such fluids are known as non-Newtonian fluids. Typical flow curves of various non-Newtonian fluids are shown in Figure 15.

Pseudoplastic flow is described by a shear stress which increases more rapidly at lower rates of shear than at higher rates of shear. Thus, the viscosity of a pseudoplastic fluid is decreased by increased rates of shear. Pseudoplastic flow curves pass through or approach the origin. The consistency of a pseudoplastic fluid is best expressed by a curve.

A plastic fluid does not begin to flow until a certain yield value of the shearing stress is exceeded; thus, a plastic flow curve does not pass through the origin, but it intersects the shearing stress axis or will if the straight part of the curve is extrapolated to the axis. When the yield value has been exceeded, any further increase in shearing stress causes a directly proportional increase in the rate of shear. The reciprocal of the slope of a plastic flow curve is known as the plastic viscosity.

Dilatant fluids exhibit an increase in resistance to flow as the rate of shear is increased. When the shear is removed, a dilatant fluid returns to its initial consistency. Materials possessing dilatant flow are usually suspensions containing a high concentration of small, deflocculated particles. Zinc oxide suspensions in water, and 40-50% starch in aqueous glycerin are dilatant. Obviously, an attempt to pass a dilatant fluid through a colloid or roller mill will increase the viscosity to the extent that the motor will be overloaded and possibly damaged.

Thixotropy is a reversible gel-sol formation with no change in volume or temperature. Thixotropy is characterized by a hysteresis loop (See Exercise 31 Gels).

As the rate of shear affects the viscosity, the method of measurement of viscosity must be considered. For a plastic system a single measurement is often misleading or worthless; a series of determinations must be made and the viscosity-rate of shear curve considered.

In Figure 16 the effect of the rate of shear on viscosity is shown for a Newtonian and a non-Newtonian fluid. The viscosity of the Newtonian fluid is unchanged by a change in the rate of shear. The non-Newtonian fluid has a marked change in viscosity with a change in rate of shear; it is very viscous at a low rate of shear and very fluid at a high rate

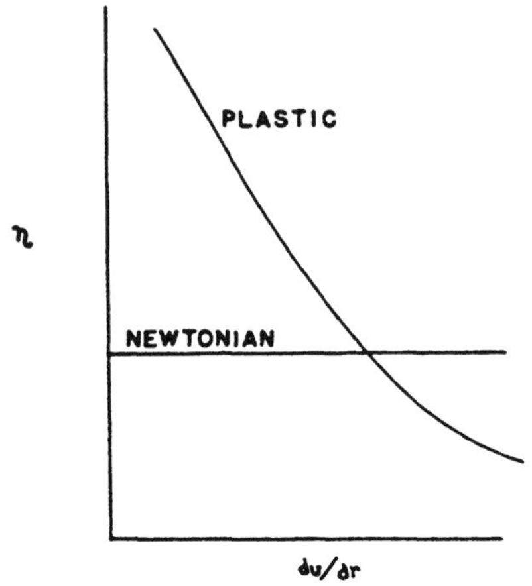

Figure 16 — Effect of rate of shear on viscosity.

of shear. Most methods of derterminining viscosity use a high rate of shear and would indicate the Newtonian fluid to be the better suspending agent. Actually this non-Newtonian fluid would be the suspending agent of choice as at the low rate of shear existing in a pharmaceutical product, it would have a higher viscosity than the Newtonian fluid.

Pharmaceutical preparations such as syrups, mucilages, and jellies have high viscosities. Viscous flow is a frictional phenomenon and, as such, is important from the chemical engineering viewpoint in pumping liquids. By controlling the viscosity of suspensions and emulsions, the separation of the phases is retarded, insuring a more uniform dose for the patient. In flavoring pharmaceuticals it has been found that increasing the viscosity slows diffusion into the taste buds and somewhat lessens unpleasant taste. Liquids of high viscosity are emptied from the stomach more slowly than liquids of low viscosity. If the amount of suspending agent and the amount of the pharmaceutical preparation are great enough so that a relatively high viscosity is maintained upon dilution with the gastric contents, drug absorption may be retarded.

Many studies have shown in man a correlation between the viscosity of blood plasma and the clinical condition. The measurement of viscosity of the plasma is as common as the measurement of the erythrocyte sedimentation rate. As a nonspecific test the viscosity of the plasma indicates the presence of organic disease and the reaction of the body to the disease. Changes in the concentrations of plasma protein are usually associated with inflammation or tissue destruction.

PROCEDURE. Absolute viscosity may be determined directly by measuring the time required for a measured volume of liquid to flow through a capillary tube under an applied pressure. The experimental determination of the absolute viscosity of a liquid is a difficult task, but the measurement of relative viscosity, the ratio of the viscosity of a liquid to that of some reference liquid such as water, is simple and adequate for most purposes. This relative viscosity multiplied by the absolute viscosity of the reference liquid will give the absolute viscosity of the liquid being measured.

With the Ostwald viscometer the pressure driving a liquid through the capillary depends on the difference in the liquid level, h, and the density, ρ, and the acceleration of gravity, g; and it is given by the expression $gh\rho_1$. If exactly the same volume of a second liquid of viscosity η_2 is introduced into the tube, the pressure driving the liquid through the tube is equal to $hg\rho_2$, where ρ_2 is the density of the second liquid.

The viscosity is proportional to the pressure and the time of efflux for the same volume, thus,

$$\frac{\eta_1}{\eta_2} = \frac{\rho_1 t_1}{\rho_2 t_1}$$

To obtain good results the apparatus must be clean and dry. Clamp the viscometer vertically so it can be easily viewed and add an exact quantity of water from a pipet. The liquid surface at the start should be as much below the center of the lower bulb as it is above the center at the end of the experiment.

A dust-free rubber tube is attached to the smaller tube, and the liquid is drawn up into the enlarged bulb and above the upper marker. The liquid is then allowed to flow down the capillary tube, and a stopwatch is started when the meniscus passes the upper mark and is stopped when it passes the lower mark. Make several check determinations of the time of outflow.

Record the temperature at which this is done. Look up in a physics-chemistry handbook the viscosity of water at this temperature.

Calculate the calibration constant K for your viscometer using the relationship

$$K = \frac{\eta}{\rho t}$$

where η is the absolute viscosity of water, ρ is the density of water at a given temperature, and t is the efflux time of the water.

A. Using the Ostwald viscometer #50 or #100 determine the viscosity of acetone. Record the temperature and viscosity.

B. Prepare approximately 200 ml of 0.2, 0.4, 0.6, and 0.8 mole fraction solutions of acetone in water. Using a Westphal balance, determine the density of each of the prepared solutions and of acetone. Determine the viscosity of each solution, tabulate, and plot the relative viscosity against the mole fraction. Plot the mole fraction as the abscissa.

The viscosity of an ideal solution is a linear function of the concentration; however, few solutions used in pharmacy are ideal. Various carbohydrate gums and derivatives are employed as suspending or dispersing agents. Being large molecules with polyfunctional grouping they are highly associated in solution with the resulting deviation from ideal behavior.

Methylcellulose is a typical example of such a thickening agent. Methylcellulose is available in several types designated according to the viscosity of a 2% aqueous solution. Methylcellulose 1500 cps, for example, is that methylcellulose which dissolved in water to form a 2% solution will yield a viscosity of 15 poises; as this solution is nonideal, a 4% solution will not have a viscosity of double, but greater than double that of a 2% solution.

C. Prepare 100 ml of a 1, 2, 3, and 4% methylcellulose solution. The instructor will indicate the viscosity type to be used. Using the Ostwald viscometer, find the absolute viscosity of each solution and tabulate.

   Very viscous solutions may require one or two additional Ostwald viscometers having larger bore capillaries. Calibration constants for each of the viscometers can be determined employing methylcellulose solutions for which the absolute viscosity and density had been previously determined by use of a smaller bore viscometer and a Westphal balance.

   Methylcellulose is soluble in cold water, but its solution becomes cloudy and may precipitate or gel if heated. Solutions are prepared by mixing the methylcellulose powder with about half the required amount of hot water and boiling for several minutes; then the remaining water is added as cold water or ice. Upon cooling or being refrigerated a clear solution is formed.

   Attempt to plot some function of the viscosity and concentration in such a manner that a linear relationship is shown.

The falling ball viscometer has been recognized as one of the most effective and accurate instruments for the one-point determination of viscosity. The Stokes law provides a theoretical basis for the use of the falling ball viscometer. Gilmont viscometers (Size No. 1 and 2) cover the range of 0.25 to 300 cp. They may be conveniently calibrated using the equation

$$K = \frac{\eta}{(\rho_b - \rho)\, t}$$

where η is the viscosity in centipoises, t is the time of descent in minutes, K is the viscometer constant, and ρ_b and ρ are the densities of the ball and liquid in g cc^{-1}, respectively. For accurate work the standard liquid should have physical properties similar to those of the liquid being measured. The viscosity is calculated by the formula

$$\eta = K(\rho_b - \rho)\, t$$

D. Using a Gilmont viscometer, determine the viscosity of glycerin and a glycerin-water mixture supplied by the instructor. Record the temperature and the viscosity.

E. Using a Brookfield viscometer, determine the viscosity of one of the methylcellulose solutions prepared in C at 0.5, 1.0, 2.5, 5, 10, 20, 50, and 100 revolutions per minute (rpm). The instructor will demonstrate the operation of the viscometer and the use of the scale readings in determining the viscosity.

Plot the viscosity on the ordinate against the revolutions per minute.

In a similar manner determine the viscosity of a syrup or glycerin. Plot the viscosity against the rpm and label each curve with the name of the solution and its rheological type.

REFERENCES

Barras, J. P. 1969. Blood rheology – General review. Bibl. Haemat. 33:277.

Braun, R. J. and E. L. Parrott. 1972. Influence of viscosity and solubilization on dissolution rate. J. Pharm. Sci. 61:175.

Davis, S. S. 1974. Is pharmaceutical rheology dead? Pharm. Acta Helv. 49:161.

Davis, S. S., B. Warburton, and J. E. Dippy. 1970. Chemical balance as a rheometer for biological fluids. J. Pharm. Sci. 57:836.

The Dow Chemical Company. 1962. Methocel. Thickener, stabilizer, film former, emulsifier, binder. Midland, Michigan.

Fry, D. L. 1969. Certain chemorheologic considerations regarding the blood vascular interface with particular reference to coronary artery disease. Supplement IV to Circulation, Vols. 39 and 40. IV-38.

Gibaldi, M. 1976. Biopharmaceutics. In The theory and practice of industrial pharmacy, 2nd ed. L. Lachman, H. A. Lieberman, and L. Kanig, Eds. Lea and Febiger, Philadelphia. Chap. 3, p. 107.

Hewitt, R. R. and G. Levy. 1971. Effect of viscosity on thiamine and riboflavine absorption in man. J. Pharm. Sci. 60:784.

Jasin, H. E., J. LoSpelluto, and M. Ziff. 1970. Rheumatoid hyperviscosity syndrome. The Am. J. of Medicine, 49:484.

Levy, G. and W. J. Jusko. 1965. Effect of viscosity on drug absorption. J. Pharm. Sci. 54:219.

Martin, A. N., J. Swarbrick, and A. Cammarata. 1969. Fundamentals of rheology. Chap. 18 in Physical pharmacy. Lea and Febiger, Philadelphia.

Martin, A. N., G. S. Banker, and A. H. C. Chun. 1964. Rheology. In Advances in pharmaceutical sciences, Vol. 1. H. S. Bean, A. H. Beckett, and J. E. Carless, Eds. Academic Press, New York. p. 1.

Merrill, E. W. 1969. Rheology of blood. Physiol. Rev. 49:863.

National Bureau of Standards. 1963. Viscometer calibrating liquids and capillary tube viscometers. Governmental Publications. Washington, D.C., Catalogue No. C 13. 44:55.

Saski, W. 1968. Effect of nonionic surface-active polymer on passage of hydrocortisone across rat intestine *in vitro*. J. Pharm. Sci. 57:836.

Schott, H. 1975. Rheology. In Remington's Pharmaceutical sciences, 15th ed. Mack Publishing Co., Easton, Pa. Chap. 24, p. 350.

Scott Blair, G. W. 1969. Elementary rheology. Academic Press, London & New York. Appendix 3: Books for further reading, with brief appraisals. p. 139.

Van Wazer, J. R., J. W. Lyons, K. Y. Kim, and R. E. Colwell. 1963. Viscosity and flow measurements: A laboratory handbook of rheology. Interscience Publishers, Inc., New York.

Rheology

Data and Conclusions

1. Give a sample of the calculations used to complete the following table:

Volume of Acetone, ml	Weight of Acetone, g	Volume of Water, ml	Weight of Water, g	Mole Fraction of Acetone in Water

2. Give a sample of the calculations used to complete the following table:

Temperature °C   Calibration constant K =

Mole Fraction of Acetone in Water	Density, g cc^{-1}	Time, sec	Relative Viscosity
0			
1.0			

3. Give a sample of the calculations used to complete the following table:

Temperature _____ °C

Percent of Methylcellulose Type_____ cp	Density, g cc^{-1}	Time, min	η_{rel} with standard of water	η	$\sqrt[8]{\eta}$
1.0					
2.0					
3.0					
4.0					

4. Attempt to plot some function of the absolute viscosity and concentration in such a manner that a linear relationship is obtained. How may this be accomplished?

5. For B, plot the relative viscosity against mole fraction. Explain the form of the curve.

6. Record your results in D in the following table:

Temperature ______°C

Percent of Glycerin	Density, g cc^{-1}	Time, min	Absolute Viscosity, cp

Did the experimental values of viscosity agree with your anticipations? Rationalize your answer.

7. Record your results in E in the following table:

Temperature_____°C

rpm	Spindle	Factor	Scale Reading	Viscosity, cp

What are the implications of your findings in the design and formulation of suspensions?

25. SOME CHARACTERISTICS OF INTERFACIAL TENSION

The molecules at the surface of a liquid are subjected to an unbalanced force of molecular attraction as the molecules of the liquid tend to pull those at the surface inward. Due to this unbalanced force a liquid tends to maintain a minimum surface area. The magnitude of this force acting perpendicular to a unit length of a line in the surface is called the surface tension. Surface tension, γ, may be defined by considering a movable bar against which a liquid film is stretched like a soap-bubble film on a wire frame where a force, f, in dynes is exerted on the length of the bar, 1, in centimeters

$$\gamma = \frac{f}{2\,1}$$

The factor 2 is introduced as there are two liquid surfaces, one at the front and another at the back. Surface tension is expressed in dynes cm^{-1}.

Conventionally, the tension that exists between a liquid and the atmosphere is called the surface tension, and the tension that exists at the interface between two immiscible liquids is known as the interfacial tension. In pharmacy it is the interfacial tension with which we are chiefly concerned.

A surface-active molecule possesses approximately an equal ratio between the polar and nonpolar portions of the molecule. When such a molecule is placed in an oil-water system, the polar groups are attracted to or oriented toward the water, and the nonpolar groups are oriented toward the oil. The surface-active molecule is adsorbed or oriented in this manner, consequently, lowering interfacial tension between the oil and water phase.

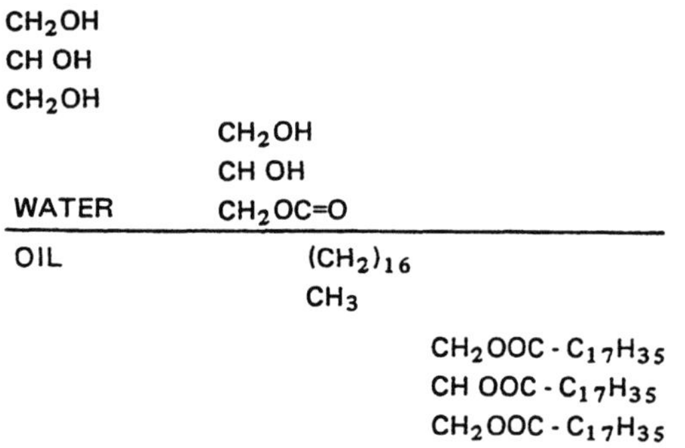

Figure 17 — Orientation of glycerol and glyceryl esters showing the influence of the ratio of polar to nonpolar groups.

If a molecule, such as glycerin, possesses a dominance of polar groups, it will not be surface active as it will dissolve in the aqueous phase and will not be oriented at the oil-water interface. If a molecule, such as glyceryl tristearate, possesses a dominance of nonpolar groups, it will not be surface active as it will dissolve in the oil phase. A molecule, such as glyceryl monostearate, which possesses approximately an equal balance between the polar and nonpolar groups will be oriented at the interface and will be surface active.

Since a surface-active agent is adsorbed or oriented at a surface or interface, it is logical that the concentration of a surface-active substance at the surface of a solution would be greater than the concentration in the bulk solution. Mathematically, such a relationship has been derived by Gibbs

$$\Gamma = -\frac{c}{RT}\frac{d\gamma}{dc}$$

where Γ is the difference in concentration of the solute in the surface layer and the bulk solution in moles cm^{-2}, and $d\gamma / dc$ is rate of change of surface tension with concentration, c, T is the absolute temperature, and R is the gas constant.

Depending on the technical use and the specific purpose for which used, these surface-active agents may be known as wetting agents, surfactants, solubilizing or emulsifying agents.

When two immiscible liquids are in contact, they tend to maintain as small surface as possible. It is therefore difficult to mix these two liquids. The addition of a proper surface-active agent will lower the interfacial tension and permit easy mixing of the immiscible ingredients. This occurs in the formation of pharmaceutical emulsions.

Surface-active agents are widely used in pharmacy. Wetting agents are added to suspensions, both oral and parenteral, to hinder caking of the particles during storage. Powdered suspensions for reconstitution contain wetting agents added to facilitate rapid suspension of the particles upon the addition of a vehicle.

Surface-active agents have been incorporated into nonemulsion ointments not only to aid in dispersing the drugs but also to facilitate removal of the ointment from the skin. Experiments have been conducted to determine if surface-active agents increase penetration from dermatological preparations. Further, from the physiological viewpoint, surface-active agents have been found to modify the effectiveness of antiseptics and the gastrointestinal absorption of drugs solubilized by means of surfactants.

Surface-active agents have been incorporated into tablets to aid in the penetration of moisture into the tablet to hasten its disintegration.

PROCEDURE. There are many methods for determining the surface tension of a single liquid; however, pharmaceutically one is normally concerned with solutions. The Wilhelmy plate pull method and the ring detachment method are best suited for determining interfacial tensions of solutions.

The most direct method for measuring the surface and interfacial tensions of solutions is the Wilhelmy plate pull method. A thin rectangular plate, usually made of glass or platinum, is suspended from one arm of a sensitive balance. The weight of the plate in air is balanced, and then a container with the liquid is raised until its surface just touches the bottom of the plate. If the plate is wetted by the liquid, a disturbance of the liquid surface occurs, resulting in an increase in surface area of the liquid. To minimize the increase of area, the plate is pulled into the liquid and, in order to restore the balance arm to its original position, a force, f, must be applied to the plate suspension. The surface work is given by the relationship

$$\text{Work} = \text{force} \times \text{distance}$$

As indicated above,

$$f = \gamma \times 2\,l$$

where l is the length of the blade. Thus, work = $\gamma \times 2\,l \times$ distance. It follows that force $\times$ distance = $\gamma \times 2\,l \times$ distance and, the surface tension is

$$\gamma = \frac{f \times \text{distance}}{2\,l \times \text{distance}} = \frac{f}{2\,l}$$

Surface tension is the downward force per unit length on the perimeter of the plate. For example, if 363.6 mg was necessary to restore equilibrium to a blade of 2.5 cm length, the surface tension is

$$\gamma = \frac{0.3636\ \text{g} \times 981\ \text{cm sec}^{-2}}{2 \times 2.5\ \text{cm}}$$

$$= 71.34 \frac{\text{g} \times \text{cm sec}^{-2}}{\text{cm}} = 71.34\ \text{dyne cm}^{-1}$$

A. Prepare a 0.1% aqueous solution of dioctyl sodium sulfosuccinate, sodium lauryl sulfate, or the surface-active agent supplied by the instructor. By use of appropriate pipets and volumetric flasks, dilute this solution to 0.05, 0.01, and 0.001% solutions.

Determine the surface tension of each of these solutuions. Tabulate your results and plot the surface tension against concentration of surface-active agent. On your graph indicate the value of the critical micelle concentration.

The du Noüy tensiometer consists of a platinum-iridium ring supported by a stirrup attached to the beam of a torsion balance. The ring is placed at the interface of two immiscible liquids and is pulled upward by turning the torsion wire, thus applying a force which is known from calibration of the instrument.

Theoretically, the force just needed to separate the ring from the interface is equal to $4\pi R\gamma$ where R is the mean radius of the ring. Doubling of the perimeter 2 R arises from the fact that there are two boundary lines between the liquid and the wire, one on the outside and one on the inside of the ring. This treatment holds for liquids with zero contact angle, a condition usually met, and for an ideal situation where the ring holds up a thin cylindrical shell of liquid before the break occurs, a condition seldom met. Actually the shape of the liquid influences the force needed to break away. The shape is a function of R^3/V and R/r where V is the volume of the liquid held up and r is the radius of the wire. The surface tension is given by the relationship

$$\gamma = \frac{f}{4\pi R} F$$

where f is the maximum force registered on the torsion balance scale and F is the correction factor due to the shape of the liquid held up. These correction factors have been evaluated by Harkins and Jordan.

Recent instruments such as the Fisher Surface Tensiomat are calibrated by the manufacturer, so the dial reading is the apparent interfacial tension. In order to obtain the true interfacial tension, the relationship used is

$$\gamma = \gamma_a F$$

where γ is the true value, γ_a is the apparent value and F is the correction factor.

The correction factor may be calculated with the equation

$$F = 0.7250 + \sqrt{\frac{0.01452\gamma_a}{C^2 (\rho_l - \rho_u)} + 0.04534 - \frac{1.679r}{R}}$$

in which C is the mean circumference of the ring, ρ_l is the density of the lower phase, and ρ_u is the density of the upper phase. For most rings the circumference is 6 cm and the radius is 0.007 inches, giving a value for R/r of 53.2. As a convenience, a curve may be drawn from the preceding equation so that the F value may be read. As the dimensions of the ring vary slightly, curves for R/r values of 50 and 60 are shown in Figure 18, so that correction factors may be found for any value of the ratio between 50 and 60 without calculation.

B. Using a du Noüy tensiometer, determine the interfacial tension between mineral oil and water at 25°. Place the water in a beaker and raise the platform until the ring is immersed approximately 10 mm in the water. Carefully add mineral oil until a layer approximately 10 mm, or deep enough to prevent the ring from entering the upper surface before the film breaks, is formed. By means of the platform, adjust the beaker until the ring is in the interface and the lever arm is in the zero position. Increase the torsion of the wire and lower the beaker, keeping the index of the lever arm at zero. The reading when the film at the interface breaks is the apparent interfacial tension.

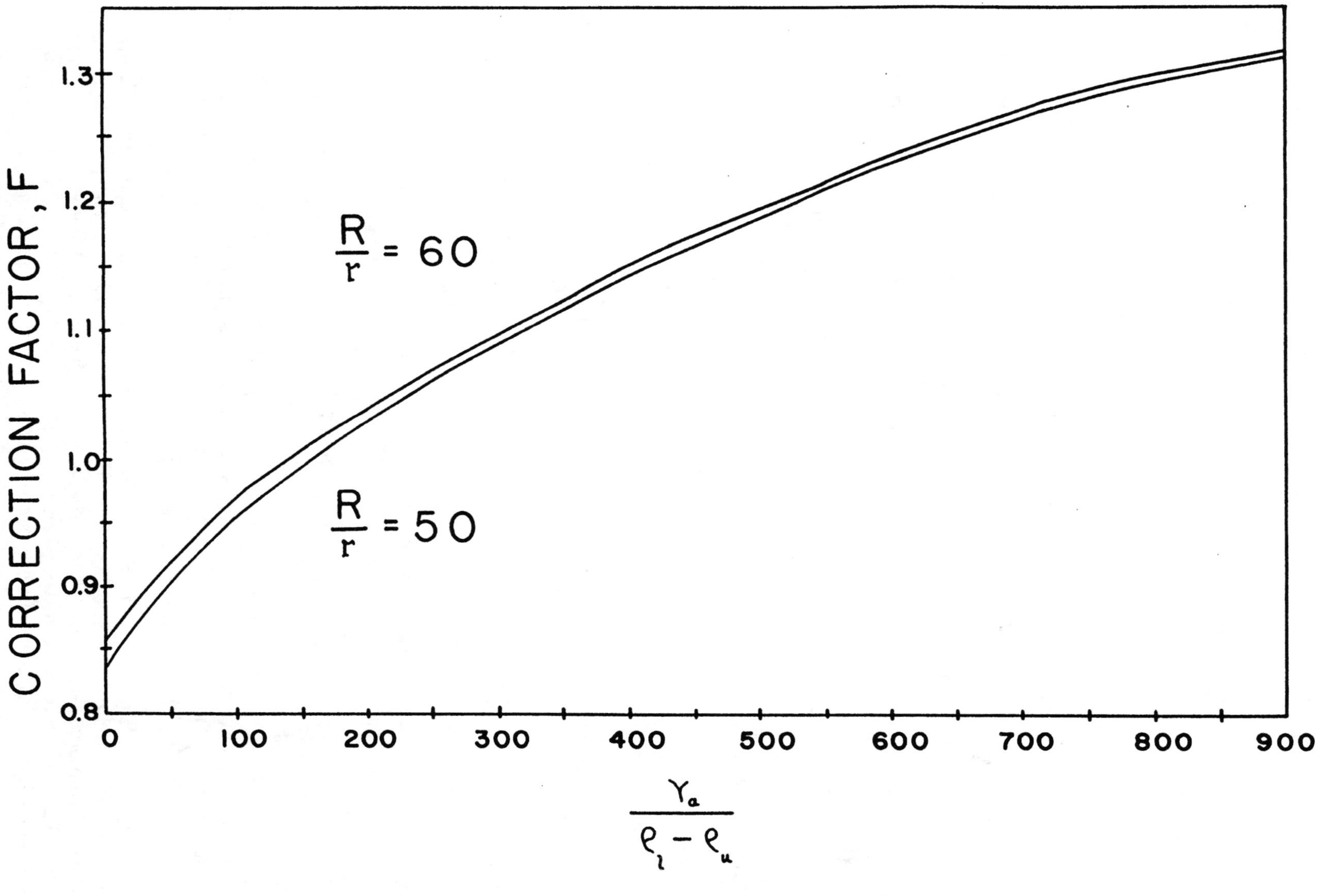

Figure 18 -- Relation of correction factor to apparent interfacial tension and densities.

The ring is cleaned with hot cleaning solution, rinsed with warm distilled water, and allowed to dry. Occasionally the ring may be passed through a Bunsen burner flame if further cleaning is required. Care must be taken that the ring is not touched with the fingers or bent.

To make a reading, attach the clean ring to the lever arm and turn the knurled knob to zero. With the screw in its uppermost position, raise the platform until the ring is approximately at the interface. Then lower the entire platform by means of the screw until the ring is just at the interface and approximately centered in respect to the container with the index at zero.

Increase the torsion by rotating the knob and simultaneously lowering the platform by means of the screw, keeping the index on zero. Maintaining the index on zero, continue this double movement until the ring breaks away from the interface. If the platform is not lowered with the pointer at zero to keep the ring horizontal, too high a reading will be obtained.

C. Using the solutions of the surface-active agent as prepared in A, determine the interfacial tension between mineral oil and each of these solutions. Tabulate your results and plot the interfacial tension against concentration of the surface-active agent.

Wetting agents are surface-active agents which are capable of lowering the contact angle between a liquid droplet and the solid surface over which it spreads and of helping in the removal of air at the solid surface and replacement of the air with the liquid. They hinder caking of particles in oral and parenteral suspensions during storage, and they facilitate the rapid dispersion of the particles of a suspension for an extemporaneous reconstitution upon the addition of a vehicle. Charcoal, magnesium stearate, sulfas, sulfur, and even a powder with as high a density (7.15 g cc^{-1}) as calomel, may float on the surface of a liquid and be difficult to disperse.

D. Using a mortar and pestle, prepare 100 ml of a 2% suspension of sulfur in water. After brief trituration of the sulfur with a small amount of water, transfer the contents to a graduate and add sufficient water to make 100 ml. Observe.

Using a mortar and pestle, prepare 100 ml of a 2% suspension of sulfur. Triturate the sulfur with 2 ml of alcohol U.S.P. and add sufficient water to make 100 ml. Observe.

Using a mortar and pestle, prepare 100 ml of a 2% suspension of sulfur. Triturate the sulfur with 10 ml of a 1% solution of dioctyl sodium sulfosuccinate and add sufficient water to make 100 ml. Observe.

E. In adjacent beakers place purified water and a 0.1% solution of dioctyl sodium sulfosuccinate. Simultaneously add approximately 1 g of powdered sulfur to each beaker and observe.

Add several drops of a 1% solution of a wetting agent to the beaker containing the water and the sulfur and observe.

When a drop of a liquid is placed on the surface of a solid or a liquid with which it is immiscible, it may spread to a film or remain as a drop. The surface tensions of the two liquids and the interfacial tension between them determine whether or not the liquid will spread. The spreading of a liquid on a solid is determined by the same factors.

The work of cohesion, W_c, is the work required to separate the molecules of the spreading liquid so it can flow over a sublayer. Spreading occurs if the attraction between two immiscible liquids or the work of adhesion, W_a, is greater than the work of cohesion. If $W_a - W_c > O$, the liquid will spread. The difference between the work of adhesion and the work of cohesion is known as the spreading coefficient. If the spreading coefficient is negative, no spreading will occur.

F. Place purified water in four adjacent petri dishes. Add a drop of benzene, chloroform, mineral oil and oleic acid, respectively, and observe.

To the petri dish to which a drop of mineral oil has been added, add several drops of a solution of a wetting agent used in E and observe.

A floating type of bath oil prevents skin dryness by spreading a thin layer of oil over the skin. A simple exercise demonstrates the spreading ability of a bath oil consisting of essentially mineral oil and 1% polyoxyethylene polyol fatty acid ester (Arlatone T).

G. Shake talcum powder on the surface of water in a petri dish. Add one drop of mineral oil near the center of the floating talc. Record your observation.

Shake talcum powder on the surface of water in a petri dish. Add one drop of mineral oil containing 1% of a spreading agent. Record your observation.

REFERENCES

Atlas Cosmetic Bulletin LD-105. High efficiency spreading agent Arlaton T. Surfactant for floating bath oils.

Cadenhead, D. A. 1969. Monomolecular films at the air-water interface. Ind. and Engineer. Chemistry, 61:22.

Carey. M. C. and D. M. Small. 1970. The characteristics of mixed micellar solutions with particular reference to bile. The Am. J. of Medicine, 49:590.

Elworthy, P. H. and J. F. Treon. 1967. Physiological activity of nonionic surfactants. In Nonionic surfactants, M. J. Schick, Ed. Marcel Dekker, Inc., New York. Chap. 28, p. 923.

Engel, R. H. and S. J. Riggi. 1969. Intestinal absorption of heparin facilitated by sulfated or sulfonated surfactants. J. Pharm. Sci., 58:706.

Felmeister, A. 1972. Relationships between surface activity and biological activity of drugs. J. Pharm. Sci., 61:151.

Fisher Instruction Manual. Surface tensiomat, Model 21. Fisher Scientific Co., Pittsburgh.

Florence, A. T. 1968. Surface chemical and micellar properties of drugs in solution. Adv. in Colloid and Interface Sci., 2:115-149.

Fort, T. and H. T. Patterson. 1963. A simple method for measuring solid-liquid contact angles. J. Colloid Sci., 18:217.

Gaines, G. L. 1966. Insoluble monolayers at liquid-gas interfaces. Interscience Publishers, New York.

Giammona, S. T. and S. Bondurant. 1965. Comparison of DuNouy tensiometer and Wilhelmy balance for measuring surface tension of pulmonary surfactant. The J. of Laboratory and Clinical Medicine, 65:329.

Gibaldi, M. and S. Feldman. 1970. Mechanisms of surfactant effects on drug absorption. J. Pharm. Sci. 59:579.

Ginn, M. E., C. M. Noyes, and E. Jungerman. 1968. The contact angle of water on viable human skin. J. Colloid and Interface Sci., 26:146.

Harder, S. W., D. A. Zuck, and J. A. Wood. 1970. Characterization of tablet surfaces by their critical surface-tension values. J. Pharm. Sci. 59:1787.

Harkins, W. D. and H. F. Jordan. 1950. A method for the determination of surface and interfacial tension from the maximum pull on a ring. J. Am. Chem. Soc., 52:1751.

Harper, H. R. and D. Seaman. 1965. The action of surface-active agents in aqueous milling processes, especially at low concentrations. Kolloid-Zeitschrift u. Zeitschrift fur Polymere, 204:83.

Kakemi, K., H. Sezaki, S. Muranishi, and A. Yano. 1970. Mechanism of drug absorption from micellar solution. I. Absorption of solubilized vitamin A from the rat intestine. Chem. Pharm. Bull., 18:1563.

Kaneda, A., K. Nishimura, S. Muranishi, and H. Sezaki. 1974. Mechanism of drug absorption from micellar solutions. II. Effect of polysorbate 80 on the absorption of micelle-free drugs. Chem. Pharm. Bull., 22:523.

Kawanishi, T., T. Seimiya, and T. Sasaki. 1970. Correction for surface tension measured by Wilhelmy method. J. Colloid and Interface Sci., 32:622.

Lawrence, C. A., C. M. Carpenter, and A. W. C. Naylor-Foote. 1957. Iodophors as disinfectants. J. Pharm. Sci., 46:500.

Martin, A. N., J. Swarbrick, and A. Cammarata. 1969. Physical pharmacy, 2nd ed., Lea and Febiger, Philadelphia. Chap. 15, Interfacial phenomena. p. 413.

Mitsui, T. and S. Takada. 1969. On factors influencing dispersibility and wettability of powder in water. J. Soc. Cosmetic Chemists, 20:335.

Penzotti, S. C. and A. M. Mattocks. 1968. Acceleration of peritoneal dialysis by surface-active agents. J. Pharm. Sci., 57:1192.

Rothen, A. 1968. Surface film techniques. In Physical techniques in biological research, 2nd ed., Vol. II, Part A. D. H. Moore, Ed. Academic Press, New York and London.

Saski, W. 1968. Effect of a nonionic surface-active polymer on passage of hydrocortisone across rat intestine *in vitro*. J. Pharm. Sci., 57:836.

Saski, W., M. Mannelli, M. F. Saettone, and F. Bottari. 1971. Relative toxicity of three homologous series of nonionic surfactants in the planarian. J. Pharm. Sci., 60:854.

Schott, H. 1972. Contact angles and wettability of packaging materials and of human skin. Am. J. Pharm. Educ., 36:232.

Sebba, F. 1972. A surface-chemical theory of cancer. J. Colloid and Interface Sci., 40:479.

Shah, D. O. 1973. Surface chemistry and its biomedical implications. In Biological horizons in surface science. L. M. Prince and D. F. Sears, Eds. Academic Press, New York and London. p. 103.

Stevenson, D. G. 1961. Mechanisms of detergency. J. Soc. Cosmetic Chemists, 12:353.

Tanford, C. 1973. The hydrophobic effect: Formation of micelles and biological membranes. John Wiley & Sons, New York.
Weintraub, H. and M. Gibaldi. 1969. Physiologic surface-active agents and drug absorption. IV. Effect of pre-micellar concentrations of surfactant on dissolution rate. J. Pharm. Sci., 58:1368.
Zografi, G. 1975. Interfacial phenomena. In Remington's Pharmaceutical sciences, 15th ed. Mack Publishing Co., Easton, Pa. Chap. 20, p. 285.

Some Characteristics of Interfacial Tension

Data and Conclusions

1. List the dimension of the ring used and the calibrated value of a single scale division.

2. What is the relationship between a gram and a dyne?

3. Complete the following chart for A:

Temperature ______ °C

Percent w/v of ____________	Scale reading, mg	γ, dyne cm^{-1}

4. Briefly, explain the principle on which the operation of the Rosano balance tensiometer is based.

5. Complete the following chart for B and C:

Percent of Surfactant, w/v	γ_a, dyne cm^{-1}	$\gamma_a/\rho_1 - \rho_2$, cc sec^{-2}	F	γ, dyne cm^{-1}

Density of lower phase ________________ g cc^{-1}

Density of upper phase ________________ g cc^{-1}

6. At what concentration of the surface-active agent used in C does the interfacial tension reach a constant value? What is the practical implication of this observation?

7. In effect, the du Noüy tensiometer measures the weight of the liquid pulled out of the plane of the interface immediately prior to the removal of the ring. In a surface tension determination 242 dynes were required to withdraw the ring from the surface of a liquid with a density of 0.825 g cc^{-1}. Calculate the volume of the liquid held.

8. In D, which provided the most ready dispersion of the sulfur?

9. Record your observation in E.

10. Record your observations in F and rationalize in terms of initial and final spreading coefficients.

11. Record your observation from C.

12. Indicate the application of principles involved in this exercise to the preparation and formulation of lotions.

26. SEDIMENTATION

A suspension is a heterogenous system containing dispersed solids of such size that they settle. Whether a pharmaceutical suspension is to be taken orally, applied topically or injected, the dispersed phase should be uniformly distributed in order to ensure the administration of a uniform dose. The rate of sedimentation or settling for a suspended phase depends on several factors which may be controlled by the pharmacist.

Assuming all dispersed particles to be spheres of uniform size and sufficiently far apart so that the movement of one does not affect neighboring particles, Stokes derived an equation expressing the rate of sedimentation or settling, dx/dt, as

$$\frac{dx}{dt} = \frac{2}{9}\frac{r^2(\rho_1 - \rho_2)g}{\eta}$$

where r is the radius of the dispersed particle, ρ_1 and ρ_2 are the densities of the internal and external phase, respectively, g is the gravitational constant, and η is the viscosity.

Sulfadiazine has a density of 1.5 g cc^{-1} and a mean particle diameter of 2.55 microns. If it is suspended in an aqueous medium having a viscosity of 15 cp, the rate of settling may be calculated.

$$\frac{dx}{dt} = \frac{2(\frac{1}{2} \times 2.55 \times 10^{-4})^2 (1.5 - 1.0)\, 980}{9 \times 0.15} = 1.18 \times 10^{-5} \text{ cm sec}^{-1}$$

Although the Stokes equation does not consider all variables which affect a suspension, it gives an approximation of the rate of settling and an appreciation of the effect which controllable factors exert on the settling rate. By reducing particle size, by increasing the viscosity, and by increasing the density of the external phase, the pharmacist may retard settling.

Suspending agents are physiologically inert substances which increase viscosity when added to suspensions. On prolonged standing, suspensions tend to cake as some crystals knit together at points of contact. A second, important function of suspending agents is to facilitate redistribution of a suspension on shaking.

When suspended particles are strongly held together, the clusters are known as agglomerates or aggregates. Caking is the aggregation of these particles into a solid mass at the bottom of the container.

When suspended particles are held together by van der Waals forces in a loose, open structure, the clusters are known as floccules or flocs.

In the literature of colloid science, the term "stable" as applied to sols and suspensions is synonymous with "deflocculated." The large fluffy clumps of a flocculated system settle rapidly and are considered to be "unstable." Accordingly, the industrial chemist and pharmacist have often believed that a suspension should be maintained in a deflocculated condition. It should be realized that deflocculated particles will settle in the presence of the most effective suspending agents with subsequential growth and fusion of these deflocculated particles. This suggests that controlled flocculation may be desirable in preventing caking of pharmaceutical suspensions.

PROCEDURE. Shake lotions, magmas, and mixtures are traditionally classified as such for convenience but are actually suspensions. Depending upon the properties of the ingredients, these products may or may not contain suspending agents. Various injectables, such as Protamine Zinc

Insulin Injection, Sterile Procaine Penicillin G Suspension, and Bismuth Subsalicylate Injection, are suspensions prepared with the necessary precautions required for parenteral use.

Suspensions such as Cortisone Acetate Ophthalmic Suspension, are even used in the eye. Among the biological products that are suspensions are Smallpox Vaccine, Alum Precipitated Diphtheria and Tetanus Toxoids and Pertussis Vaccine Combined, and Rabies Vaccine.

A liquid preparation containing finely divided substances in suspension intended for external application without friction is a shake lotion.

A. Prepare 60 ml of White Lotion N. F.

Since its introduction into the N. F. about half a century ago, Calamine Lotion has been popular with the laity. Its evolution shows the increasing trend of pharmacy to use newer ideas and to constantly seek to improve medicinal products. The following have been more recent formulations.

B. Prepare 60 ml of Calamine Lotion U. S. P. XIV.

Calamine	8 g
Zinc oxide	8 g
Polyethylene glycol 400	8 g
Polyethylene glycol 400 monostearate	2 g
Water	90 ml

Heat the polyethylene glycol 400 monostearate to 70° on a water bath. Add the water, previously heated to boiling, to the monostearate. Stir until the temperature drops to 40°. Mix the zinc oxide and the calamine in a mortar and make a paste with the polyethylene glycol 400. Gradually add the cooled monostearate dispersion and continue trituration until a uniform suspension is formed.

C. Prepare 60 ml of Calamine Lotion U. S. P.

Calamine		8 g
Zinc oxide		8 g
Glycerin		2 ml
Bentonite Magma		25 ml
Calcium Hydroxide Solution	q. s.	100 ml

Dilute the bentonite magma with an equal volume of calcium hydroxide solution. Mix the powders intimately with the glycerin and about 10 ml of the diluted magma, triturating until a smooth paste is formed. Gradually incorporate the remainder of the diluted magma. Finally add enough calcium hydroxide solution to make 100 ml.

Place each of the calamine lotions in a two-ounce bottle after examination and allow to sit until next period as part of your evaluation of the lotions.

Any dosage form should be prepared so that the patient can easily measure an amount and have the same dose or amount of active ingredient each time. This is especially important with internal medication, but by no means is it to be neglected in the preparation of topical medicinals.

Many shake lotions, after being shaken, will settle before the patient can conveniently measure out the medication. A suspending agent may be added to increase the viscosity and retard sedimentation. Methylcellulose has found wide use for this purpose in both internal and external preparations.

D. Prepare 60 ml of the following:

Sulfur, ppt.		2.5 g
Camphor		2.5 g
Alcohol		20 ml
Rose Water	q. s.	60 ml

Dissolve the camphor in the alsohol and triturate with the sulfur. Gradually, with trituration, add the rose water.

E. Repeat D but include 2% methylcellulose 1500 cp. Compare the sedimentation rate of the two lotions.

Magmas are thick aqueous suspensions of freshly precipitated inorganic substances in a colloidal or very fine state of subdivision generally intended for internal use. Two popular magmas are Milk of Bismuth and Milk of Magnesia. A mixture is an aqueous or hydro-alcoholic liquid containing fine particles intended for internal use. Brown Mixture is an example of this class.

F. Prepare 250 ml of Milk of Bismuth N. F.

G. Prepare 100 ml of Kaolin Mixture with Pectin N. F. XIII. After completing the preparation, under the supervision of the instructor, pool the preparations of the class and pass the mixture through a colloid mill.

In selecting a suspending agent one must consider incompatibilities, viscosity desired, appearance, and ease of preparation. Such factors will limit the acceptable suspending agents and the final choice will be determined by actually preparing and observing the products.

H. Evaluate several suspending agents against the following control:

Calamine		5.0 g
Purified water	q. s.	100 ml

Prepare similar products using as suspending agents: 2% acacia, 2% sodium carboxymethylcellulose, medium type, 2% methylcellulose, 1500 cp, 1% tragacanth, and a suspending agent assigned by the instructor.

Place each of these preparations and the control in the same size test tube or graduated cylinder and shake simultaneously. Set aside and record the sedimentation by measuring the height of the sediment after 5, 15, 45 and 90 minutes have elapsed.

Plot the height of the sediment in millimeters against time. Evaluate the suspending agents.

I. Prepare 75 ml of a solution of an anionic flocculating agent:

Potassium dihydrogen phosphate, anhydrous		0.4 g
Purified water	q. s.	75 ml

Prepare 200 ml of a 0.5% sodium methylcellulose, 1500 cp, solution.

Prepare 100 ml of a 1.0% sodium methylcellulose, 1500 cp, solution.

Assemble five 100-ml graduated cylinders and number them consecutively. Add 10.0 g of bismuth subnitrate to each graduated cylinder. To the first cylinder add sufficient purified water to make 100 ml of suspension.

To the second cylinder add 25.0 ml of the solution of the anionic flocculating agent prepared previously and sufficient purified water to make 100 ml of suspension.

To the third cylinder add 25.0 ml of the solution of the anionic flocculating agent and a sufficient volume of 0.5 methylcellulose, 1500 cp, solution to make 100 ml.

To the fourth cylinder add 25.0 ml of the solution of the anionic flocculating agent and a sufficient volume of 1.0% methylcellulose, 1500 cp, solution to make 100 ml.

To the fifth cylinder add 25.0 ml of purified water and sufficient volume of the 0.5% methylcellulose, 1500 cp, solution to make 100 ml.

Stopper the graduated cylinders and invert several times to disperse the bismuth subnitrate. Allow the suspensions to remain undisturbed. Measure and record the height of the sedimentation volume intially and after 15, 60, and 120 minutes. Measure and record the height of the sedimentation volume after one week.

The Helipath attachment used with the Brookfield viscometer helps in measuring the settling behavior of suspensions. The instrument consists of a slowly rotating T-bar spindle, which while descending into suspension encounters new undisturbed material as it rotates. The dial reading of the viscometer measures resistance to flow that the spindle encounters. Taking rheograms at various time intervals gives information of the suspension stability. This technique is most useful for measurement of shear stress in suspensions with a high solid content and a high viscosity.

J. Combine several preparations from B and let the lotion stand in a beaker for one week. Similarly let preparations from C stand for one week.

By means of the Helipath attachment for the Brookfield viscometer, determine the rate of settling of the particles by plotting the dial readings as ordinates against the number of turns of the spindle as abscissa. Make a dozen readings. Record the data.

REFERENCES

Akers, R. J. 1972. Zeta potential and use of electrophoretic mass transport analyzer. American Laboratory, 4:41.

Bondi, J. V., R. L. Schnaare, P. J. Niebergall, and E. T. Sugita. 1973. Effect of adsorbed surfactant on particle-particle interactions in hydrophobic suspensions. J. Pharm. Sci., 62:1731.

Brookfield Engineering Laboratories. The Brookfield Helipath Stand. Data Sheet 051-B. Stoughton, Mass.

Carstensen, J. T. and K. S. E. Su. 1970. Sedimentation kinetics of flocculated suspensions. I. Initial sedimentation region. J. Pharm. Sci., 59:666. II. Sedimentation below the critical height. 59:671. III. Effect of ζ-potential. 1972. 61:1999.

Chiou, W. L., and S. Riegelman. 1971. Pharmaceutical applications of solid dispersion systems. J. Pharm. Sci., 60:1281.

The Dow Chemical Company. 1962. Methocel. Thickener, stabilizer, film former, emulsifier, binder. Midland, Michigan.

Ecanow, B., B. Gold, and C. Ecanow. 1969. Newer aspects of suspension theory. Am. Perfumer and Cosmetics, 84:27.

Ecanow, B., B. Gold, R. Levinson, H. Takruri, and W. Stanaszek. 1969. Conceptual clarification of the coagulation and flocculation phenomena. Am. Perfumer and Cosmetics, 84:30.

Ecanow, B., R. Grundman, and R. Wilson. 1966. Flocculation and coagulation. Am. J. Hosp. Pharm., 23:404.

Ecanow, B. and H. Takruri. 1970. Flocculation theory and polysorbate 80 sulfaguanidine suspensions. J. Pharm. Sci., 59:1848.

Haines, B. A., Jr. and A. N. Martin. 1961. Interfacial properties of powdered material; caking in liquid dispersions I. Caking and flocculation studies. J. Pharm. Sci., 50:228, and II. Electrokinetic phenomena. J. Pharm. Sci., 50:753.

Heyd A. and D. J. Dhabhar. 1975. Enhancing fluidity of concentrated antacid suspensions. J. Pharm. Sci., 64:1697.

Hiestand, E. N. 1964. Theory of coarse suspension formulation. J. Pharm. Sci. 53:1.

Hiestand, E. N. 1972. Physical properties of coarse suspensions. J. Pharm. Sci., 61:268.

Hiestand, E. N., W. I. Higuchi, and N. F. H. Ho. 1976. Theories of dispersion techniques. In The theory and practice of industrial pharmacy, 2nd ed. L. Lachman, H. A. Lieberman, and J. L. Kanig, Eds. Lea and Febiger, Philadelphia. Chap. 4, p. 141.

Higuchi, W. I. and A. P. Simonelli. 1975. Particle phenomena. In Remington's Pharmaceutical sciences, 15th ed., Mack Publishing Co., Easton, Pa. Chap. 23, p. 340.

Jones, R. D. C., B. A. Matthews, and C. T. Rhodes. 1970. Physical stability of sulfaguanidine suspensions. J. Pharm. Sci., 59:518.

Kennon, L. and G. K. Storz. 1976. Pharmaceutical suspensions. In The theory and practice of industrial pharmacy, 2nd ed. L. Lachman, H. A. Lieberman, and J. L. Kanig, Eds. Lea and Febiger, Philadelphia. Chap. 5, p. 162.

La Mer, V. K. and T. W. Healy. 1963. Adsorption-flocculation reactions of macromolecules at the solid-liquid interface. Reviews of Pure and Applied Chemistry, 13:112.

Martin, A. N. 1961. Physical chemical approach to the formulation of pharmaceutical suspensions. J. Pharm. Sci., 50:513.

Martin, A. N., J. Swarbrick, and A. Cammarata. 1969. Coarse dispersions: Suspensions, emulsions and semisolids. Chap. 19 in Physical pharmacy. Lea and Febiger, Philadelphia.

Matthews, B. A. and C. T. Rhodes. 1968. Some studies of flocculation phenomena in pharmaceutical suspensions. J. Pharm. Sci., 57:569.

Matthews, B. A. and C. T. Rhodes. 1969. The use of comparative analysis of sedimentation and Brownian motion as a guide to suspension formulation. Pharm. Acta Helv., 45:52.

Matthews, B. A. and C. T. Rhodes. 1970. Use of the Derjaguin, Landau, Verwey, and Overbeek theory to interpret pharmaceutical suspension stability. J. Pharm. Sci., 59:521.

Nash, R. A. 1965. The pharmaceutical suspension. Part I. Drug and Cosmetic Industry, 97:843. and 1966. Part 2. 98:39.

Pattison, K. L. and J. L. Lichtin. 1967. Suspensions by controlled flocculation. Am. J. Pharm. Ed. 31:528.

Polon, J. A. 1970. The mechanisms of thickening by inorganic agents. J. Soc. Cosmetic Chemists, 21:347.

Short, M. P. and C. T. Rhodes. 1973. A study of the formulation of steroidal suspensions. Canadian J. Pharm. Sci., 8:46.

Tingstad, J. E. 1964. Physical stability testing of pharmaceuticals. J. Pharm. Sci., 53:955.

Tingstad, J., J. Dudzinski, L. Lachman, and E. Shami. 1973. Simplified method for determining chemical stability of drug substances in pharmaceutical suspensions. J. Pharm. Sci., 62:1361.

Wilson, R. G. and B. Ecanow. 1963. Powdered particle interactions: Suspension flocculation and caking I, II, III, and IV. J. Pharm. Sci., 52:757, 1031, 53:782, 913.

Sedimentation

Data and Conclusions

1. The order of mixing the ingredients of a prescription is often important to the pharmacist. Illustrate, with at least three examples, the necessity of a correct order of mixing.

2. Why is White Lotion freshly prepared?

3. Which of the calamine lotions do you personally believe to be the best. Why? What is the purpose of each ingredient in the calamine lotions?

4. Did the inclusion of a suspending agent improve the lotion of sulfur and camphor in D and E?

5. Outline the process used for preparing the magma in F. Give the equations for the reactions which occurred.

6. Give the purpose of each ingredient in Kaolin Mixture with Pectin.

7. Complete the following chart according to the experimental value obtained in H:

		Sediment in cm at Time in min			
Suspending Agent	Percent	5	15	45	90
Water (control)					
Acacia					
Sodium CMC, Med.					
MC, 1500 cp					
Tragacanth					

8. What are the advantages of a synthetic dispersing agent, such as methylcellulose, over a natural gum?

9. How is a solution of methylcellulose properly prepared? What is meant by the "1500 cp" of the methylcellulose used?

10. What fundamental force is responsible for the settling of a suspension? This same force acts on a colloidal dispersion yet it does not settle. Explain.

Substance	Density, g cc^{-1}	Diameter of Particles, μm
Ammoniated mercury U. S. P.	5.2	1.19
Bismuth subcarbonate U. S. P.	6.86	0.16
Bismuth subnitrate N. F.	4.93	1.93
Mercury sulfide	8.10	2.24
Sulfanilamide	1.4	14.4
Sulfadiazine U. S. P.	1.5	2.55
Sulfur U. S. P.	2.07	11.1
Sulfur, colloidal	2.07	0.73
Zinc oxide U. S. P.	5.47	0.31

11. Compare the rates of settling of sulfur and colloidal sulfur in water.

12. What is the rate of settling of the bismuth subcarbonate particles in the following?

Bismuth subcarbonate	10 g
Methylcellulose 25 cp	2 g
Distilled water q. s.	100 ml

13. If sulfanilamide is to be suspended in a medium with a density of approximately one so that it settles at a rate of 1 cm day^{-1}, what viscosity would be required?

14. In an aqueous preparation containing particles of sulfadiazine U.S.P. what viscosity would be necessary so that the rate of sedimentation would be 1 cm hr^{-1}?

15. In a calamine lotion, what would be the rate of settling if the viscosity of the preparation were 50 cps?

16. Complete the following table for I:

	Height of Sediment in cm in				
Time	Water	Anionic agent	Anionic agent and 0.5% MC	Anionic agent and 1.0% MC	0.5% MC
0					
15 min					
60					
120					
1 wk					

17. From the data tabulated in 16 for each interval of time calculate the ratio, $H_{ultimate}/H_{original}$, for the five suspensions.

18. Explain what caused the results observed in I and the values calculated in 17.

19. What is the significance of controlled flocculation in the preparation of pharmaceutical suspensions?

20. Record the data from J.

Number of Turns of Spindle	Dial Reading

Which of the two formulations for calamine lotion appears more stable in regard to sedimentation? (See article by J. E. Tingstad in J. Pharm. Sci., 53:955, 1964.)

27. BLENDING OF IMMISCIBLE LIQUIDS

An emulsion is a system of two immiscible substances, one of which is dispersed in globular form throughout the other substance. The substance divided into small globules is known as the dispersed, internal, or discontinuous phase. The phase in which the globules are scattered is called the dispersing, external, or continuous phase.

Microemulsions are stable dispersions of spherical droplets having a diameter of approximately 1400 Å in another immiscible liquid. As the size of the droplet is less than one-fourth the wave length of white light, light may pass through the microemulsion; however, it is not necessarily transparent and often exhibits Tyndall scattering. A distinction may be made between a micellar solution and a microemulsion. In a micellar solution the dispersed phase is in equilibrium with a saturated solution of the molecular units composing the micelle. In a microemulsion the internal phase is not in equilibrium with the external phase, and as there are no molecular species of the dispersed phase in the external phase, there is no critical micelle concentration in this phase.

When two immiscible liquids, such as oil and water, are in contact, interfacial tension causes each liquid to maintain as small a surface as possible. If two immiscible liquids are shaken together, the liquids break up into small droplets, greatly increasing the total surface area of each liquid. The increased energy associated with the increased surface area is supplied by the mechanical energy of agitation. The work of emulsion formation, W, may be expressed

$$W = \gamma\, dS$$

where γ is the interfacial tension and dS is the change in surface area.

As the interfacial tension is a measure of the force to be overcome in mixing two immiscible liquids, any substance which lowers interfacial tension will facilitate the preparation of an emulsion as less mechanical energy need be expended in breaking up and dispersing the internal phase. For example, if a pharmacist is to emulsify 100 ml of liquid petrolatum with an initial surface area of 300 cm² so that the average radius of the dispersed oil globule is 1 micron, the work of emulsification may be calculated. The volume of each spherical oil globule is

$$V_i = \frac{4\pi r^3}{3} = \frac{4\pi(10^{-4})^3}{3} = 4.19 \times 10^{-12} \text{ cc}$$

The number of oil globules in 100 ml of mineral oil is $100/4.19 \times 10^{-12}$ or 2.39×10^{13}. Each spherical globule has a surface area

$$S_i = 4\pi r^2 = 4\pi(10^{-4})^2 = 12.57 \times 10^{-8} \text{ cm}^2$$

The total surface area of the dispersed phase is the product of the number of globules and the surface area of an individual globule or 30.0523×10^5 cm². The interfacial tension between liquid petrolatum and water is 57 dyne cm^{-1}. The work of emulsification is

$$W = \gamma\, dS = 57\,(3{,}005{,}230 - 300) = 17.1 \times 10^7 \text{ ergs}$$

Ergs may be converted to joules by dividing by 10^7 so the work of emulsification is 17.1 joules. Joules, in turn, may be changed to calories by dividing by 4.184; the work of emulsification is 4.1 calories.

If 1% Tween 65 is added to the system, the interfacial tension between the liquid petrolatum and water is lowered to 3 dyne cm^{-1}. The work of emulsification is then about 1/20 as great as that necessary to disperse the oil phase in the absence of a surface-active agent

$$W = \gamma dS = 3(3{,}005{,}230\text{-}300) = 9 \times 10^6 \text{ ergs}$$

The work of emulsification with Tween 65 is 0.2 calories.

In addition to facilitating emulsion formation, an emulsifying agent stabilizes an emulsion. The surface energy associated with the dispersed globules exists as potential energy in the emulsion. As such a system is thermodynamically unstable, the less energy associated with the surface of the dispersed phase, the more stable the emulsion.

A surface-active substance is one which collects or is absorbed at an interface and in doing so lowers interfacial tension. To be surface-active the molecule must possess approximately an equal balance between the hydrophilic and hydrophobic structures within the molecule. A surface-active molecule collects at an oil and water interface so that its nonpolar or hydrophobic portion will be oriented toward the oily phase, and the polar or hydrophilic portion will be oriented toward the aqueous phase.

Not only does this adsorption at the interface lower interfacial tension, but a film is thus formed about the globule of the internal phase. If pure oil and water are shaken, the globules formed collide and coalesce into progressively larger particles until two layers have completely separated. If an emulsifying agent has been adsorbed about an oil globule and has formed a condensed, rigid film, coalescence of two colliding globules is prevented by the adsorbed film, and greater emulsion stability results.

Reduction of interfacial tension is probably the most important factor in preparing an emulsion; however, the rigidity of the adsorbed film of the emulsifying agent is of prime importance in the stability of an emulsion. The stability of an emulsion can be determined only by a size-frequency analysis; if the growth of average particle size is rapid, the emulsion is not stable.

Upon standing, the emulsified oil globules of an O/W emulsion may rise to the surface because of the difference in the densities of the phases; this is known as creaming. If the adsorbed film of the emulsifying agent is rigid and condensed, it will prevent coalescence, and upon being shaken the internal phase will be redispersed.

The type of emulsion formed depends mainly on the relative solubilities of the emulsifying agent in the two liquids. The phase in which the emulsifying agent is more soluble generally becomes the external phase. For example, sodium oleate is water-soluble and will form an O/W emulsion with water as the continuous phase. A divalent soap such as calcium oleate is oil-soluble and will form a W/O emulsion with oil as the external phase. Polyoxyl 40 stearate is water-soluble and forms an O/W emulsion.

Blending of immiscible liquids and the reduction of particle size of the globules of the internal phase is most commonly accomplished in the retail pharmacy by a mortar and pestle. A Waring Blendor may be used to prepare extemporaneous emulsions, but it should not be used with high viscosity emulsions and emulsions that contain a foaming agent, as unwanted air would be incorporated into the preparation. Generally, the passage of an emulsion through a hand homogenizer will improve an emulsion and reduce the size of the dispersed globules.

Large multistage homogenizers such as the Manton Gaulin type are commonly used industrially for preparing pharmaceutical emulsions. Colloid mills which force the emulsion between a stator and rotor separated by a variable distance also are used on a manufacturing scale. The equipment used depends somewhat on the properties of the individual formulation. For example, a high-speed mixer, such as a Homo-Mixer fitted with paddles and scraper blades in a kettle, may be used to prepare an excellent emulsion of medium viscosity.

PROCEDURE. In preparing an extemporaneous emulsion, using acacia as an emulsifying agent, a primary emulsion consisting of 4 parts of oil, 2 parts of water, and 1 part of acacia is prepared.

The high viscosity of this mixture hinders coalescence as the oil droplets move less rapidly and allows more time for the emulsifying agent to become properly oriented. After a good primary emulsion has been formed by rapid trituration in a mortar, it may be diluted with water as required with further trituration.

In one method of preparing emulsions using gums, 1 part of the emulsifying agent is mixed thoroughly with 4 parts of the internal phase, and then 2 parts of the external phase is added all at once with rapid trituration. After one or two minutes of trituration, a crackling sound indicates the formation of a good primary emulsion. This method, in which the water is added at once to the previously mixed gum and oil, is known as the Continental method.

After the formation of the primary emulsion, other ingredients may be added gradually with trituration. Electrolytes in high concentrations may crack an emulsion. Any electrolyte should be added lastly in as high a dilution as possible. Alcoholic solutions tend to dehydrate and precipitate acacia as well as other hydrophilic colloids and should be added as diluted as possible.

Employing the same ratio of gum, oil and water, a different order of mixing may be used. When the internal phase is added gradually with trituration to the external phase containing the emulsifying agent, the process is known as the English method. If, while adding the 4 parts of oil gradually with trituration, the mixture becomes too viscoid, a little water may be added with constant trituration after which the addition of the oil in divided portions is continued.

A. Prepare 100 ml of Mineral Oil Emulsion N. F. by the Continental method. Stain a sample of the emulsion with amaranth and examine under a microscope. Draw a sketch. Measure the smallest and largest globule.

   By means of a hand homogenizer, homogenize half of the emulsion, stain, and examine microscopically for globular size and uniformity. Draw a sketch and compare with the sketch of the original emulsion.

B. Prepare 100 ml of Mineral Oil Emulsion N. F. by the English method. Stain a sample of the emulsion with amaranth and examine microscopically. Measure the smallest and largest globule.

C. Prepare 100 ml of a Mineral Oil emulsion using tragacanth instead of acacia. Usually, about ten times as much acacia is used as tragacanth. Homogenize and examine microscopically. Compare with the homogenized emulsion containing acacia.

D. Allow all emulsions to remain undisturbed for three weeks in order to compare the influence of homogenization on creaming of an emulsion.

Emulsion of low viscosity may be prepared by shaking in a bottle. For example, 2 parts of volatile oil are placed in a dry bottle with 1 part of powdered acacia and mixed thoroughly. Two parts of water are added at once and the bottle is shaken vigorously and intermittently. The remaining ingredients are then added in divided portions with shaking. More gum is employed in the bottle method to increase the viscosity.

E. Prepare 60 ml of a paraldehyde emulsion:

Paraldehyde	20 ml
Acacia, in fine powder	3 g
Peppermint water q. s.	60 ml

Place the powdered acacia in a dry bottle, add the paraldehyde, mix thoroughly, add 10 ml of peppermint water, stopper, and agitate briskly until an emulsion forms. Then gradually add sufficient peppermint water to make the product measure 60 ml and mix thoroughly.

F. Prepare 60 ml of a liniment by shaking equal volumes of olive oil and lime water in a bottle. Determine by the dilution method the type of emulsion formed.

Add 1.0 ml of hydrochloric acid to 30 ml of the emulsion. Record any change.

Emulsions containing gelatin cannot be prepared by use of the mortar and pestle but must be homogenized. Although gelatin is a good film-forming substance, it does not appreciably lower interfacial tension, so the mechanical energy supplied by the pestle and mortar is not adequate for emulsion formation. Many other natural and synthetic gums such as agar, karaya, and methylcellulose act similarly.

G. Prepare 100 ml of an emulsion containing Pharmagel A:

Pharmagel A	8.0 g
Tartaric acid	0.6 g
Syrup	100.0 ml
Vanillin	40.0 mg
Alcohol	60.0 ml
Water q. s.	500 ml
Mineral oil	500 ml

Place the Pharmagel A and the tartaric acid in 300 ml of water, allow to stand for 5 minutes, then heat until the gelatin is dissolved. Raise and maintain the temperature at 100° for 20 minutes to hydrolyze the gelatin. Cool to 50°, add the syrup, the alcoholic flavor and enough water to make 500 ml. Add 500 ml of oil, mix, and homogenize several times.

Add 10 ml of acacia mucilage to 20 ml of the above emulsion. Mix and note the results.

Add 15 ml of a 2% methylcellulose, 1500 cp solution to 20 ml of the above emulsion. Mix and note the results.

H. Prepare 100 ml of an emulsion containing Pharmagel B by replacing the Pharmagel A and tartaric acid in G with Pharmagel B and sodium bicarbonate. Phenol red indicator or pHydrion paper may be used to determine the amount of sodium bicarbonate required to adjust to the proper pH.

Add 10 ml of acacia mucilage to 20 ml of the above emulsion. Mix and note the results.

Add 15 ml of a 2% methylcellulose, 1500 cp solution to 20 ml of the above emulsion. Mix and note the results.

The pharmaceutical class of preparations known as Emulsions, as found in the official books, is composed of O/W emulsions intended for internal use. Actually, emulsions are widely used as cosmetics, such as vanishing and cold creams, as well as in washable ointments.

I. Prepare 100 g of the following vanishing cream:

Stearic acid	25.0 g
Triethanolamine	2.0 g
Glycerin	12.0 g
Purified water	61.0 g

Using a water bath, melt the stearic acid. Dissolve the glycerin and triethanolamine in the water and heat to 70°. With gentle stirring so that air is not incorporated, add the aqueous phase to the melted stearic acid. Save for future exercise.

J. Prepare 30 g of a brushless shave cream:

Stearic acid	12.5 g
Span 60	2.5 g
Tween 60	1.0 g
White petrolatum	110.0 g
Propylene glycol	5.0 ml
Purified water	67.0 ml
28% Ammonium hydroxide solution	2.0 ml
Lavender oil	0.15 ml

Melt the stearic acid, Span, Tween, and petrolatum and bring to 80°. Heat the propylene glycol and water to 80°. Add the ammonium hydroxide to the aqueous phase and quickly add the oily phase with moderate agitation. Stir until the temperature drops to 55°. Add the lavender oil and mix thoroughly.

Certain colloidal solids may be used to make emulsions. Pharmaceutically, they are limited to aluminum hydroxide gel, magnesium hydroxide and trisilicate, and bentonite and other colloidal clays. Bentonite has a rather unusual ability to form either O/W or W/O emulsions depending on the order of mixing. If oil is added last to a bentonite suspension, an O/W emulsion is formed. If water is added last to an oil and bentonite suspension, a W/O emulsion is formed.

K. Prepare the following emulsion:

Calamine	3.0 g
Zinc oxide	3.0 g
Olive oil	24.0 ml
6% Bentonite in Lime Water	24.0 ml

Record your method of preparation. Determine the type of emulsion that formed.

L. Prepare 60 ml of the following:

Cottonseed oil	30 ml
Milk of Magnesia	30 ml

Mix in a bottle. Determine the type of emulsion that formed.

To half of the emulsion add 1 ml of oleic acid. Compare with the original emulsion.

REFERENCES

Anderson, R. A. and C. E. Chow. 1967. The distribution and activity of benzoic acid in some emulsified systems. J. Soc. Cosmetic Chemists, 18:207.

Balsam, M. S. and E. Sagarin. 1972. Cosmetics. Science and technology. 2nd ed. Vol. 1 and Vol. 2. Wiley-Interscience, New York.

Barry, B. W. 1969. The control of oil-in-water emulsion consistency using mixed emulsifiers. J. Pharm. Pharmacol., 21:533.

Becher, P. 1965. Emulsions: Theory and practice. 2nd ed. Reinhold Publishing Corp., New York.

Carey, M. C. and D. M. Small. 1970. The characteristics of mixed micellar solutions with particular reference to bile. The Am. J. Medicine, 49:590.

Davies, J. T. 1964. Emulsions. In Recent progress in surface science. Vol. 2. J. F. Danielli, K. G. A. Pankhurst, and A. C. Riddiford, Eds. Academic Press, New York and London. p. 129.

Garrett, E. R. 1962. Prediction of stability in pharmaceutical preparations. VIII. Oil-in-water emulsion stability and the analytical ultracentrifuge. J. Pharm. Sci., 51:35.

Garrett, E. R. 1965. Stability of oil-in-water emulsions. J. Pharm. Sci., 54:1557.

Geyer, R. P. 1973. Fluorocarbon-polyol artificial blood substitutes. New England J. Medicine, 289:1077.
Groves, M. J. and D. C. Freshwater. 1968. Particle-size analysis of emulsion systems. J. Pharm. Sci., 57:1273.
Kakemi, K., H. Sezaki, S. Muranishi, H. Ogata, and K. Giga. 1972. Mechanism of intestinal absorption of drugs from oil in water emulsions. II. Absorption from oily solutions. Chem. Pharm. Bull., 20:715.
Kimizuka, H., L. G. Abood, T. Tahara, and K. Kaibara. 1972. Adsorption kinetics of surface active agent at an interface. J. Colloid and Interface Sci., 40:27.
Knoechel, E. and D. Wurster. 1959. Investigation of stability in emulsions of varying viscosities. J. Am. Pharm. Assoc., Sci. Ed., 48:1.
Lissant, K. J., Ed. 1974. Emulsions and emulsion technology (in two parts). Part I & Part II. Marcel Dekker, Inc. New York.
Martin, A. M., J. Swarbrick, and A. Cammarata. 1969. Coarse dispersions: Suspensions, emulsions and semisolids. Chap. 19 in Physical pharmacy. Lea and Febiger, Philadelphia.
Meng, H. C. 1974. Fat emulsions. In Total parenteral nutrition. P. L. White and M. E. Nagy, Eds. Publishing Sciences Group, Inc., Acton, Massachussetts. Chap. 5, p. 155.
Mittal, K. L. 1971. Conceptual clarification of the terms used to describe emulsion behavior. J. Soc. Cosmetic Chemists, 22:815.
Mittal, K. L. and R. D. Vold. 1972. Effect of the initial concentration of emulsifying agents on the ultracentrifugal stability of oil-in-water emulsions. J. Am. Oil Chemists' Society, 49:527.
Mulley, B. A. 1974. Medicinal emulsions. In Emulsions and emulsion technology. K. J. Lissant, Ed. Part I. Marcel Dekker, Inc. New York. Chap. 6, p. 291.
Nixon, J. R., R. S. Ul Haque, and J. E. Carless. 1971. The phase diagram of cetomacrogol 1000-water-benzaldehyde in the presence of gallate antioxidants. J. Pharm. Pharmacol. 23:1.
Patel, N. K. and J. M. Romanowski. 1970. Heterogeneous systems. II. Influence of partitioning and molecular interactions on *in vitro* biologic activity of preservatives in emulsions. J. Pharm. Sci., 59:372.
Prince, L. M. 1974. Microemulsions. In Emulsions and emulsion technology. Part I., K. J. Lissant, Ed. Marcel Dekker, Inc. New York. Chap. 3, p. 125.
Rieger, M. M. 1976. Emulsions. In The theory and practice of industrial pharmacy. 2nd ed. L. Lachman, H. A. Lieberman, and J. L. Kanig, Eds. Lea and Febiger, Philadelphia. Chap. 6, p. 184.
Saski, W. and M. H. Malone. 1960. A technique for the evaluation of emulsion stability. J. Pharm. Pharmacol., 12:523.
Sherman, P. 1968. Emulsion science. Academic Press, New York.
Schmolka, I. R. 1970. Theory of emulsions. Federation Proceedings, 29:1717.
Shinoda, K. 1967. The correlation between the dissolution state of nonionic surfactant and the type of dispersion stabilized with the surfactant. J. Colloid and Interface Sci., 24:4.
Shotton, E. and S. S. Davis. 1968. The influence of emulsifier concentration on the rheological properties of an oil-in-water emulsion stabilized by an anionic soap. J. Pharm. Pharmacol. 20:439.
Shotton, E. and S. S. Davis. 1968. The use of the Coulter Counter for the particle size analysis of some emulsion systems. J. Pharm. Pharmacol. 20:430.
Shotton, E. and R. F. White. 1960. Rheology of acacia – Stabilized emulsions. J. Pharm. Pharmacol., 12, Suppl. 108 T.
Shotton, E. and K. Wibberley. 1960. The emulsifying properties of gum acacia. J. Pharm. Pharmacol., 12, Suppl. 105 T.
Swarbrick, J. 1975. Coarse dispersions. In Remington's Pharmaceutical sciences, 15th ed. Mack Publishing Co., Easton, Pa. Chap. 22, p. 322.
Talman, F. A. J. and E. M. Rowan. 1970. An examination of some oil-in-water emulsions by electron microscopy. J. Pharm. Pharmacol. 22:535.
Vold, R. D. and K. L. Mittal. 1972. Effect of age on ultracentrifugal stability of liquid petrolatum-water emulsions. J. Pharm. Sci., 61:769.
Weddenburn, D. L. 1964. Preservation of emulsions against microbial attack. In Advances in pharmaceutical sciences, Vol 1. H. S. Bean, A. H. Beckett, and J. E. Carless, Eds. Academic Press, London and New York. p. 195.
Wretlind, A. 1974. Fat emulsions. In Parenteral nutrition in acute metabolic illness. H. A. Lee, Ed. Academic Press, London and New York. Chap. 5, p. 77.

Blending of Immiscible Liquids

Data and Conclusions

1. Sketch the microscopic view of the Mineral Oil Emulsion before and after homogenization. Record and compare the globule size before and after homogenization.

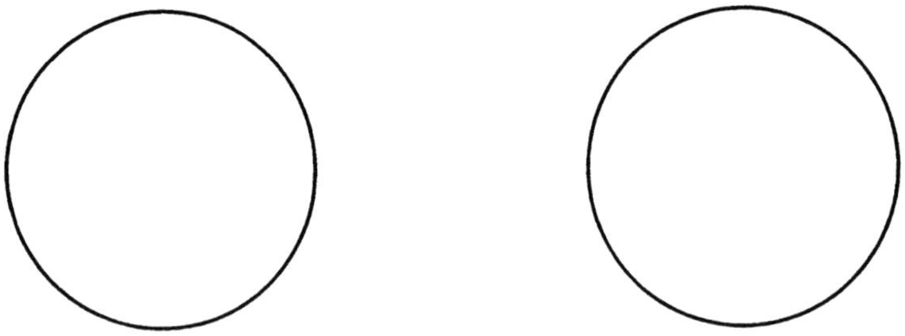

2. Compare the English and the Continental method of preparing an emulsion. How does the globular size differ in a given formulation prepared by both methods?

3. How readily does tragacanth form a mineral oil emulsion? Compare the size and uniformity of emulsified globules prepared with acacia against an emulsion prepared with tragacanth.

4. May Mineral Oil Emulsion be prepared by the bottle method?

5. What type of emulsion is formed when equal amounts of olive oil and Calcium Hydroxide Solution are shaken? What occurs when an acid is added in F? Explain.

6. Compare what occurs when acacia mucilage is added to the emulsions containing Pharmagel A and Pharmagel B. Explain. Define "coacervation."

7. Compare what occurs when methylcellulose solution is added to the emulsions containing Pharmagel A and Pharmagel B. Explain.

8. Draw a sketch comparing the initial and a later size-frequency distribution curve of an unstable emulsion.

9. Name the emulsifying agent in the vanishing cream prepared in I. Give an equation for its formation.

10. Name the emulsifying agents in the shaving cream prepared in J.

11. Record your method of preparation of the emulsion in K. What type of emulsion did you form? Explain what would occur if an acid were added.

12. What type of emulsion does a mixture of equal amounts of cottonseed oil and milk of magnesia form? What occurs when oleic acid is added?

13. List the official substances that are used as suspending agents.

14. Considering emulsifying agents as substances that markedly lower interfacial tension, list the official emulsifying agents. What concentration of each is generally employed in preparing an emulsion?

15. List the substances that are used to flavor the official emulsions. Give the concentration of each flavoring agent.

16. What factor(s) limit the use of soaps in pharmaceutical products?

17. What mechanism(s) stabilize an emulsion formed with acacia?

18. How would you physically distinguish between:

a. an emulsoid and a suspensoid?

b. O/W and W/O emulsion?

c. a suspension and a colloidal dispersion?

d. a suspending agent and an emulsifying agent?

19. An O/W emulsion is prepared by two methods. In Method A the emulsion is prepared with a mortar and pestle, and the diameter of the oil globules is found to be 20 microns; the viscosity of the emulsion is increased to 1000 cp by the addition of an inert suspending agent.

    In Method B the emulsion as produced by the mortar and pestle is homogenized to yield an average oil globule diameter of 2 microns with a viscosity of 100 cp.

    Calculate the rate of creaming of each emulsion.

20. With intravenous fat emulsions in combination with carbohydrate a large amount of nutritional energy may be given in a small volume of isotonic fluid through a peripheral vein in contrast to larger volumes of concentrated glucose solution which has to be given through a central vein catheter. Why is there no commercial intravenous fat emulsion in the United States?

28. SOME CHARACTERISTICS OF SURFACE-ACTIVE AGENTS

A surface-active molecule possesses approximately an equal ratio between the polar and non-polar portions of the molecule. When such a molecule is placed in an oil-water system, the polar groups are attracted to or oriented toward the water, and the nonpolar groups are oriented toward the oil. The surface-active molecule is adsorbed or oriented in this manner, consequently, lowering interfacial tension between the oil and water phase.

Realizing that a surface-active agent is adsorbed at an interface and by assuming that it is adsorbed in a monomolecular layer, the amount of emulsifying agent required to emulsify a given volume of a liquid to a certain globular size may be calculated. The molecular weight and the cross-sectional area occupied by a molecule of the emulsifying agent must be known.

Sodium lauryl sulfate has a molecular weight of 288 g $mole^{-1}$ and a cross-sectional area of 22 $Å^2$ (22×10^{-16} cm^2). If 100 ml of oil is emulsified to an average globular diameter of 1 micron, the amount of sodium lauryl sulfate required may be calculated. The volume of each dispersed spherical oil globule is

$$V_i = \frac{4}{3}\pi r^3 = \frac{4}{3}\pi(\tfrac{1}{2} \times 10^{-4})^3 = 0.524 \times 10^{-12} \text{ cc}$$

The number of globules per cc is

$$\frac{1 \text{ cc}}{\text{Volume of a Globule}} = \frac{1}{0.524 \times 10^{-12}} = 1.91 \times 10^{12} \text{ globules}$$

The surface area of an individual dispersed globule is

$$S_i = 4\pi r^2 = 4\pi(\tfrac{1}{2} \times 10^{-4})^2 = 3.14 \times 10^{-8} \text{ cm}^2$$

The total surface area of all the globules in 1 cc of oil is the product of the surface area of the individual globule and the number of globules in 1 cc or

$$3.14 \times 10^{-8} \times 1.91 \times 10^{12} = 6 \times 10^4 \text{ cm}^2$$

The number of molecules of sodium lauryl sulfate adsorbed at the surface of all of the dispersed oil globules from 1 cc of oil is equal to the total surface area divided by the cross-sectional area of the emulsifying agent or

$$\frac{6 \times 10^4}{22 \times 10^{-16}} = 2.72 \times 10^{19} \text{ molecules}$$

The moles of sodium lauryl sulfate required per 1 cc of oil is equal to the total number of molecules adsorbed at the interface divided by the Avogadro number or

$$\frac{2.72 \times 10^{19}}{6.02 \times 10^{23}} = 0.45 \times 10^{-4} \text{ moles}$$

To emulsify 100 cc of oil 0.0045 moles of sodium lauryl sulfate is required. The weight of sodium lauryl sulfate to be used is the product of the moles and the molecular weight or

$$0.0045 \times 288 = 1.3 \text{ g}$$

Substances in which the ability to lower interfacial tension resides in the anion are known as anionic surface-active agents. Duponol C and Aerosol OT are anionic surfactants. Cationic surface-active agents are those in which the ability to lower interfacial tension resides in the cation. Cationic surface-active agents, such as Zephiran chloride and Phemerol chloride, are not used as emulsifying agents but primarily as antibacterial agents. Nonionic surface-active agents, such as Tween 80 and octyl phenoxy polyethoxyethanol, appreciably lower interfacial tension but do not ionize.

Although it is relatively easy to predict the type of emulsion that will be formed by use of an ionic emulsifying agent, it is more difficult to predict the type of emulsion that will be formed by a mixture of nonionic emulsifying agents. The hydrophile-lipophile balance or HLB method is useful for expressing the hydrophilic and hydrophobic characteristics of an emulsifying agent. An arbitrary scale has been set up, and the HLB values have been determined experimentally. Equations have been derived which permit the calculation of HLB values of a surface-active agent based on its composition. The HLB values of Spans range from 1.8-8.6, indicating oil-soluble or dispersible molecules. A high HLB value indicates water dispersibility or solubility; the HLB values of the Tweens range from 9.6-16.7. The technological application of a surface-active agent falls within a certain HLB range. For example, those substances that have an HLB value of 8-18 are suitable for preparation of O/W emulsions.

In the formation of emulsions, usually a blend of an emulsifier with a low HLB value and an emulsifier with a high HLB value will produce a more stable emulsion than the use of a single emulsifier with the correct HLB value.

The HLB numbers are additive so that the HLB value of a blend of emulsifying agents may be calculated. For example, the HLB value of a 60% Tween 80 and 40% Arlacel 80 is

	HLB		Fraction of Emulsifier		
Arlacel 80	4.3	X	0.4	=	1.7
Tween 80	15.0	X	0.6	=	9.0
					10.7

Certain HLB values are required to form the most efficient emulsions of various oil phases (See Appendix: Required HLB Values). To form an O/W emulsion of stearyl alcohol and petrolatum, HLB values of 14 and 10.5, respectively, are required. If one were to prepare an ointment base,

Stearyl alcohol	25 g
White petrolatum	25 g
Propylene glycol	12 g
Emulsifier	3 g
Purified water	35 g

the correct combination of emulsifiers for an O/W emulsion could be calculated. The required HLB value of the oil phase is found

	HLB		Fraction of Oil Phase		
Stearyl alcohol	14	X	25/50	=	7.0
White petrolatum	10.5	X	25/50	=	5.25
					12.25

An emulsifier combination with an HLB value of 12.2 is optimum for producing a stable O/W emulsion. Using a mixture of Arlacel 80 and Polysorbate 80, the fraction of each to be used in the mixture may be determined. If α represents the fraction of the total emulsifier combination composed of Polysorbate 80, then $(1 - \alpha)$ is the fraction representing Arlacel 80. The sum of these is to give a total HLB value of 12.25, therefore,

$$4.3(1-\alpha) + 15\alpha = 12.25$$

$$\alpha = 0.74 \text{ or } 74\% \text{ Polysorbate } 80$$

The emulsifying mixture consists of 74% Polysorbate 80 and 26% Arlacel 80. The total concentration of a blend of nonionic emulsifiers is approximately 20% of the internal phase. The emulsifier with the low HLB value is generally dissolved in the oil phase and warmed to 70 - 75°. The emulsifier with the high HLB value is dissolved in the aqueous phase and warmed to the same temperature as the oily phase. In forming the emulsion, the oily phase is added to the aqueous phase with constant stirring until the emulsion has cooled.

PROCEDURE. The surface orientation of molecules can be demonstrated by simple procedures. In fact, by employing careful technique, the area occupied by a surface-oriented molecule may be measured with a minimum of equipment.

A. Place approximately 5 g of pure stearic acid on the surface of hot water in a beaker. The fatty acid will melt to a lens-shaped drop. Allow the water to cool. When the stearic acid has solidified, remove it without disturbing the surfaces and allow it to dry.

   With a few drops of water, attempt to wet the bottom of the cake which solidified in contact with water. Record your observation. Add a few drops of water to the top of the cake which solidified in contact with the air and attempt to wet this surface. Record your observation.

B. Using equal volumes of heavy mineral oil and distilled water, prepare 100 ml of an O/W emulsion using a blend of Span 85 and Tween 85 as the emulsifying agent (See Appendix: Average HLB Values of Some Surface Active Agents and Required HLB Values). Record the proportion and amounts of each used.

   Using equal volumes of heavy mineral oil and distilled water, prepare 100 ml of a W/O emulsion using a blend of Span 85 and Tween 85. Record the proportion and amount of each used.

The concept of HLB values is useful and has had success in practical formulation of emulsions, but it has limitations. The HLB system gives no information as to the concentration of surface-active agents required. Calculations such as shown above are helpful, but the optimum amount of the blend of emulsifiers must be experimentally determined. Inversion of an emulsion may occur when the amount of the emulsifier is increased. Stable O/W emulsions of mineral oil with cetyl alcohol-polyoxyethylated cetyl alcohol ether combinations have been reported with HLB numbers as low as 1.9. Stable O/W emulsions of mineral oil with surface-active agent combinations having HLB values of 3.9 have also been reported. The emulsions were thixotropic and creamed to a limited extent.

Regardless of the HLB number, at times the procedure and order of mixing may be the factors in determining the type of emulsion formed.

C. By the various procedures given, prepare emulsions using the formula:

Mineral Oil	70.0 ml
Sorbitan monooleate (HLB = 4.3)	5.0 ml
Purified water	25.0 ml

1. Place the oil and the emulsifier into a mortar. While triturating with a pestle, add the water. Pass the emulsion through a hand homogenizer. Determine and record the type of emulsion formed.

2. Without prior mixing, add all ingredients to the hand homogenizer and pass through the homogenizer. Determine and record the type of emulsion formed.

3. Place the oil and emulsifier into a Waring blender. With the blender operating, gradually add the water. Determine and record the type of emulsion formed.

4. Place the oil, emulsifier and water into the Waring blender. Operate the blender. Determine and record the type of emulsion formed.

5. Decrease the concentration of oil to less than 60% of the total volume. By any procedure you select, try to prepare a W/O emulsion. Determine and record the type of emulsion formed.

As it has been demonstrated, equipment and procedure influence emulsification. Under given conditions an O/W emulsion will be more easily formed when glass equipment is used, but a W/O emulsion will be more easily formed when water-repellant plastic equipment is used. Perhaps the relative wetting tendency of the oil and water determine which phase is to become the external phase. Emulsions containing a given amount of water and an emulsifier behave differently with respect to coalescence depending on whether the oily phase consists of an aromatic or an aliphatic hydrocarbon. Davis has proposed that the type of emulsion is related to the relative rate at which the oil and water droplets coalesce.

Although emulsions are defined as two-phase systems in which the adsorption of the emulsifier at the interface promotes stability, emulsions are more complex. As the solubility of emulsifiers is often low, there may be a formation of a liquid-crystal phase.

REFERENCES

Buchanan, A. S., G. M. Laycock, and A. Shulman. 1969. Action of central nervous system stimulant and depressant drugs in the intact animal. Part 4. Surface activity of drugs with central stimulant depressant, or dual stimulant-depressant action. European J. of Pharmacology, 7:60.

Carriere, G. 1964. Classification of emulsifiers. Am. Perfumer and Cosmetics, 79:27-69.

Collett, J. H. and R. Withington. 1973. A quantitative approach to the *in vitro* availability of drugs from some non-ionic surfactant solutions. J. Pharm. Pharmacol. 25:723.

Danziger, R. G., A. F. Hofmann, L. J. Schoenfield, and J. L. Thistle. 1972. Dissolution of cholesterol gallstones by chenodeoxycholic acid. New England J. Medicine, 286:1.

Florence, A. T. 1968. Surface chemical and micellar properties of drugs in solution. Advances in Colloid and Interface Science, 2:115-149.

Florence, A. T. and J. A. Rogers. 1971. Emulsion stabilization by non-ionic surfactants: Experiment and theory. J. Pharm. Pharmacol., 23:153-169 and 233-251.

Fox, C. 1974. Cosmetic emulsions. In Emulsions and emulsion technology. K. J. Lissant, Ed. Marcel Dekker, Inc., New York. Chap. 13, p. 701.

Friberg, S. and L. Mandell. 1970. Influence of phase equilibria on properties of emulsions. J. Pharm. Sci., 59:1001.

Friberg, S. and I. Wilton. 1970. Liquid crystals – The formula for emulsions. Am. Perfumer and Cosmetics, 85:27.

Gibson, J. W. 1969. Comparative antibacterial activity of hexachlorophene in different formulations used for skin disinfection. J. Clin. Path., 22:90.

Griffin, W. C. 1954. Calculation of HLB values of non-ionic surfactants. J. Soc. Cosmetic Chemists, 5:249.

Gump, W. S. 1969. Toxicological properties of hexachlorophene. J. Soc. Cosmetic Chemists, 20:173.

Humphreys, K. J., G. Richardson, and C. T. Rhodes. 1968. The effect of a non-ionic surfactant upon the antifungal activity of benzoic acid. J. Pharm. Pharmacol., 20: Suppl., 4S.

Kensit, J. G. 1975. Hexachlorophene: Toxicity and effectiveness in prevention of sepsis in neonatal units. J. of Antimicrobial Chemotherapy, 1:263-272.

Lin, T. J. 1970. Surfactant location and required HLB. J. Soc. Cosmetic Chemists, 21:365.

McDonald, C. 1970. Hydrophilic-lipophilic balance values and solubility parameters. The Canadian J. Pharm. Sci., 5:81.

Mulley, B. A. 1964. Solubility in systems containing surface-active agents. In Advances in pharmaceutical sciences. H. S. Bean, A. H. Beckett, and J. E. Carless, Eds. Vol. I. Academic Press, London and New York. p. 86.

Redinger, R. N. and D. M. Small. 1972. Bile composition, bile salt metabolism and gallstones. Arch. Intern. Med., 130:618.

Riegelman, S. and G. Pichon. 1962. A critical re-evaluation of factors affecting emulsion stability. Am. Perfumer and Cosmetics, 77:31.

Rosevear, F. B. 1968. Liquid crystals: The mesomorphic phases of surfactant compositions. J. Soc. Cosmetic Chemists, 19:581.

Saski, W., M. Mannelli, M. Saettone, and F. Bottari. 1971. Relative toxicity of three homologous series of nonionic surfactants in the planarian. J. Pharm. Sci., 60:854.

Schick, M. J., Ed. 1967. Nonionic surfactants. Marcel Dekker, Inc., New York.

Schott, H. 1969. Hydrophile-Lipophile balance and micelle formation of nonionic surfactants. J. Pharm. Sci., 58:1131.

Schumacher, G. E. 1969. The bulk compounding technology of liquids and semi-solids. Am. J. Hospital Pharm., 26:70-99.

Shinoda, K. and H. Saito. 1969. The stability of O/W type emulsions as functions of temperature and the HLB of emulsifiers: The emulsification by PIT - method. J. Colloid and Interface Sci., 30:258.

Sturm, R. N. 1973. Biodegradability of nonionic surfactants: Screening test for predicting rate and ultimate biodegradation. J. Am. Oil Chemists' Society, 50:159.

Swisher, R. D. 1970. Surfactant biodegradation. Marcel Dekker, Inc., New York.

Zografi, G. 1967. An approach to the teaching of factors influencing emulsion formation. Am. J. Pharm. Ed., 31:206.

Some Characteristics of Surface-Active Agents

Data and Conclusions

1. What was observed when you attempted to wet the upper surface of the stearic acid cake?

2. In B how much and what percent of Span 85 and Tween 85 did you use to prepare an O/W emulsion of mineral oil and water? Show your calculations.

3. In B how much and what percent of Span 85 and Tween 85 did you use to prepare a W/O emulsion of mineral oil and water? Show your calculations.

4. Why are Spans and Tweens used in blends rather than as single emulsifying agents?

5. Record your data from C.

Procedure	Emulsion Type	Conclusion

6. To what value do most good surface-active agents lower interfacial tension?

7. Calculate the amount of sodium lauryl sulfate required to emulsify 100 ml of oil to an average globular diameter of 5 microns.

8. Calculate the amount of sodium lauryl sulfate required to emulsify 100 ml of oil to an average globular diameter of 25 microns.

9. What influence does the amount of emulsifying agent have on the globular size of an emulsion?

10. Formulate an anhydrous ointment base containing 1 part beeswax, 12 parts petrolatum, 5 parts mineral oil and 1 part lanolin so that the ointment will readily absorb water, forming a W/O emulsion.

11. Give the HLB values that are optimum for wetting agents, W/O emulsifying agents, solubilizing agents, O/W emulsifying agents and detergents.

12. By means of a diagram show the form in which the excess emulsifying agent (sodium oleate) exists in an O/W emulsion.

13. What is "solubilization"?

14. How would you prepare a clear, antiseptic liquid containing 1% hexachlorophene?

PLASTIC SYSTEMS

29. SUPPOSITORIES

Crystalline solids have molecules or ions oriented so that a particle has a fixed number of plane surfaces inclined to one another at definite and characteristic angles and possesses a definite geometric form. Such a solid is an isotropic system. When stress is applied to an isotropic system, deformation occurs. If the deformation disappears entirely on release of the stress, the system is said to be elastic. Properties of an elastic system are studied by a stress-strain curve.

An amorphous substance is not isotropic, but it is not random because, although the distance between molecules or ions varies, there does exist a network of particles. A plastic system is one in which an external force must be applied to cause deformation or flow of the mass and in which no complete recovery is observed, after release of the stress. The force required to start a plastic flow is termed the yield value. The yield value represents the force required to convert a static system into a dynamic system. This change involves the breaking of bonds between constituent particles in the static system, either in selective planes of deformation or else in all directions with deflocculation accompanied by an increase in particular movement. Suppositories, ointments, and gels are plastic systems.

Suppositories are medicated solid bodies intended for insertion into body cavities such as the rectum, vagina, and urethra. The common vehicles are theobroma oil, substituted theobroma oil, glycerinated gelatin, surface-active bases, and polyethylene glycols. Theobroma oil is widely used in the extemporaneous preparation of suppositories. A rectal theobroma oil suppository is tapered and weighs approximately 2 g; a vaginal theobroma oil suppository is globular or oval and weighs approximately 5 g. A female urethral theobroma oil suppository is pencil shaped and tapered, weighing about 2 g; a male urethral suppository is twice as long.

Theobroma oil suppositories melt at body temperature, and the drug is leeched or partitioned from the molten oil phase. The release of a drug from glycerinated gelatin or polyethylene glycol is not dependent on the temperature as the suppository is soluble in the aqueous mucous secretions.

Some suppositories prepared by pharmaceutical manufacturers are not plastic systems but are compressed solids. Floraquin, Sultrin, and Terramycin Vaginal Tablets are compressed tablets of a shape which facilitates their use as a suppository.

Theobroma oil is composed of a mixture of triglycerides consisting of liquid triglycerides trapped in a network of solid triglycerides. The facts, that the entire structure is not uniform and that the entrapped liquid triglyceride molecules may migrate to a limited extent, prevent theobroma oil from having a sharp melting point. The structure of theobroma oil known as the beta form is the most stable and melts at approximately 35°.

If theobroma oil is overheated in preparing suppositories, all crystalline structures are destroyed. Quick cooling of the overheated theobroma oil results in the theobroma oil solidifying in the less stable polymorphic forms which melt at lower temperatures around 23-25°. Such a suppository would not be firm enough for use at room temperature. Upon standing, such a suppository would spontaneously revert to the more stable beta form. The time required for such a gradual conversion is variable depending on the conditions of manufacture and storage, as well as on the effect of the incorporated drug. Since an extemporaneous prescription must be rapidly available, one cannot wait for this conversion to occur. To maintain the overheated theobroma oil suppository as a solid at room temperature, wax or a suitable high melting-point substance might be added; however, this is not an acceptable method, because upon standing the theobroma oil will revert to the beta form, which in the presence of the wax would produce a suppository that would not melt at body temperature.

The proper procedure in preparing theobroma oil suppositories by the fusion method is to melt the theobroma oil over a water bath until it is liquid enough to pour yet still retains beta crystal nuclei. The remaining beta crystals will serve as nuclei about which the cooling theobroma oil may pattern its crystal structure, and thus solidify in the desired form which is solid at room temperature but melts at body temperature.

Suppositories may be classified within three clinical groups: (a) those used for local effect in the rectum, vagina or urethra, (b) those for relief of constipation, and (c) those used as a vehicle for drugs to be absorbed into the blood stream. In infants and in unconscious and debilitated patients the rectal route replaces the oral route of administration. The rectal route also avoids possible degradation of a drug by the enzymatic activity or pH of the gastrointestinal tract.

In medical literature there is uncertainty of the validity of intrarectal administration of systemically-active drugs. A modern pharmacist should be capable of evaluation of the relative merits of a suppository as a dosage form for drugs. To be available for rectal absorption a drug must be released from the suppository base. In general the rate of diffusion of the drug from the base to the mucosa is the limiting step as subsequent diffusion is very rapid. The availability of the drug is dependent on the physico-chemical properties, e.g., solubility, physical state, partition coefficient, of the drug and on the properties, e.g., melting point, solubility, interfacial tension, of the suppository base. If the release from the suppository base is fast, a high concentration gradient of the drug is present in the rectal fluid and favors passive diffusion into the capillaries of the submucosa, which connects to the hemorrhoidal veins. According to the pH-partition theory of absorption, a pH which results in a large fraction of the drug existing in the un-ionized form favors absorption. With the limited volume of rectal fluid, which contains no buffers, it is the drug which determines the pH in the rectal cavity.

PROCEDURE. The hand method of preparing theobroma oil suppositories has the advantage that it requires no special equipment, all material is divided into the prescribed number of suppositories, and a small number can be made faster than by the fusion method.

The procedure for making suppositories by hand is:

1. Shred or grate the theobroma oil with a kitchen grater. Excessive melting may be avoided by holding the theobroma oil in a piece of paper.
2. Weigh out the required amount of shredded theobroma oil.
3. Weigh out and thoroughly mix the finely divided medicaments in a mortar.
4. Add an equal amount of the grated theobroma oil to the drugs and triturate until uniformly mixed. Continue to add the remainder of the theobroma oil in geometric proportions until all has been added and well mixed.
5. Triturate until a cohesive, plastic mass is formed. Remove the mass from the mortar and knead with the hands for a minute or so until plastic; then form into a crude cylinder. If one desires, the mass may be kneaded through a piece of filter paper.
6. Using a pill tile and a small roller, form a uniform cylinder the diameter of the completed suppository. Excessive pressure will cause the cylinder to split; insufficient pressure will cause the cylinder to be uneven or hollow.

7. Place the cylinder against a measuring device and mark off the prescribed number of suppositories. Using a razor blade, carefully cut off the segments. If properly cut, one end will become the base of the completed suppository.
8. Shape the remaining end of the segment to a tapered point.

Suppositories may be prepared by the cold compression method. The drugs and the theobroma oil are mixed as in the hand method. This mixture is placed in the cylinder of the suppository machine and chilled in a refrigerator. After chilling, the cylinder is fitted into the machine and pressure is applied by means of a handle to force the mixture into the molds.

The mold is calibrated by mixing the drug required for the suppositories with an insufficient amount of theobroma oil to fill the cavities. Then, after this mixture has been forced into the die cavities, more theobroma oil is forced into the cavities until they are filled. The finished suppositories are removed and weighed. The difference between the weight of the finished suppositories and the weight of the drug is the weight of the theobroma oil to be used for the number of suppositories molded.

A. Using the hand method, prepare six rectal theobroma oil suppositories containing 1% Mercurochrome. The incorporation of the dye is facilitated by adding 0.5 ml of purified water to the dye. The viscous liquid formed may then be thoroughly incorporated into the theobroma oil. Save these suppositories for a future exercise.

B. The instructor will demonstrate the operation of the Whitall-Tatum and the Applebaum suppository machines. Using one of these machines, prepare six 0.6 g aspirin suppositories. Record the method of calibration and the amount of each ingredient used.

Heat is used in preparing polyethylene glycol, gelatin, and theobroma oil suppositories. The hot process using theobroma oil is:

1. The calculated amount of grated theobroma oil is melted in a casserole on a water bath at low temperature.
2. The medicaments are triturated until finely divided and added to the molten theobroma oil.
3. The mixture is stirred until it has cooled so that the viscosity is noticeably increased and is poured immediately in an uninterrupted stream into a mold.
4. The filled mold is placed in a refrigerator for several minutes, and any excess material is sliced from the base of the suppository.
5. After a total of fifteen minutes in the refrigerator, the mold is removed and the sections of the mold are separated. The suppositories may be removed by slight pressure.

Generally if the mold has been properly cared for, no lubricant is necessary. To maintain a mold it should be washed with a hot detergent solution after each prescription to avoid pits. Hard instruments should not be used to remove suppositories from the mold, as they damage the polished surface of the mold.

To calibrate a mold, mix the drug for one suppository with insufficient molten cocoa butter to fill the cavity and pour into the mold. Add enough molten theobroma oil to fill the cavity. Allow the suppository to harden and remove from the mold. The difference in weight between the finished suppository and the drug is the amount of theobroma oil required per suppository.

C. Using theobroma oil, prepare by the fusion method six 100 mg bismuth subgallate rectal suppositories. Record your calibration data.

D. Using theobroma oil, prepare by the fusion method six 100 mg bismuth subgallate rectal suppositories. Heat the theobroma oil to 40-50°. Compare the overheated suppositories with those prepared in C.

E. By the fusion method, prepare and save three of the following rectal suppositories:

Mercurochrome	1%
Polyethylene glycol 1540	33%
Polyethylene glycol 6000	46%
Polyethylene glycol 400	20%

F. By the fusion method, prepare and save three of the following rectal suppositories:

Mercurochrome	1%
Span 40	90%
Water	9%

G. By the fusion method, prepare and save three of the following rectal suppositories:

Mercurochrome	1%
Tween 61	89%
Glyceryl monolaurate	10%

H. Using the hand method, prepare and save three of the following rectal suppositories:

Mercurochrome	1%
Glyceryl monostearate	10%
Theobroma oil	85%
Purified Water	4%

I. Using the hand method, prepare and save three of the following rectal suppositories:

Mercurochrome	1%
Cholesterol	2%
Theobroma oil	92%
Purified water	5%

J. Prepare six 1% Mercurochrome glycerinated gelatin suppositories. The U. S. P. method is:

Drug and Purified Water	10%
Gelatin, granular	20%
Glycerin	70%

Thoroughly mix the drug and sufficient water so the mixture constitutes 10% by weight of the finished suppository. Add the glycerin and mix well. Add the gelatin, mix well, avoiding the incorporation of air, and heat on a steam bath until the gelatin has dissolved. Pour in an uninterrupted stream into an unchilled and unlubricated mold. Allow to stand at room temperature until firm. Open and remove the suppositories. If necessary, the suppositories may be dusted with a minimum of talc.

K. Compare the characteristics of the seven suppository bases containing 1% Mercurochrome. Record the appearance and consistency of each.

Place water at body temperature in seven test tubes. Place a suppository of each of the bases containing 1% Mercurochrome into a test tube and record your observations and the time at which any changes occurred.

L. The effect of the suppository base on bioavailability of salicylate from a rectal suppository is determined by the administration of a suppository containing 600 mg of aspirin, and the collection of urine specimens at 2-hour intervals.

Prepare accurately a suppository containing 600 mg of powdered aspirin in the base (theobroma oil; polyoxyethylene (4) sorbitan monopalmitate; or a mixture of 34% polyethylene glycol 1540, 46% polyethylene glycol 6000 and 20% polyethylene glycol 400) assigned by the instructor.

On the day preceding the laboratory period the student voids his or her bladder upon arising and collects a urine specimen to be used as a blank. A suppository is inserted, and a minimum volume of 250 ml of water is taken. Food may be ingested as desired, but no salicylates should be ingested. Defecation should be avoided. Urine specimens are collected every two hours for fourteen hours. The volumes of the urine specimens are measured and recorded, and aliquots are retained in test tubes for analysis in the laboratory. The 14- to 24- hours urine specimens are pooled, the volume is measured, and the specimen is analyzed.

Each aliquot of urine specimen is diluted with water so the salicylate concentration is from 0.1 to 0.5 mg per ml. The dilution depends on the volume of urine, but it is usually from 2- to 5-fold.

To 1.0 ml of diluted urine specimen 5.0 ml of color reagent is added. In each 100 ml of aqueous solution the color reagent contains 4 g of ferric nitrate $[Fe(NO_3)_3 \cdot 9H_2O]$, 4 g of mercuric chloride and 12 ml of N hydrochloric acid. The clear, supernatant liquid is placed in a cuvette and the absorbance is determined using a spectrophotometer at 540 nm. The urine specimen which was collected upon arising is diluted in the same manner, and 1.0 ml of the diluted specimen is mixed with 5.0 ml of the color reagent to provide a blank for each analysis. A standard absorption curve relating the absorbance to concentration of salicylate is provided by the instructor.

Record the time interval of the specimen collected, the volume of each specimen, the absorbance, and the milligrams of salicylate excreted per time interval. Plot the cumulative amount excreted against time. Plot the amount excreted per time interval against time.

REFERENCES

Burt, R. A. P. and A. H. Beckett. 1971. The absorption and excretion of pentazocine after administration by different routes. Br. J. Anaesth. 43:427.

Feldman, S. 1975. Bioavailability of acetominophen suppositories. Am. J. Hosp. Pharm., 32:1173.

Goldstein, A., L. Aronow, and S. M. Kalman. 1974. Principles of drug action: The basis of pharmacology. 2nd ed., John Wiley & Sons, New York, pp. 143-149.

Lieberman, H. A. and J. Anschel. 1976. Suppositories. In The theory and practice of industrial pharmacy. L. Lachman, H. A. Lieberman, and J. L. Kanig, Eds., 2nd ed., Lea and Febiger, Philadelphia, Chap. 8, p. 245.

Parrott, E. L. 1971. Salicylate absorption from rectal suppositories. J. Pharm. Sci., 60:867.

Parrott, E. L. 1973. Student experiments in pharmaceutical technology. VII. Preparation and evaluation of suppository formulations. Am. J. Pharm. Ed. 37:39.

Parrott, E. L. 1975. Influence of particle size on rectal absorption of aspirin. J. Pharm. Sci., 64:878.

Plaxco, J. M., C. B. Free, and C. R. Rowland. 1967. Effect of some nonionic surfactants on the rate of release of drugs from suppositories. J. Pharm. Sci. 56:809.

Saidman, L. J. and E. I. Eger II. 1973. Uptake and distribution of thiopental after oral, rectal and intramuscular administration: Effect of hepatic metabolism and injection site blood flow. Clinic. Pharmacol. Therapeut. 14:12.

Senior, N. 1974. Rectal administration of drugs. In Advances in pharmaceutical sciences. H. S. Bean, A. H. Beckett, and J. E. Carless, Eds., Vol. 4, pp. 363-433. Academic Press, London and New York.

Sevelius, H., R. Runkel, A. Pardo, E. Ortega, J. Varady, and E. Segre. 1973. Naproxen suppository: Tissue response and comparative bioavailability. Europ. J. Clinical Pharmacol., 6:22.

Takuho, T., H. Matsumaru, S. Tsuchiya, and M. Hiura. 1973. Studies on absorption of suppositories. IV. Effect of buffer reagents on absorption of sulfonamides. Chem. Pharm. Bull. 21:1440.

The United States Pharmacopeia. 19th rev. 1975. Suppositories. pp. 703-704.

Suppositories

Data and Conclusions

1. Record the weight of theobroma oil and Mercurochrome used in preparing the suppositories in A.

2. Record the method of calibration and the amounts of ingredients used in preparing six 0.6 g aspirin suppositories in B.

3. Compare the two batches of bismuth subgallate suppositories made in C and D. Explain this difference.

4. What are polyethylene glycols? What is the significance of the number associated with each polyethylene glycol?

5. What system is formed when glyceryl monostearate is mixed with water and theobroma oil? Is an oil-soluble drug released rapidly or slowly from such a system?

6. For various suppository bases containing 1% Mercurochrome, complete the following table:

Base	Appearance	Consistency	Observation in Water at 37°	Speed of Release

7. Which of the bases in 6 would be suitable for rapid release of a water-soluble drug?

8. What factor must be considered in choosing gelatin to be used in preparing a glycerinated gelatin medicinal suppository?

9. An oil-soluble drug has a molecular weight of 165 g $mole^{-1}$. The fusion method is employed to prepare a 2 g theobroma oil suppository containing 300 mg of the oil-soluble drug. Assuming the melting point of theobroma oil is 34° and the molal freezing-point depression constant of theobroma oil to be 6, calculate the temperature at which the suppository will melt.

10. List the offical suppositories.

11. The pH of the blood and rectal fluid is 7.3 and 7.0, respectively. Utilizing the pH-partition theory, rationalize the availability of aspirin (pK_a = 3.5) for absorption when administered rectally.

12. Record the data from L. Show a sample calculation.

Time Interval	Ml of Urine	Dilution	Absorbance	Concentration	Mg Excreted

13. Compare the cumulative milligrams excreted-time curve with those of other students who used different suppository bases. What conclusion can you make concerning the effect of suppository bases on rectal absorption?

30. OINTMENTS

An ointment is a semisolid preparation intended for external application with rubbing; it may be a vehicle for a drug or it may serve as a protective or emollient. Physically, an ointment may be considered as a plastic system such as Petrolatum, Polyethylene Glycol Ointment and Sulfur Ointment, or as an emulsion system such as Rose Water Ointment and Hydrophilic Ointment.

A cream is a soft, cosmetically acceptable O/W or W/O emulsion ordinarily used topically. A paste is an ointment-like preparation intended for external use. A paste may be a single-phase gel, e.g., hydrated pectin, or a fatty paste, e.g., Zinc Oxide Paste, U. S. P., which consists of a thick, stiff ointment that does not flow at body temperature, and therefore serves as a protective coating over the area of application.

Pharmaceutically, ointment bases are classified as oleaginous, absorptive, emulsion, and water-soluble bases. The oleaginous ointments consist of hydrocarbon and glyceride bases. In addition to being stable and inert, the hydrocarbons are bland and have a wide range of melting points which permit blending to form an ointment base of any consistency. As the degree of unsaturation of the acids in glycerides increases, they are more prone to rancidity. From the viewpoint of the patient, oleaginous bases have the disadvantage of being greasy and difficult to remove from the skin; from the viewpoint of the pharmacist, they have the disadvantage of being unable to absorb aqueous liquids. Therapeutically, oleaginous ointments hinder the loss of heat from inflamed areas and prevent drainage from congested, oozing lesions.

Absorptive bases are those which are anhydrous but still readily absorb appreciable amounts of aqueous liquids. For example, Hydrophilic Petrolatum is anhydrous, yet water may be readily incorporated by virtue of the cholesterol present forming a W/O emulsion.

Emulsions used as ointment bases may be either W/O or O/W emulsions. Generally, the O/W or washable ointment base is more readily accepted by the patient because of its esthetic appeal and ease of removal. The washable emulsion base absorbs serous discharges from a lesion and allows the heat in inflamed areas to be easily dissipated. Hydrophilic Ointment, Neobase, Unibase, Multibase, and Dermabase are examples of O/W emulsions; Rose Water Ointment and Hydrous Wool Fat are W/O emulsions.

Although some water-dispersible ointment bases are often listed under the classification of water-soluble ointment bases, polyethylene glycol ointment bases are the only widely used truly water-soluble bases. The polyethylene glycols range from liquids to waxy solids, which permits blending until an ointment of a desired consistency is obtained. As there is the possibility of complex formation between polyethylene glycol and certain drugs, especially phenolic compounds, care must be observed in formulations containing these substances. A strong tendency toward complex formation may retard the release of a drug from the ointment base and even alter the activity of the drug.

A primary requirement for topical therapy is that the drug incorporated in the ointment base reach the surface of the skin at an adequate rate and in a sufficient amount. The efficacy of a drug applied topically is often dependent on the composition of the base. Many of the effects ascribed to a vehicle are consequences of two diffusional processes. The drug must diffuse from the bulk of the vehicle to the surface of the skin, and then it must penetrate the horny layer of the skin. The process, which occurs more slowly, may determine the overall effectiveness of the ointment. The two processes are closely related and dependent upon the physical properties of the drug, vehicle and barrier.

PROCEDURE. Ointments may be prepared by the technique of mechanical mixing, by the use of heat, by the aid of a solvent which facilitates incorporation of the drug, and by complex or chemical interaction.

In the pharmacy mechanical blending is accomplished by use of the mortar and pestle or a slab and a spatula. Generally, the mortar and pestle are preferred when a liquid is to be incorporated or a very stiff and a soft ointment are being mixed. Before adding the drug to the ointment base, it must be in as fine a state of subdivision as practical. It is advisable to use a small amount of a levigating agent to aid in reducing the particle size of insoluble drugs. The levigating agent should be chosen so that it is similar to the base being used. For example, if an oleaginous base is being employed, mineral oil is a satisfactory levigating agent. If a water-dispersible base is being used, glycerin is a suitable levigating agent. Sulfur Ointment illustrates the proper use of a levigating agent.

Industrially, paint mills and roller mills are used to insure reduction of particle size in ointments. Ophthalmic ointments which must not contain particles greater than 2 μ are usually processed in a ball mill.

A. Prepare 30 g of Sulfur Ointment U. S. P.

B. Prepare 30 g of Zinc Oxide Paste U. S. P. The instructor will collect the ointment prepared by the class and demonstrate the operation of an ointment mill.

Ointments are prepared by the fusion method when they contain solid, fusible materials. The simplest procedure is to place all of the ingredients together and melt them simultaneously. Heating should be carried out over a water bath or in a steam kettle.

If the drug is insoluble, it is sifted as a fine powder into the molten base which is stirred until it congeals to insure uniformity. If an aqueous phase is to be added to the molten oily phase, the aqueous phase is heated to the same temperature prior to blending. The final blend is stirred gently, avoiding the incorporation of air, until congealed. It is not generally advisable to attempt to cool the ointment rapidly, because the higher melting point ingredients may separate on the surface of the vessel.

C. Prepare and save for future use 100 g of Cold Cream U. S. P.

D. Prepare and save for future use 100 g of Polyethylene Glycol Ointment U. S. P.

E. Prepare and save for future use 100 g of Hydrophilic Ointment U. S. P.

F. Prepare and save for future use 100 g of White Ointment U. S. P.

G. Develop a formula for and prepare 100 g of stearic acid vanishing cream. Save for future exercise.

A solvent may be used, as in the instance of Epinephrine Bitartrate Ophthalmic Ointment, to dissolve a drug insuring uniform distribution throughout the base. Diluted Alcohol is used to soften the pilular Belladonna Extract prior to incorporation in Belladonna Ointment, chloroform is used to soften Chrysarobin prior to incorporation in Chrysarobin Ointment.

H. Prepare 30 g of Belladonna Ointment N. F. XI

Chemical or complex interaction between a drug and an adjuvant may alter the properties of the drug so that it will more readily be incorporated into the base. In the preparation of Iodine Ointment, the formation of the triiodide ion, which dissolves in glycerin, illustrates this technique.

I. Prepare 30 g of Iodine Ointment N. F. X

No one ointment base is satisfactory for all drugs. From the pharmaceutical aspect, a single base cannot be used for all drugs because of incompatibilities and difficulties of incorporation.

J. Prepare about 10 g of 5% ointments of the following drugs:

1. Peruvian Balsam
2. Coal tar
3. Ichthammol
4. Phenol
5. Salicylic acid

in the following bases:

1. Hydrophilic Ointment
2. Polyethylene Glycol Ointment
3. Cold Cream
4. White Ointment
5. Vanishing Cream

Prepare a chart comparing the ease of incorporation, compatibilities, stability, and other remarks pertinent to the evaluation of the five bases for these five drugs.

Percutaneous absorption is the penetration of a medicinal compound from the surface of the skin into and through the skin into the blood stream. A medicinal compound that is percutaneously absorbed must penetrate consecutively through a surface film of the emulsified lipids, the stratum corneum, the skin barrier, the stratum germinativum, and the dermis into the blood vessels. Colaizzi has reported an uncomplicated procedure using the rabbit to demonstrate the effect of the ointment base on percutaneous absorption.

K. Each group of students will be provided with a white rabbit weighing approximately 3 kg. The rabbit has been fasted for 12 hours prior to the exercise. By use of animal clippers or a depilatory remove the hair from both ears and from the dorsal area between the forelegs and the hind-legs on both sides of the spine. During the exercise the rabbit is to receive no food or water.

Each group of students will use 10% salicylic acid in an ointment base (Hydrophilic Ointment, White Ointment or Polyethylene Glycol Ointment) assigned by the instructor. Weigh 5.0 g of the assigned ointment and spread it uniformly over the surface of a 8 X 8 cm sheet of aluminum foil. Affix the foil with the ointment side in contact with the shaven back of the rabbit by means of adhesive tape. To assure intimate contact between the ointment and the skin, the assembly is covered with two elastic bandages.

A zero time sample of blood is withdrawn from the marginal ear vein. The rabbit is placed in a restrainer. The ear is rubbed briskly to increase its blood supply until the marginal vein becomes distended. Then a small artery clip is placed on the vein near the base of the ear, and a puncture is made 1-2 cm above the clip with a blood lancet. A rapid succession of drops of blood should issue from the puncture upon withdrawal of the lancet. The blood is drawn into a 1 cc syringe fitted with a 1-inch hypodermic needle and containing an anticoagulant (0.1 ml of heparin, 5000 units per ml). When 0.5 ml of blood has been collected, the clamp is removed and a piece of gauze is held on the puncture until bleeding ceases.

The specimen composed of 0.5 ml of blood and 0.1 ml of anticoagulant solution is added to 5.0 ml of color reagent in a centrifuge tube. In each 100 ml of aqueous soltuion the color reagent contains 4 g of ferric nitrate [$Fe(NO_3)_3 \cdot 9H_2O$], 4 g of mercuric chloride and 12 ml of N hydrochloric acid. The centrifuge tube is shaken for several seconds to insure that the precipitated protein is finely dispersed. The tube is then centrifuged at approximately 6000 X g for two minutes. After centrifuging the supernatant liquid is filtered through a small filter into a cuvette. The absorbance of the solution is measured at 540 nm using a suitable blank. The zero time blood specimen serves as a control, and the absorbance is subtracted from the absorbance of subsequent blood specimens.

Blood specimens are withdrawn at ½, 1, 2, and 3 hours after the application of the ointment and analyzed for salicylate. A standard absorption curve relating the absorbance to concentration of salicylate is provided by the instructor.

Record the time interval of the specimen collected and absorbance. Plot the blood concentration expressed in milligram percent against time in hours.

Ophthalmic ointments must be absolutely grit free. It is advisable that ophthalmic ointments be sterile. Petrolatum is often used as a base as it is stable, chemically unreactive, and readily sterilized by heating at 150° for one hour. Ophthalmic ointments must be packaged in collapsible ointment tubes with an ophthalmic tip. Any collapsible ointment tube may be filled in the following steps:

1. Place the ointment in the center of a square piece of paper at least as long as the ointment tube to be filled.
2. Roll the ointment tightly in the paper so that a thin cone is formed.
3. Insert this cone as far as possible into the uncapped, empty tube.
4. Lay the tube on a flat surface, and with a broad spatula held almost flat gradually push the ointment toward the apex of the cone of paper within the tube. Continue advancing the spatula along the paper and along the tube, flattening it until the ointment extrudes from the tip of the tube.
5. Pressing firmly with the spatula on the flattened lower portion of the tube, rapidly jerk the paper from the tube.
6. Replace the cap, trim the lower end of the tube if necessary, and fold over at least once.
7. Place the clip over the folded end so that all folds are covered by the clip and by means of a crimper, crimp the clip firmly into place.

L. Develop a formulation and prepare 5 g of a sterile ophthalmic ointment containing 1000 units of potassium penicillin G per g.

REFERENCES

Allenby, A. C., N. H. Creasey, J. A. G. Edginton, J. A. Fletcher, and C. Schock. 1969. Mechanism of action of accelerants on skin penetration. Br. J. Derm., 81, Supplement 4, 47.

Blank, I. H. 1969. Transport into and within the skin. Br. J. Derm., 81, Supplement 4, 4.

Bowman, F. and S. Holdowsky. 1959. Sterility of antibiotic ophthalmic ointment. J. Am. Pharm. Assoc., Sci. Ed. 48:95.

Colaizzi, J. L. 1970. A laboratory experiment for biopharmaceutics: Percutaneous absorption. Am. J. Pharm. Education 34:185.

Crowell, W. J. 1963. The mechanics of the three roll mill. Am. J. Hospital Pharm. 20:289.

Idson, B. 1975. Percutaneous absorption. J. Pharm. Sci. 64:901.

Ostrenga, J., C. Steinmetz, and B. Poulsen. 1971. Significance of vehicle composition. I. Relationship between topical vehicle composition, skin penetrability, and clinical efficacy. J. Pharm. Sci. 60:1175.

Ostrenga, J., C. Steinmetz, B. Poulsen, and S. Yett. 1971. Significance of vehicle composition. II. Prediction of optimal vehicle composition. J. Pharm. Sci. 60:1180.

Roberts, M. S. and R. A. Anderson. 1975. The percutaneous absorption of phenolic compounds: The effect of vehicles on the penetration of phenol. J. Pharm. Pharmac. 27:599.

Wurster, D. E. 1972. Some practical applications of percutaneous absorption theory. Chapter XI in Advances in Biology of Skin, Vol. XII. Pharmacology and the Skin. W. Montagna, E. J. van Scott, and R. B. Stoughton, Eds. Appleton-Century-Crofts, New York Educational Division, Meredith Corporation.

Ointments

Data and Conclusions

1. Pharmaceutically classify ointment bases.

2. Distinguish between Lanolin and Wool Fat.

3. When should a rubber spatula be used in preparing ointments? Give specific examples.

4. Give your formulation and describe in detail the method of preparation of a stearic and vanishing cream. Calculate how much of the stearic acid was saponified.

5. Give your formulation and describe in detail the method of preparation of a sterile ophthalmic ointment containing 1000 units of penicillin per g.

6. Complete your evaluation of the following bases for the listed drugs:

Bases	Drugs				
	Peruvian Balsam	Coal Tar	Ichthammol	Phenol	Salicylic Acid
Hydrophilic Ointment					
Polyethylene Glycol Ointment					
Cold Cream					
White Ointment					
Vanishing Cream					

7. An anhydrous base is desired which will readily incorporate aqueous liquids forming an W/O emulsion. The base is to contain 5% beeswax, 60% petrolatum, and 25% mineral oil. Suggest how this might be done.

8. When petrolatum is an ingredient in a prescription, what petrolatum must be used?

9. List the advantages of collapsible ointment tubes. When can tubes not be used?

10. Devise a physical method by which the ease of release of a drug from an ointment base could be determined.

11. Give the reaction responsible for rancidity in a triglyceride containing linoleic acid. Why are the final products undesirable?

12. Record the data from K. Show a sample calculation.

Time, hr	Absorbance	Concentration, mg %

Compare the blood concentration-time curve with those of other groups which used different ointment bases. What conclusions can you make concerning the effect of ointment bases on percutaneous absorption?

31. GELS

A gel is a semirigid system in which the movement of the dispersing medium is restricted by an interlacing network of particles or solvated macromolecules of the dispersed phase. The increased viscosity caused by the interlacing and the consequential internal friction is responsible for the semisolid state.

As a hot, colloidal dispersion of gelatin cools, the gelatin macromolecules lose kinetic energy. With a reduction of kinetic energy or thermal agitation, the gelatin macromolecules are associated through dipole-dipole interaction into elongated or threadlike aggregates. The size of these association chains increases to the extent that the dispersing medium is held in the interstices among the interlacing network of gelatin macromolecules, and the viscosity increases to that of a semisolid. Gums, such as agar, Irish moss, algin, pectin and tragacanth, form gels by the same mechanism as gelatin.

Occasionally, the interaction between the particles of the dispersed phase is so great that on standing, the dispersing medium is squeezed out in droplets. The shrinkage of a gel with a simultaneous extrusion of liquid is known as syneresis.

Bentonite is a colloidal hydrated aluminum silicate which is insoluble in water. Bentonite, Laponite, and Veegum are a montmorillonite type of clay in which the units in the structure of the clay are held together by weak O-O association. In the presence of water, these weak O-O associations are broken to an extent, and the clay imbibes water. With the imbibition of water into its structure, the clay swells and effectively the particles spread out and interfere with each other, resulting in an increased viscosity. The amount of free water is reduced as the water dipole is oriented in some manner with the swollen particle and is not free to move at random. At a concentration of 5% bentonite the sum of these two effects produces a gel.

Thixotropy is a reversible gel-sol formation with no change in volume or temperature. Bentonite magmas may form a semirigid gel, which on shaking will revert to a sol. This sol upon standing will re-form to a gel. Thixotropy is a type of non-Newtonian flow and is used pharmaceutically in cough gels, veterinary mastitis ointments, and Sterile Procaine Penicillin G with Aluminum Stearate Suspension to retard the sedimentation of insoluble particles.

Gels have been used as ointments. Jelene or Plastibase is a combination of mineral oils and heavy hydrocarbon waxes with a molecular weight of approximately 1300. The liquid hydrocarbons are held in a matrix of submicroscopic interstices. The rate of cooling such hydrocarbon mixtures seems to affect the gel structure and the final properties of the gel. Mineral oil gels made with aluminum monostearate differ according to the rate of cooling.

Some of the block polymers of surface-active agents derived solely from propylene oxide and ethylene oxide, e.g., Pluronic F-127, lend themselves to the formulation of satisfactory gels suitable for application to a burn wound or abraded skin area.

Suitably plasticized methacrylic gels are used in dentistry as tissue conditioners. They have been shown to be capable of carrying and releasing medicaments used in the treatment of certain lesions of the oral mucosa, and they have been used successfully as periodontal dressings.

PROCEDURE. Gels made from natural products, such as tragacanth and algin, vary in consistency according to the variation in different batches of the natural product. Synthetic materials often are more uniform and yield a reproducible consistency and a more presentable gel.

The United States Patent 2,798,053 describes useful carboxylic polymers obtained when a carboxylic monomer, e.g., acrylic acid or maleic acid, is copolymerized with certain proportions of a polyalkenyl polyether of a polyhydric alcohol containing more than one alkenyl ether grouping per molecule and the parent polyhydric alcohol contains at least four carbon atoms and at least three hydroxyl groups. The resulting polymers are nearly insoluble in water and in most common organic solvents, and they are resistant to hydrolytic degradation of the cross-linkages by strong alkali and acid. Such polymers resemble and are superior to natural gums. They are useful in a variety of formulations including dentifrices, surgical gels, creams, bulk laxatives, ion-exchange resins and as carriers in sustained action medication.

Carbomer 934P is a polymer of acrylic acid cross-linked with a polyfunctional agent. Carbomer N. F. is recognized as an emulsifying agent and a suspending agent. The primary thickening of Carbomer is based on neutralization and the subsequent repulsion of like charges; however, thickening may occur due to hydrogen bonding without neutralization. With the aid of an agitator, Carbopol 934 at pH 3 disperses readily in water, forming a colloidal dispersion with a low viscosity. When neutralized, a gel is formed. Solutions of potassium or sodium hydroxide, sodium carbonate, ammonia, borax, or an amine may be used to adjust the pH.

During vigorous agitation air bubbles are incorporated into an aqueous Carbopol 934 dispersion. Since the dispersion does not gel until neutralized, any bubble formed prior to neutralization can escape from the dispersion. Therefore, instead of neutralizing the dispersion immediately after the polymer and water are mixed, neutralization is delayed until the air bubbles have escaped. The cavitation produced by an ultrasonic unit is effective in removing both dissolved and undissolved air.

The viscosity of the gel increases logarithmically with an increase in pH to a maximum. When sodium hydroxide is used to adjust the pH, a maximum in viscosity is reached at pH 5.6 and maintained until pH 10, after which further increase in alkalinity results in a marked decrease in the viscosity. This plateau in the viscosity-pH curve permits the choice of pH within a wide range with no effect on the consistency of the gel.

Carbopol 934 gels maintain their consistency over a range of pH 5 to 11. They may be autoclaved without loss of viscosity, and the sterilized gels may be of value in controlling the excoriation around fistulas and surgical incisions.

A. Prepare 100 g of a 1% Carbopol 934 gel using 5% sodium hydroxide solution to adjust the pH. Measure the initial pH and viscosity. Add 0.5 ml of the sodium hydroxide solution. Measure the pH and viscosity after each addition. Add the alkaline solution until the gel formed liquifies. Determine the pH at which this occurs. Using semilogarithmic paper, plot the viscosity as ordinate against the pH.

B. Prepare 100 g of an ephedrine gel as follows:

Ephedrine base, hydrous	1.0 g
Carbopol 934	1.0 g
Eucalyptol	0.1 ml
Methyl salicylate	0.01 ml
Pine Needle oil	0.01 ml
Purified water	98.0 ml

Place 70 ml of water in a Waring Blendor, add the Carbopol 934, and blend for 10 seconds. Allow to stand until the entrapped air is released. Transfer to a beaker. Add eucalyptol, methyl salicylate, and Pine Needle Oil and mix with a stirring rod. Dissolve the ephedrine in 28 ml of water and gradually add to the dispersion in the beaker with constant stirring.

Determine the pH and viscosity of the gel formed. Place the gel in collapsible ointment tubes.

Several hydrophilic nonionic surface-active agents form gels when added in sufficient concentrations to water or aqueous systems. The solubilization of oily ingredients and the gelation make them useful in pharmaceutics and cosmetics.

C. Prepare a simple clear gel using Brij 78 or surface-active agent assigned by the instructor as follows:

Brij 78	35.0 g
Purified water	65.0 ml

Heat the Brij 78 to 90° and the purified water to 95°. Add the water to the Brij with agitation. Pour when cooled to 80°.

D. Prepare 400 g of a 5% bentonite gel. Allow the bentonite magma to remain undisturbed until the next laboratory period; then, measure the thixotropy of the gel. Using a Brookfield RVF Viscometer, measure the torque at 0.5, 1.0, 2.5, 5, 10, 20, 50, and 100 rpm and immediately after reaching this speed, measure the torque at 50, 20, 10, 5, 2.5, 1.0, and 0.5 rpm. Plotting the torque in dynes cm as the abscissa, draw two curves – one upward and another downward. The latter should be a straight line. The area between the two curves, a thixotropic hysteresis loop, is a measure of the thixotropy of the system.

E. Prepare 400 g of 6% bentonite gel. Determine the thixotropic hysteresis loop. Compare it with that of a 5% bentonite gel.

Starch Glycerite is a gel prepared by heating starch, glycerin, and water at 140° until the starch membranes rupture and the mass becomes translucent and gel-like. Cold water is used to prepare the original starch paste, as hot water causes starch to form lumps. During preparation, the temperature must be high enough to disperse the starch but not high enough to char the starch or decompose the glycerin.

Aluminum Hydroxide Gel is a suspension of colloidal aluminum hydroxide. Dilute solutions of sodium carbonate and potassium and aluminum sulfate react to form aluminum hydroxide. Since ions decrease the zeta potential and coagulate a colloidal suspension, the sodium and potassium ions are removed by washing or by dialysis.

F. Prepare 30 g of Starch Glycerite N. F.

G. Prepare Aluminum Hydroxide Gel U. S. P. Dissolve 30 g of sodium carbonate monohydrate in 120 ml of hot water and filter. Dissolve 24 g of ammonium alum in 60 ml of hot water and filter into the carbonate solution with constant stirring. Add 120 ml of hot water and allow the gas to dissipate. Dilute to 800 ml with cold water. Collect and wash the precipitate and suspend it in 60 ml of purified water flavored with 0.01% peppermint oil and preserved with 0.1% sodium benzoate.

H. Prepare the following gel which is similar to Ortho-Gynol Vaginal Jelly:

Ricinoleic acid	0.70 ml	Glycerin	5.00 ml
Glacial acetic acid	0.33 ml	Acacia	0.53 g
Hydroxyquinoline sulfate	0.02 g	Tragacanth	3.00 ml
Boric acid	3.00 g	Perfume	0.02 ml
Propylparaben	0.05 g	Purified water	81.00 ml

Determine your method of preparation and the pH of the gel.

REFERENCES

Adams, I. and S. S. Davis. 1973. The formulation and sterilization of a surgical gel based on carboxypolymethylene. J. Pharm. Pharmacol. 25:640.

Addy, M. and W. H. Douglas. 1975. A chlorhexidine-containing methacrylic gel as a periodontal dressing. J. Periodontology 46:465.

Bernstein, H. B. and M. Barr. 1955. Thixotropic measurements of bentonite suspensions. J. Am. Pharm. Assoc., Sci. Ed. 44:375.

Blacow, N. W., Ed. 1972. Martindale. The extra pharmacopoeia. 26th ed. The Pharmaceutical Press, London, England. p. 1076

Block, J. H., E. B. Roche, T. O. Soine, and C. O. Wilson. 1974. Inorganic medicinal and pharmaceutical chemistry. Chapter 8: Gastrointestinal agents. Lea and Febiger, Philadelphia.

Brown, H. P. 1957. Carboxylic polymers. United States patent 2,798,053 assigned to the B. F. Goodrich Company, New York.

B. F. Goodrich Chemical Company, a division of The B. F. Goodrich Company. Carbopol Water-Soluble Resins. Service Bulletin GC-36. Cleveland. pp. 7 and 36.

Discher, C. A. 1964. Modern inorganic pharmaceutical chemistry. John Wiley and Sons, Inc., New York. Chapter 10: Physical phenomena in pharmaceutical practice. I. Amorphous silica, insoluble hydrous oxides, soluble silicates. Chapter 11: Physical phenomena in pharmaceutical practice. II. Relationship between structure and use; the insoluble silicates.

Dittmar, C. A. 1957. A new water soluble polymer for cosmetic compounding. Drug and Cosmetic Industry, 81:446, 532.

Fischer, E. K. 1953. Colloidal dispersions. John Wiley and Sons, Inc., New York.

Foster, S., D. Wurster, T. Higuchi, and L. Busse. 1951. A pharmaceutical study of jelene ointment base. J. Am. Pharm. Assoc., Sci. Ed. 40:123.

ICI United States Inc. 1975. Atlas products for cosmetics and pharmaceuticals. Wilmington, Delaware. p. 36.

Lang, W. 1972. Thickening cosmetics without neutralization. Drug and Cosmetic Industry 110:52 (No.4).

Lin, T. J. 1969. Bubble formation in hydroalcoholic gels. J. Soc. Cosmetic Chemists 20:795.

Lin, T. J. 1971. Mechanism and control of gas bubble formation in cosmetics. J. Soc. Cosmetic Chemists, 22:323.

Neumann, B. S. and K. G. Sansom. 1970. *Laponite* clay – A synthetic inorganic gelling agent for aqueous solutions of polar organic compounds. J. Soc. Cosmetic Chemists, 21:237.

Ober, S., H. Vincent, D. Simon, and K. Frederick. 1958. A rheological study of procaine penicillin G depot preparations. J. Am. Pharm. Assoc., Sci. Ed. 47:667.

Saski, W. 1960. A new concept of ephedrine gel formulation. Drug Standards 28:79.

Schmolka, I. R. 1972. Artificial skin. I. Preparation and properties of Pluronic F-127 gels for treatment of burns. J. Biomed. Mater. Res. 6:571.

Schneiderwirth, H. J. and P. W. Wilcox. 1947. Thixotropic mineral gels and their therapeutic possibilities. J. Am. Pharm. Assoc., Sci. Ed., 36:402.

Secard, D. L. 1962. Carbopol pharmaceuticals. Drug and Cosmetic Industry, 90:28.

Gels

Data and Conclusions

1. Complete the following chart concerning a 1% Carbopol 934 dispersion:

Volume of Alkali Added	pH	Viscosity
0		

2. Complete the following table:

	5% Bentonite	6% Bentonite
Torque Upward curve		
Downward curve		
Area of hysteresis loop		

3. Explain the gel formation between Carbopol 934 and ephedrine.

4. What is the pH of the contraceptive gel prepared in H? What range of pH is commonly satisfactory for such preparations?

5. Why is a hot solution used in preparing Aluminum Hydroxide Gel? How does the particle size influence the therapeutic effectiveness?

6. Aluminum Hydroxide Gel is used as an antacid and as a protective coating for inflamed and ulcerated gastric areas. Explain why the gel does not produce alkalosis and does not interfere with the enzymes which function only in an acidic medium.

7. Discuss the effect electrolytes may have on a gel.

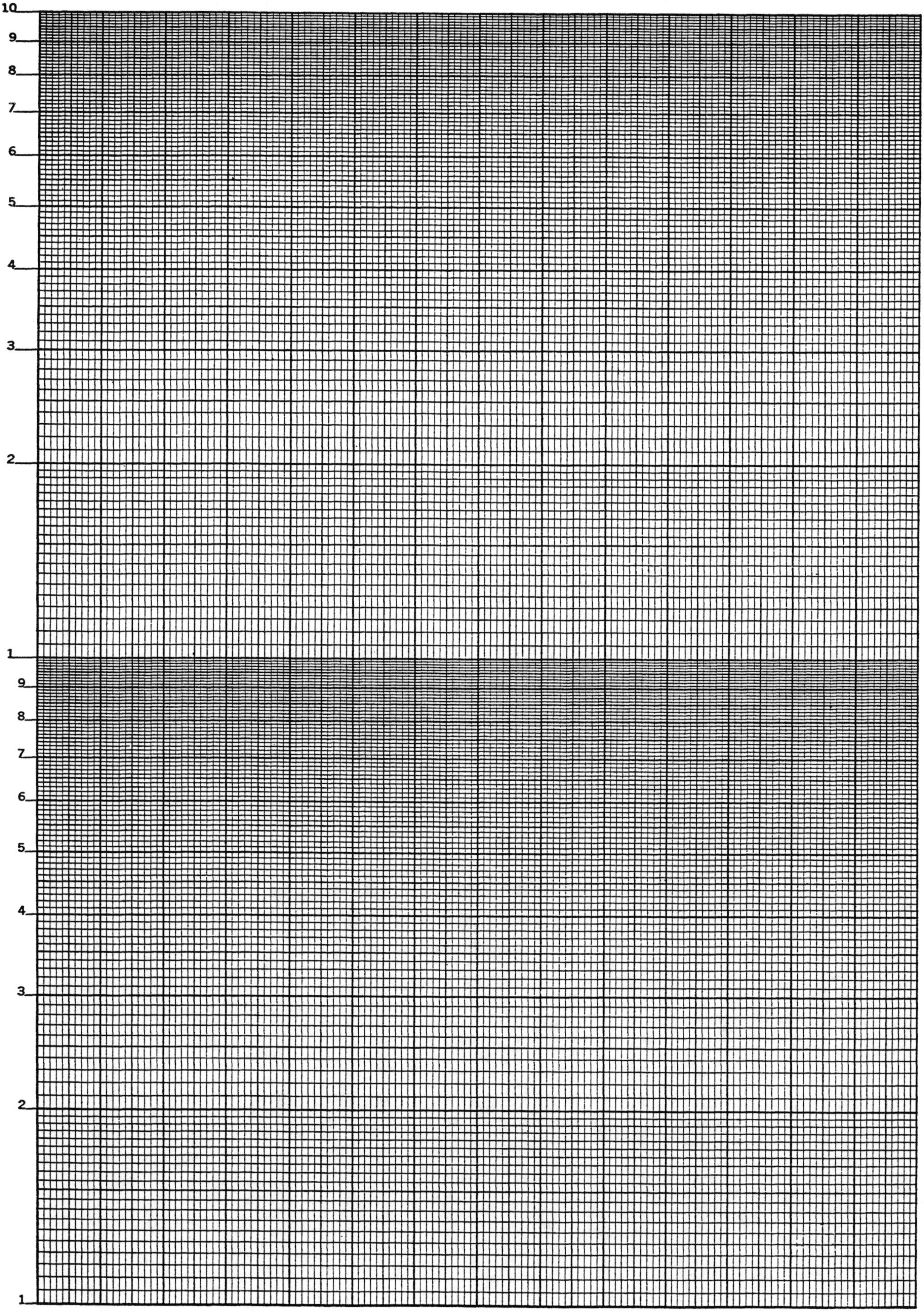
10
9
8
7
6
5
4
3
2
1
9
8
7
6
5
4
3
2
1

APPENDIX

REPRESENTATION OF EXPERIMENTAL DATA

The values of each experimental measurement should include all the certain digits and only the first doubtful digit of the number. Such significant figures indicate the precision of a measurement. If the experimental weight of a powder is recorded as 14.0 g, this indicates that the most probable weight is between 13.7 and 14.3 g. If the experimental weight is recorded as 14.00 g, it indicates that the weight lies between 13.97 and 14.03 g. If the concentration in a solution is 0.0062 moles $liter^{-1}$, the zeros are not significant because they indicate the decimal point, and they express nothing about the precision of the measurement. There are only two significant figures, and the precision and magnitude are best shown by writing the value as 6.2×10^{-3} indicating that the most probable value is between 6.25×10^{-3} and 6.15×10^{-3} moles $liter^{-1}$.

Experimental data may be represented by a table, a graph, or an equation. In the functional table used in the physical sciences, the corresponding values of an independent variable x and a dependent variable y are tabulated side by side. The table should be clearly titled and each column should have a heading giving the name and units of the quantity listed. Tables I and II are typical tables.

Table I – The Relation of Pressure, Temperature, and Volume of 1 Mole of an Ideal Gas

Pressure	Temperature	Volume
0.37 atm	100°K	22.4 liter
0.75	200	22.4
1.0	58	5.0
1.0	125	10.0
1.0	240	20.0
1.0	273	24.0
1.0	360	30.0
1.12	300	22.4
1.50	400	22.4
2.0	273	12.0
4.0	273	6.0

Table II – Serum Level of Theophylline as a Function of Time After the Intravenous Injection of 0.5 g of Theophylline

Time	Concentration
2 hr	0.80 mg/100 ml
4	0.52
6	0.32
8	0.20
10	0.13

In pharmaceutical science it is generally advantageous to plot the data, draw a representative smooth curve, and read the information directly from the curve at the desired points. One of the most important advantages of the graph is that the curve may reveal maxima, minima, inflection points, and other significant features which might be overlooked in a table (see Exercise 24: Viscosity). Tedious or impossible mathematical operations can be performed on the curve. Direct differentiation may be performed by drawing tangents to the curve, and integration may be accomplished by determining the area under a curve.

The first step in preparing a satisfactory graph is to select the correct graph paper. Rectangular coordinate paper is satisfactory for most purposes (see Exercise 7: Some Properties of Solids or Exercise 25: Some characteristics of Interfacial Tension). Semilogarithmic paper is convenient when one of the coordinates is to be the logarithm of an observed variable (see Exercise 24: Rheology). If both coordinates are logarithms of variables, log-log paper may be used. When the functional relationship is unknown, various types of papers are tried until one is found which yields approximately a straight line. Another special paper which has triangular coordinates may be used (see Exercise 23: Characteristics of Colloidal Dispersions).

The independent variable is conventionally plotted along the x-axis or abscissa. The scale is chosen so that the coordinates of any point can be easily and rapidly read. The scale should be numbered so the curve covers the entire graph paper, and the geometrical slope is approximately unity. The variable should be chosen so that the curve approaches a straight line.

The name and the units of each quantity should be given along each axis. Each plotted point should be surrounded by a circle or a suitable symbol. The size of the symbol should correspond to the precision of the measurement.

After the points are plotted, the best smooth curve is drawn through the points. In general, inflections or discontinuities will be absent; however, in some instances an inflection is useful in interpretation, e.g., the inflection in a cooling curve aids in defining the freezing point. The end points should not be emphasized as they are often the least accurate points on the graph. The

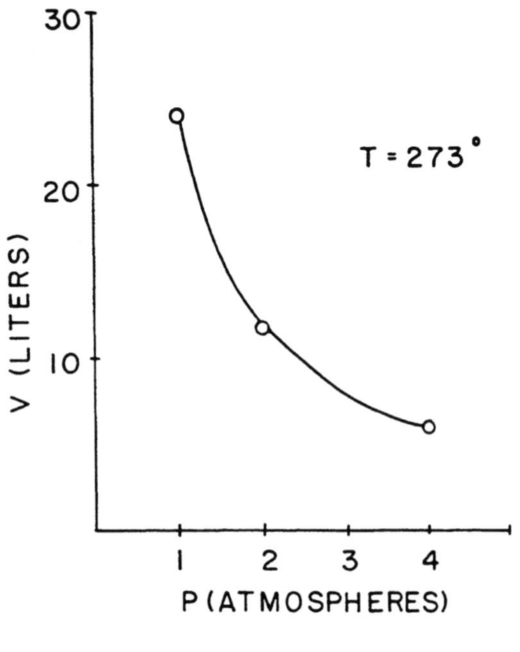

Graph 1 – Volume of one mole of an ideal gas vs pressure at a constant temperature.

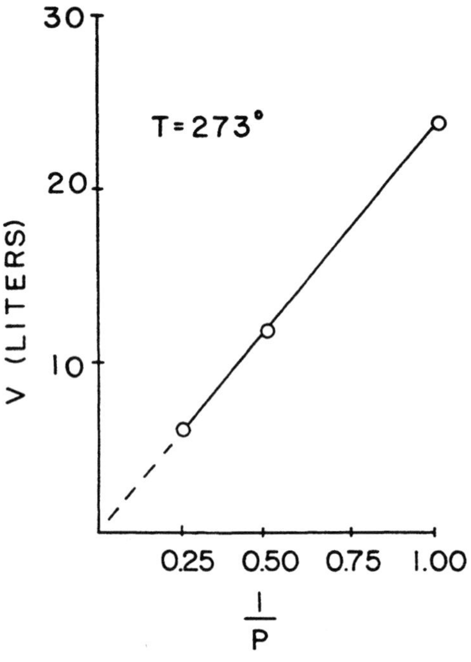

Graph 2 – Volume of one mole of an ideal gas vs reciprocal of pressure at constant temperature.

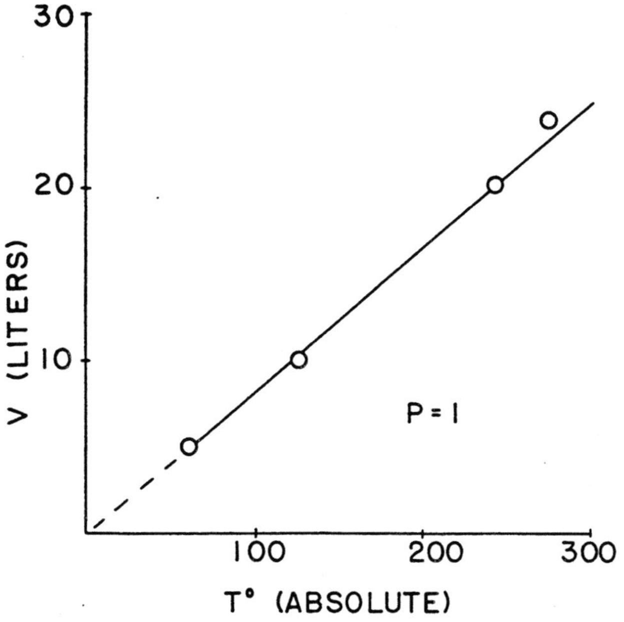

Graph 3 — Volume of one mole of an ideal gas vs temperature at a constant pressure.

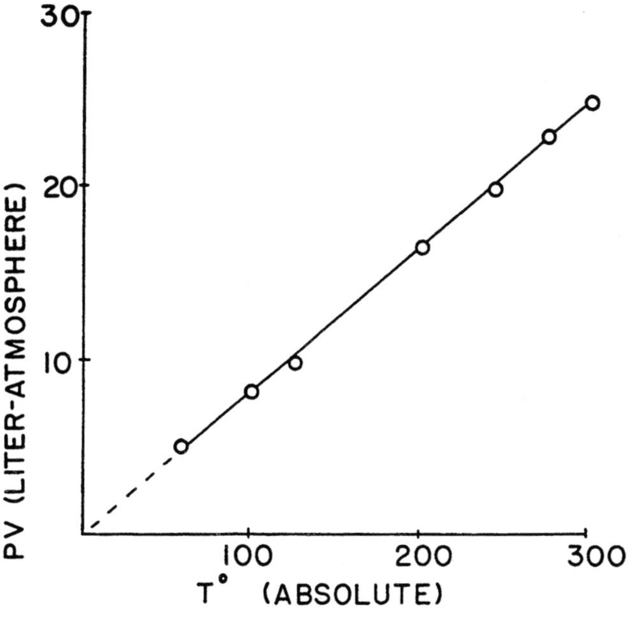

Graph 4 — Relation of volume pressure, and temperature of one mole of an ideal gas.

graph should have a caption which describes the purpose of the plot. Various graphic representations of the data given in Table I are shown above. Notice how the variables in Graph 1 may be arranged to obtain a straight line as plotted in Graph 2.

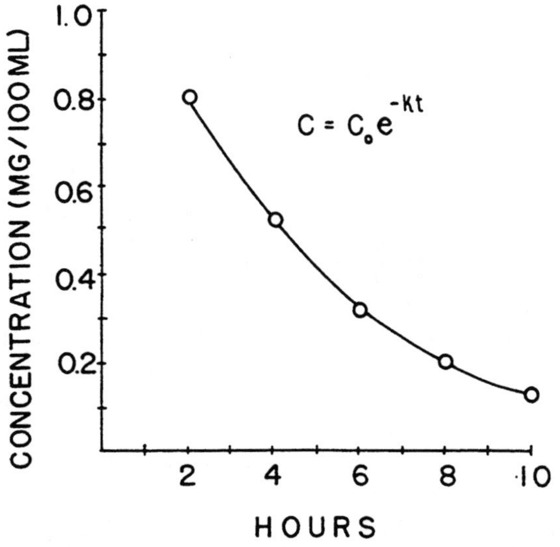

Graph 5 — Serum level vs time after intravenous injection of 500 mg of theophylline.

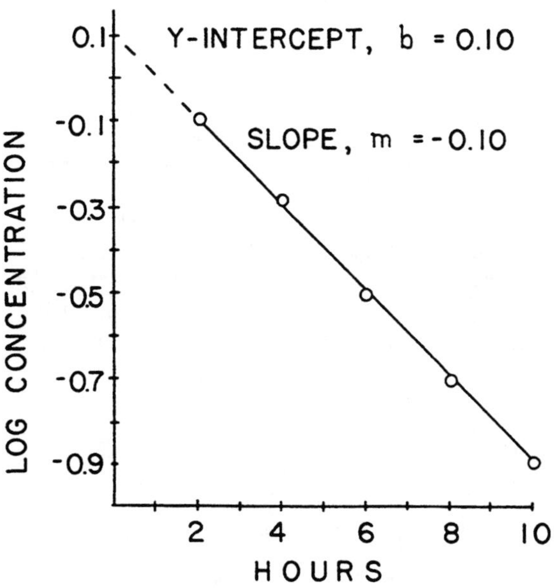

Graph 6 — Serum level vs time after intravenous injection of 500 mg of theophylline.

The data in Table II is plotted in Graph 5 and 6. The semilog plot is the more convenient of the two graphs.

A third variable may be treated on a two-dimensional graph by plotting several curves on a single sheet of paper. In accelerated stability studies of pharmaceutical solutions, the stability constant may be plotted against pH as shown in Graph 7. Three separate curves are plotted at three different temperatures. Thus, basic similarity of the curves and the effect of temperature on degradation are brought out more forcefully than by plotting each curve on a separate paper.

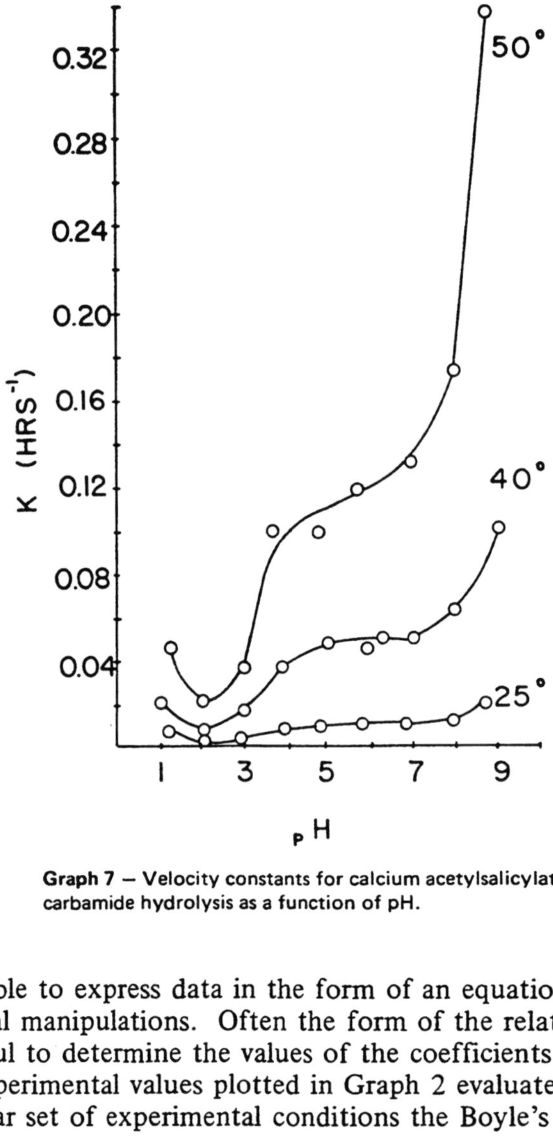

Graph 7 – Velocity constants for calcium acetylsalicylate carbamide hydrolysis as a function of pH.

It is generally desirable to express data in the form of an equation which is compact and convenient for mathematical manipulations. Often the form of the relationship between the variables is known, and it is useful to determine the values of the coefficients in the equation. For example, the slope of the experimental values plotted in Graph 2 evaluate the k_1 of Boyle's equation so that for this particular set of experimental conditions the Boyle's equation is

$$V = \frac{K_1}{P} = \frac{24}{P}$$

Similarly, from Graph 3 the experimental points permit the evaluation of the constant of Charles' equation

$$V = k_2 T = 0.082\,T$$

Graph 4 illustrates the consideration of all three variables in a manner yielding a straight line. This may be expressed as the ideal gas equation for 1 mole

$$PV = RT = 0.082\,T$$

and provides a graphical method of evaluating the gas constant R (see Appendix: Gas Constant).

If the form of the relationship between the variables is not known, the data is plotted and compared with known functions. By proper selection and substitution of variables a straight line graph may be obtained.

The graphic method of evaluation constants in a linear equation is extremely useful. In a first-order rate process a graph of concentration against time produces a curved line as shown in Graph 5; however, if the logarithm of concentration is plotted on rectangular coordinate paper as a function of time, a straight line is obtained as shown in Graph 6. Using the general equation of a straight line,

$$y = mx + b$$

for a first-order rate process the equation becomes

$$\log C = -\frac{kt}{2.3} + \log C_O$$

When the experimental data is plotted, a straight line verifies the validity of the linear equation. The slope of the line is calculated from the coordinate x_1, y_1 and x_2, y_2 of two widely separated points on the line

$$m = \frac{y_2 - y_1}{x_2 - x_1} = \frac{k}{2.3} = \frac{\log C_2 - \log C_1}{t_2 - t_1}$$

If from Graph 6 the 2 and 8 hours points are selected, the slope is

$$m = \frac{-0.1 - (-0.698)}{2 - 8} = -0.10$$

The slope of the line as determined from the graph multiplied by 2.3 evaluates the specific rate constant k; therefore, $k = 0.23\ hr^{-1}$. The constant b, which in the case of a first-order rate process represents $\log C_O$, is numerically equal to the intercept on the y-axis for $x = 0$. At times it may be more convenient to use the determined value of the slope and the coordinates of one point on the line to calculate the constant b

$$b = y_1 - mx_1 = \log C_O$$

$$b = -0.1 - (-0.1 \times 2) = 0.1$$

which compares favorably with the value read directly from the graph. As the constants have now been evaluated, the general equation for this example of a first-order rate process is

$$\log C = \frac{-0.23t}{2.3} + 0.1 = -0.1t + 0.1$$

A method of averages may be used to determine the constants. From two experimental points the constants in a linear equation can be calculated. Usually several experimental points are available, and different values for the constants will be obtained when different experimental points are used in the calculations. In the method of averages all experimental points are used. The correct values of the constants m and b are those that make the sum of the differences between the values of y_c calculated from the empirical equation and the experimentally determined values y_i equal to zero,

$$(y_i - y_c) = mx + b - y_i$$

Therefore, if there are r constants, the $(y_i - y_c)$ values may be divided into r groups with $(y_i - y_c) = 0$ for each group. The groups are selected to contain nearly the same number of experimental values; however, different methods of choosing the groups will lead to different values for the constants. If there are n items in a group, the summation is

$$\Sigma (y_i - y_c) = m\Sigma x_i + kb - \Sigma y_i = 0$$

If the data in Table III is divided into two groups, e.g., (2, 4 and 6 hours) and (8 and 10 hours), the two equations are

$$12\,m + 3\,b - (-0.876) = 0$$

$$18\,m + 2\,b - (-1.585) = 0$$

The values of m and b are calculated from these simultaneous equations to be

$$m = -0.10$$

$$b = 0.11$$

The graphic method and the method of averages give different values of the constants, depending on the judgment of the individual. The method of least squares gives a unique set of values for the constants, and the values of y calculated by using the constants found by this method are the most probable values of the observations, assuming a normal distribution of error. Accordingly, the probability of obtaining the observed value y_i is a maximum when $\Sigma\,(y_i - \bar{y})^2$ is a minimum. The principle of least squares states that the best representative curve is that for which the sum of the $(y_i - \bar{y})$ values is a minimum,

$$S = \Sigma\,(x_i m + b - y_i)^2$$

$$S = m^2\Sigma x_i^{\,2} + 2bm\Sigma x_i - 2m\Sigma x_i y_i + nb^2 - 2b\Sigma y_i + \Sigma y_i^2$$

The required conditions for a minimum are

$$\frac{\sigma S}{\sigma m} = 0 = 2m\Sigma x_i^2 + 2b\Sigma x_i - 2\Sigma y_i x_i$$

$$\frac{\sigma S}{\sigma b} = 0 = 2m\Sigma x_i + 2bn - 2\Sigma y_i$$

To calculate the constants it is necessary to calculate Σx_i, Σy_i, Σx_i^2, and $\Sigma x_i y_i$ as shown in Table III. Upon substituting these values the preceding equations become

$$30\,m + 30b + 18.74 = 0$$

$$30\,m + 5b + 2.41 = 0$$

and by solving simultaneously

$$m = -0.1$$

$$b = 0.1$$

Calculations by the method of least squares is time-consuming and is reserved for data that has a high degree of precision.

Table III – Calculations Required to Apply the Method of Least Squares to the Experimental Data of Table II

	Time x	Concentration C	log C y	x^2	xy
1	2 hr	0.80 mg/100 ml	-0.0947	4	- 0.194
2	4	0.52	-0.2840	16	- 1.136
3	6	0.32	-0.4949	36	- 2.970
4	8	0.20	-0.6990	64	- 5.592
5	10	0.13	-0.8861	100	- 8.861
Σ	30		-2.4609	220	-18.743

EXPONENTS

Small numbers are conveniently manipulated by expressing the numbers as powers of 10. For example, 0.00015 may be expressed as 1.5×10^{-4}. The first part is the coefficient and the second is the exponential factor of 10.

An exponent is a symbol written above and to the right of another symbol denoting how many times the latter is repeated as a factor.

The properties of exponents are:

1. In the process of multiplication, exponents are added and the coefficients are multiplied.

$$a^x a^y = a^{x+y}$$

$$1.5 \times 10^{-4} \times 5 \times 10^{2} = 7.5 \times 10^{-2}$$

2. A product raised to a power is equal to the product of each factor raised to the given power.

$$(ab)^x = a^x b^x$$

$$(1.5 \times 6)^2 = (1.5^2)(6^2) = 81$$

3. When an exponent is raised to a power, the exponent and the power are multiplied

$$(a^x)^y = a^{xy}$$

$$(\pi^2)^{4/3} = \pi^{8/3}$$

4. If $a \neq 0$, the negative exponent of a number is equal to the reciprocal of that number raised to the positive exponent

$$a^{-x} = \frac{1}{a^x}$$

$$125^{-1/2} = \frac{1}{125^{1/2}} = 0.089$$

5. In the process of division, exponents are subtracted and coefficients are divided

$$\frac{a^x}{a^y} = a^{x-y}$$

$$\frac{28 \times 10^6}{6 \times 10^{23}} = 4.67 \times 10^{-17}$$

LOGARITHMS

The logarithm of a positive number, N, to a given positive base, b, other than 1, is the exponent of the power, x, to which the base must be raised to equal the number

$$N = b^x \text{ or } \log_b N = x.$$

Thus, in the exponential form, $100 = 10^2$ and in the logarithmic form, $2 = \log_{10} 100$.

While any positive number, except 1, may be chosen as a base of a system of logarithms, two bases are most commonly used. The common logarithms use the base 10 and are designated as log. The natural logarithms use as a base the irrational number e (2.71828) and are designated as ln. Multiplying the common logarithm by 2.303 converts it to the natural logarithm

$$2.303 \log N = \ln N.$$

A logarithm consists of an integer known as the characteristic, and a decimal known as the mantissa. The characteristic determines the position of the decimal point in the number; the mantissa determines the actual digits and is independent of the decimal point.

The characteristic of a number may be found using the following rules:

1. The characteristic of any number greater than 1 is one less than the number of digits before the decimal point.
2. The characteristic of any number less than 1 is negative and is found by subtracting from 9 the number of ciphers between the decimal point and the first significant digit, and writing - 10 after the result.

The common logarithms of the same sequence of digits have the same mantissa. To find the mantissa in a four-place logarithm table, look in the column marked N for the first two digits and pick the column headed by the third digit—the mantissa is the number appearing at the intersection of this row and column.

For example, to find log 229 using a four-place logarithm table, first determine the characteristic which is 1 less than the number of digits before the decimal or 2. The mantissa is found by following the row after the number 22 until it intersects with the column under 9 or .3598. The log 229 = 2.3598.

When the characteristic is negative, it is often more convenient to use an equivalent form, writing the characteristic as the difference of two positive numbers of which the second is a multiple of 10. Thus, a -1 is equivalent to 9 - 10, and a -12 is equivalent to a 8 - 20.

For example, to find the log 0.0229, first determine the characteristic which is found by subtracting 1 from 9, and writing -10 after the result. The mantissa is found exactly as shown in the previous example. The logarithm may be expressed

$$\log 0.0229 = 8.3598 - 10 = -2 + 0.3598 = -1.6402.$$

To find the number corresponding to a given logarithm, the process is reversed. The number found is known as the antilogarithm. The sequence of digits of the given mantissa is found in the table, and the proper position for the decimal point in this sequence of digits is determined by the given characteristic.

For example, if the log N = 0.6990, examination of the logarithm tables shows the antilogarithm to be 500. The characteristic shows that there is one digit before the decimal. Thus, the number is 5.

The logarithm of the reciprocal of a number is equivalent to the negative logarithm of the number

$$\log \frac{1}{N} = \log 1 - \log N = -\log N.$$

The negative logarithm of a number can be found by subtracting the logarithm of the number from 10.0000-10.

For example, to determine -log (5 X 10^{-5}) first find the logarithm and subtract from 10.0000-10,

$$\log (5 \times 10^{-5}) = \log 5 + \log 10^{-5} = 0.6990 + (5.000 - 10) = 5.6990 - 10$$

$$\begin{array}{r} 10.0000 - 10 \\ \underline{5.6990 - 10} \\ 4.3010 \end{array}$$

Thus, - log (5 X 10^{-5}) = 4.3010.

If the negative logarithm is known, reversal of the previous operation will provide the number. For example, if - log N = 6.8, multiply by -1 to obtain log N = -6.8, then convert this logarithm to one with a positive mantissa by adding to 10.0000 - 10, and find the antilogarithm

$$\begin{array}{r} 10.0000 - 10 \\ \underline{-\ 6.8 \qquad\quad} \\ 3.2000 - 10 \end{array}$$

$$\log N = 3.2000 - 10$$

$$N = 0.000000158 \text{ or } 1.58 \times 10^{-7}.$$

Calculations are often simplified by using the properties of logarithms. Three properties of logarithms taken to the same base are:

1. The logarithm of a product is equal to the sum of the logarithms of its factors.

   $$\log AB = \log A + \log B$$

   $$\log (525 \times 27) = \log 525 + \log 27 = 2.7202 + 1.4314 = 4.1516$$

   Using four-placed logarithm tables the antilogarithm of .1516 is 142 and from the characteristic the number corresponding to this multiplication is 1.42 X 10^4.

2. The logarithm of a quotient is equal to the logarithm of the dividend minus the logarithm of the divisor.

   $$\log \frac{A}{B} = \log A - \log B$$

   $$\log \frac{4.7 \times 10^{-5}}{1.9 \times 10^{-3}} = \log (4.7 \times 10^{-5}) - \log (1.9 \times 10^{-3})$$

   $$\begin{array}{lr} \log 4.7 = & 0.6721 \\ \log 10^{-5} = & \underline{-5 \qquad} \\ & -4.3279 \end{array}$$

   $$\log 1.9 = 0.2788$$

$$\log 10^{-3} = \underline{-3}$$
$$-2.7212$$

$$\log \frac{4.7 \times 10^{-5}}{1.0 \times 10^{-3}} = -4.3279 - (-2.7212) = -1.6067$$

$$\begin{array}{r} 10.0000 - 10 \\ \underline{-1.6067} \\ 8.3933 - 10 \end{array}$$

Antilog .3933 = 247 and with a characteristic of -2 the number is 0.0247.

3. The logarithm of a power of a number is equal to the exponent times the logarithm of the number.

$\log A^p = p \log A$

$\log 2.7^{0.3} = 0.3 \log 2.7 = 0.3 \times 0.4314 = 0.1294$

Antilog .1294 = 135 and with a characteristic of 0 the number is 1.35.

TRIGONOMETRIC TERMS

The following definitions are based on the right angle triangle ABC:

$$\text{sine } \alpha = \frac{\text{opposite side}}{\text{hypotenuse}} = \frac{a}{c}$$

$$\text{cosine } \alpha = \frac{\text{adjacent side}}{\text{hypotenuse}} = \frac{b}{c}$$

$$\text{tangent } \alpha = \frac{\text{opposite side}}{\text{adjacent side}} = \frac{a}{b}$$

$$\text{cotangent } \alpha = \frac{\text{adjacent side}}{\text{hypotenuse}} = \frac{b}{a}$$

$$\text{secant } \alpha = \frac{\text{hypotenuse}}{\text{adjacent side}} = \frac{c}{b}$$

$$\text{cosecant } \alpha = \frac{\text{hypotenuse}}{\text{opposite side}} = \frac{c}{a}$$

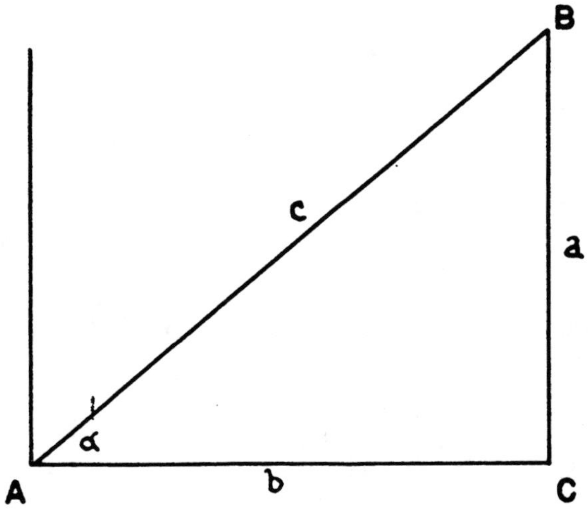

DIFFERENTIATION

DEFINITIONS. A variable is a quantity that may have different values. A constant is a quantity that retains the same value throughout any given system.

A variable, y, is said to be a function of another variable, x, if for every one of some set of values of x, there corresponds a value of y. Mathematically, the statement "y is a function of x" is written $y = f(x)$ which is read "y is the f of x."

LIMIT OF A VARIABLE AND OF A FUNCTION. The concept of a limit is essential to understanding the differential. Consider a bead with a hole strung on a wire so that the bead is movable. Let a black spot on the wire represent a fixed point whose abscissa is a. The statement, "the variable x approaches the constant a," is analogous to the bead moving along the wire. Permit the bead to come closer to the spot than 0.1 mm. Then mark off on each side of the spot 0.1 mm intervals. Move the bead until it gets between the marks and never let it out again. It may now be said that the bead comes and remains closer than 0.1 mm to the spot.

The intervals or increments can be made as small as one desires, and the bead enters and remains inside this interval. At no time is there any consideration that the bead will actually coincide with the black spot—nothing has been said to imply that x is eventually equal to a. There is no interest in having $x = a$; it is what is going on close to a that is of interest.

To expand further on the concept of a limit, consider the equation

$$x_n = \frac{n}{n+1}$$

where $x_1 = \frac{1}{2}, x_2 = \frac{2}{3}, x_3 = \frac{3}{4}, \ldots$

If these points are plotted along the x-axis, it appears that x is approaching 1. If this is a fact, one must be able to surround 1 by an interval as small as desired so that eventually all the remaining plotted points will all fall inside the interval.

Choose an interval of width 2/100 of which 1 is the middle point. Now, one expects the differences

$$1 - \frac{1}{2}, 1 - \frac{2}{3}, 1 - \frac{3}{4}, \ldots 1 - \frac{n}{n+1}$$

will become and remain less than 1/100. To see whether or not they will, consider

$$1 - \frac{n}{n+1} = \frac{n+1-n}{n+1} = \frac{1}{n+1}.$$

Evidently, $\frac{1}{n+1} < \frac{1}{100}$ if $n + 1 > 100$, that is, if $n > 99$. It can be said with certainty that $1 - x_n$ will be numerically less than 1/100 provided only that n is greater than 99. Thus, the difference in question eventually becomes and remains numerically less than 1/100. Symbolically, this may be stated, using vertical bars to mean abstract values,

$$|1 - x_n| < 1/100 \qquad \text{for all } n > 99.$$

This does not mean that x is approaching 1; it says that x eventually differs from 1 by less than 1/100 and that x might eventually reach 999/1000 and still satisfy this equation.

It must be assured that the difference between 1 and x will become and remain less than any arbitrarily small positive number. Determine if $|1 - x_n|$ will be less than some arbitrarily small number, e = 1/N.

Now

$$|1 - x_n| = 1 - \frac{n}{n+1} = \frac{1}{n+1}$$

will be less than e = 1/N if n + 1 > N = 1/e. For brevity using symbols,

$$|1 - x_n| < e = 1/n \quad \text{for all} \quad n > \frac{1}{e} - 1 = N - 1.$$

Now it is certain that x approaches 1 (written $x \longrightarrow 1$) since no matter how small an interval al (of width 2e) is chosen to surround 1, all values, after a certain one, assumed by x fall inside this interval. This certain value of x depends only on the size of the interval chosen. This discussion should clarify what is meant by the statement "that x is approaching a value" so that the limit of a function may now be discussed.

Consider y as a function of x defined by the equation

$$y = \frac{2x^2 - 2x}{x - 1}$$

The interest lies in what happens to y as x approaches 1. If x = 1 is substituted in the equation, it takes the meaningless form 0/0, which is not defined. Examine the values of x tabulated and notice that it appears that y is approaching 2.

x	1.1	1.01	1.001	1.0001	1.00001
y	2.2	2.02	2.002	2.0002	2.00002

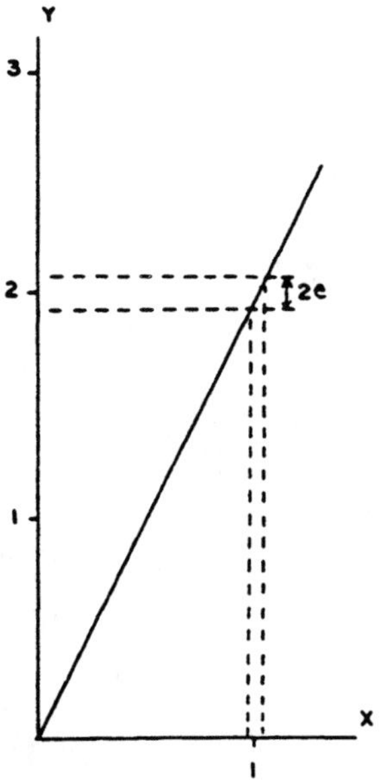

To test this observation, note that

$$y = \frac{2x(x-1)}{x-1} = 2x$$

for every value of x except x = 1. Thus,

$$|y - 2| = |2x - 2| = 2|x - 1|$$

can be arbitrarily small by taking x close to 1.

This may also be interpreted graphically. When drawn, the equation is that of a straight line with a single point omitted. The omitted point has an abscissa of 1 for which y is not defined.

Draw a horizontal strip of width 2e. All points in this strip have ordinates that differ from 2 by less than e. From where these horizontal lines intersect the curve, draw vertical lines to intersect the x-axis.

When the value of any point between 1 and the intersections on the x-axis is substituted for x in the equation, the resulting value of y will differ from 2 by less than e. It is then said that the limit of y is 2 as x approaches 1. This illustrates that the function y may be a limit as x approaches some particular value, although the function may be undefined for the value of x in question.

If y = f(x) is a function of x and if y approaches b as x approaches a, the limit of y is b as x approaches a and is written

$$\lim_{x \to a} y = b \quad \text{or} \quad \lim_{x \to a} f(x) = b.$$

The limit of a function may now be defined. If y = f(x) is a function of x, than y is said to have a limit, b, as x approaches a, provided that the numerical value of the difference between y and b becomes and remains less than any arbitrarily assigned small positive number for all values of x close enough, but not equal, to a.

Expressed symbolically, the limit of f(x) is said to be b as x approaches a if for any preassigned number $e > 0$ there exists a number $\delta > 0$ such that for $0 < |x - a| < \delta$ so that $|f(x) - b| < e$.

It must be emphasized that this definition and the idea of a limit has nothing to do with the value of the function y for x = a. It must be recognized that x may approach a in any manner.

VARIABLES BECOMING INFINITE. A variable is said to become infinite if it becomes and remains larger than any arbitrarily given number. Consider the function for which a graph is given

$$y = \frac{2}{x}.$$

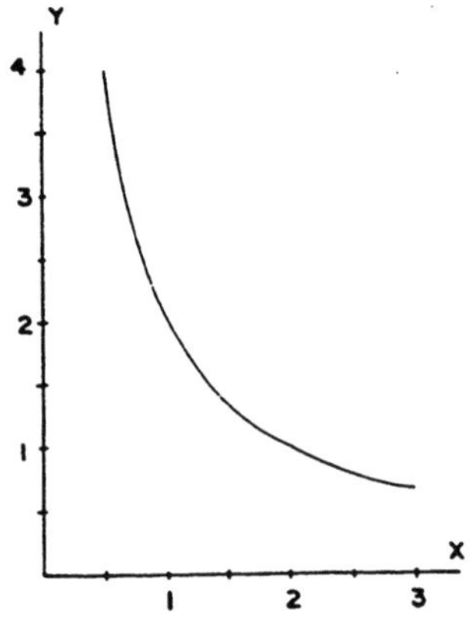

When x approaches 0, the function, y = 2/x, has no limit but may be numerically as large as desired by making x close enough to 0. It is said that "y becomes infinite as x approaches 0" and it is symbolically written

$$y \to \infty \quad \text{as} \quad x \to 0.$$

This says that y is a variable which becomes and remains numerically greater than any number we care to assign, or "y increases numerically without limit." It is not to be erroneously thought that ∞ represents some very large, although unknown, number.

DERIVATIVE. An understanding of the derivative is essential to the discussion and comprehension of the rates of change in many pharmaceutical functions. Perhaps the simplest way to investigate the properties of any function is to consider its curve. For example, the curve $y = \frac{1}{2}x^2$ is a continuous curve for all values of x. It can be shown that the curve has a tangent for every point on the curve.

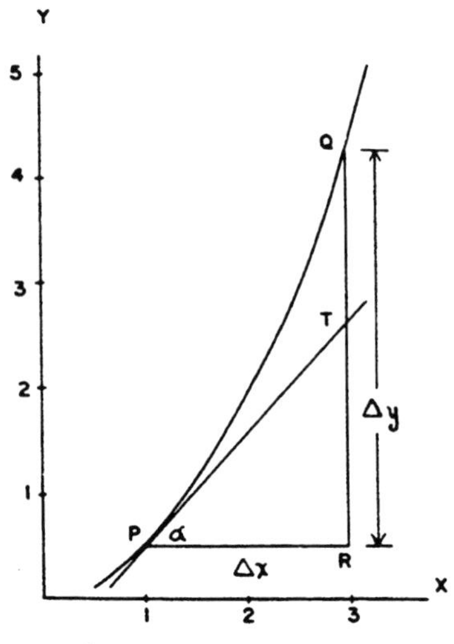

The tangent to the curve at point P (1, ½) is defined as follows: Let P be a fixed point on the curve and Q any other point on the curve. The tangent at P is the limiting position PT of the secant PQ as Q approaches P along the curve from either side of P. Draw PR parallel to the x-axis and RQ parallel to the y-axis.

This definition is equivalent to saying that the limit of the variable angle RPQ is a fixed angle α as Q approaches P along the curve; and if $\alpha \neq 90°$, this is equivalent to saying that the limit of RQ/PR = tan RPQ as Q approaches P along the curve.

Returning to point P (1, ½) of the curve $y = \frac{1}{2}x^2$, designate the distance PR by Δx (read delta x and to be considered as a single symbol, not as a product) and the distance RQ by Δy. Then Q has the coordinates $(1 + \Delta x, \frac{1}{2} + \Delta y)$, and tan RPQ = $\Delta y/\Delta x$. Note that as Q is to the right and above P, RQ and RP are positive, but if Q is to the left and below P, then RQ and PR are negative; however, in both cases RQ/PR = $\Delta y/\Delta x$ is positive.

If Q approaches P from either side of the curve, Δx approaches O. So, if $\Delta y/\Delta x$ has a limit as Δx approaches O, this limit must be tan α. Suppose Q is the point (2, 2). Then, the value $\Delta y/\Delta x$ may be determined,

$$\Delta x = \text{abscissa of Q minus abscissa of P} = 2 - 1 = 1$$
$$\Delta y = \text{ordinate of Q minus ordinate of P} = 2 - \tfrac{1}{2} = 3/2$$

and

$$\frac{\Delta y}{\Delta x} = \frac{3}{2} \div 1 = \frac{3}{2}$$

Other values of $\Delta y/\Delta x$ are tabulated:

Abscissa of P	Abscissa of Q	Δx	Ordinate of P	Ordinate of Q	Δy	$\frac{\Delta y}{\Delta x}$
1	2	1.0	0.5	2.0	1.5	1.5
1	1.5	0.5	0.5	1.125	0.625	1.25
1	1.1	0.1	0.5	0.605	0.105	1.05
1	1.01	0.01	0.5	0.51005	0.01005	1.005
i	1.001	0.001	0.5	0.5010005	0.0010005	1.0005

It appears that $\Delta y/\Delta x$ is approaching 1. To find the ordinate of Q we need only to replace x by $1 + \Delta x$ in the equation $y = \frac{1}{2}x^2$,

$$\text{ordinate of Q} = \tfrac{1}{2}(1 + \Delta x)^2 = \tfrac{1}{2}(1 + 2\Delta x + \Delta x^2)$$
$$= \tfrac{1}{2} + \Delta x \tfrac{1}{2} + \Delta x^2$$

To find Δy we subtract from this ordinate of Q the ordinate of P or ½

$$\Delta y = \Delta x + \tfrac{1}{2}\Delta x^2$$

Thus

$$\frac{\Delta y}{\Delta x} = 1 + \tfrac{1}{2}\Delta x$$

and

$$\lim_{\Delta x \to 0} \frac{\Delta y}{\Delta x} = \lim_{\Delta x \to 0} (1 + \tfrac{1}{2}\Delta x) = 1$$

It is now certain that the curve has a tangent at P and the direction, since its slope is 1, is an angle of 45° with the horizontal.

Other points, P, may be investigated. Suppose P has the coordinates (x, y). For any point Q on the curve the coordinates are $(x + \Delta x, y + \Delta y)$. Again tan RPQ $= \Delta y/\Delta x$, and it can be determined if $\Delta y/\Delta x$ has a limit as Δx approaches the 0.

As before placing the coordinates of Q in the equation one obtains

$$y + \Delta y = \tfrac{1}{2}(x + \Delta x)^2 = \tfrac{1}{2}x^2 + x\Delta x + \tfrac{1}{2}\Delta x^2.$$

To find Δy subtract the ordinates of P from the ordinate of Q giving

$$\Delta y = x\Delta x + \tfrac{1}{2}\Delta x^2.$$

So that

$$\frac{\Delta y}{\Delta x} = x + \tfrac{1}{2}\Delta x$$

and therefore

$$\lim_{\Delta x \to 0} \frac{\Delta y}{\Delta x} = \lim_{\Delta x \to 0} (x + \tfrac{1}{2}\Delta x) = x.$$

Since it is known that $\lim_{\Delta x \to 0} \frac{\Delta y}{\Delta x}$ is tan α, at any given point on the curve tan α is equal to the abscissa of that point.

The remarks made may be generalized. Given a function, $y = f(x)$, that is continuous and single-valued throughout an interval, say $a \leqq x \leqq b$, the slope of the tangent may be found for any point. Let a point be P (x, y) and let Q be another point on the curve. The coordinates of Q are $(x + \Delta x, y + \Delta y)$. To calculate the ordinate of Q, replace x by $x + \Delta x$, obtaining

$$y + \Delta y = f(x + \Delta x)$$

To find Δy, subtract the ordinate of P from this ordinate

$$\Delta y = f(x + \Delta x) - f(x)$$

Hence

$$\frac{\Delta y}{\Delta x} = \frac{f(x + \Delta x) - f(x)}{\Delta x}$$

and therefore

$$\lim_{\Delta x \to 0} \frac{\Delta y}{\Delta x} = \lim_{\Delta x \to 0} \frac{f(x + \Delta x) - f(x)}{\Delta x}$$

RATE OF CHANGE OF A FUNCTION. The function $y = \tfrac{1}{2}x^2$ may be regarded from a different viewpoint by a chemist or a pharmacist. Instead of a graphical interpretation, they would be interested in how fast y increases with an increasing x. Examination of the curve shows that near $x = 0$, the curve rises slowly and y changes slowly with increasing x, whereas for large values of x the curve rises rapidly and y changes rapidly with increasing x. The rate of change of the function y is not a constant but varies with x.

To find the average rate of change of y between $x = 1$ and $x = 2$, compute the number of units change in y and divide by the number of units change in x. When $x = 1$ and $y = \tfrac{1}{2}$ and when $x = 2$ and $y = 2$, the change in y is $\Delta y = 2 - \tfrac{1}{2} = 3/2$. The change in x is $\Delta x = 1$. The average rate of change of y between the two values of x is

$$\frac{\Delta y}{\Delta x} = \frac{3}{2} \div 1 = \frac{3}{2}$$

Then $\frac{\Delta y}{\Delta x}$ is the average rate of change of y between the original and new values of x. This average rate of change of y approaches 1 as a limit as the interval Δx is made to approach 0. This limit is called the instantaneous rate of change of y at the point where x = 1 or at the point (1, ½).

The rate of change of y at any point (x, y) of the function $y = \frac{1}{2}x^2$ may be found. The original value of x is x and the original value of y is $y = \frac{1}{2}x^2$. The new value of x is $x + \Delta x$ and the new value of y is

$$y + \Delta y = \tfrac{1}{2}(x + \Delta x)^2$$

The change in y is

$$\Delta y = x\Delta x + \tfrac{1}{2}\Delta x^2$$

and

$$\frac{\Delta y}{\Delta x} = x + \tfrac{1}{2}\,\Delta x.$$

Therefore, the rate of change of y at the point (x, y) is

$$\lim_{\Delta x \to 0} \frac{\Delta y}{\Delta x} = x.$$

In general, the average rate of change of the function y = f(x) between two values of x is simply the new value of y minus the original value of y divided by the new value of x minus the original value of x,

$$\frac{\Delta y}{\Delta x} = \frac{f(x + \Delta x) - f(x)}{\Delta x}$$

and the rate of change of y at the point (x, y) is

$$\lim_{\Delta x \to 0} \frac{\Delta y}{\Delta x} = \lim_{\Delta x \to 0} \frac{f(x + \Delta x) - f(x)}{\Delta x}$$

The result is expressed in number of units change in y per unit change in x.

DERIVATION OF A FUNCTION. The calculations involved in finding the slope of the tangent line to a curve and in calculating the rate of change of a function are exactly the same. The difference is in terminology and viewpoint. These two examples have been given to introduce a concept. A general process and definition entirely independent of these examples may now be introduced.

Let y = f(x) be a function that is single-valued and continuous in the interval $a \leq x \leq b$. Let (x, y) be any particular pair of numbers satisfying the equation, y = f(x) and having x in the specified interval. Then

1. Let x receive an increment Δx. Replace x by $x + \Delta x$, obtaining a new value of y

$$y + \Delta y = f(x + \Delta x)$$

2. Subtract the original value of y from the new value of y to obtain Δy

$$\Delta y = f(x + \Delta x) - f(x)$$

3. Form the quotient

$$\frac{\Delta y}{\Delta x} = \frac{f(x + \Delta x) - f(x)}{\Delta x}$$

4. Take the limit of this quotient as x approaches 0. The result is denoted by $\frac{dy}{dx}$ and is called the derivative of y with respect to x at the point (x, y).

$$\frac{dy}{dx} = \lim_{\Delta x \to 0} \frac{\Delta y}{\Delta x} = \lim_{\Delta x \to 0} \frac{f(x + \Delta x) - f(x)}{\Delta x}$$

The process of finding a derivative is called differentiation. The symbol $\frac{dy}{dx}$ is only to be regarded as a single symbol and is on no account to be thought of as a quotient of two numbers dy and dx. It is important to note that $\frac{dy}{dx}$ means the derivative at the particular point whose coordinates are (x, y). The derivative is independent of geometric considerations.

If the derivative of a function is positive at a given point, the function is increasing in the neighborhood of this point, if the derivative is negative, the function is decreasing in the neighborhood.

General rules for differentiation of algebraic functions are:

1. If $y = x^n$ then $\frac{dy}{dx} = nx^{n-1}$

   $y = x^3$ then $\frac{dy}{dx} = 3x^2$

2. The derivative of any constant is zero.

$$\frac{dc}{dx} = 0$$

3. The derivative of the sum of any finite number of functions is the sum of the derivatives of the separate functions. Thus,

$$\frac{d(a + b)}{dx} = \frac{da}{dx} + \frac{db}{dx}$$

$$y = x^2 + x^{-1/3} \text{ then } \frac{dy}{dx} = 2x - \frac{1}{3}x^{-4/3}$$

4. The derivative of the product of two functions is the first times the derivative of the second plus the second times the derivative of the first. Thus,

$$\frac{d(ab)}{dx} = a\frac{db}{dx} + b\frac{da}{dx}$$

$$y = x^2(x^3 + x + 5)$$

$$\frac{dy}{dx} = x^2(3x^2 + 1) + 2x(x^3 + x + 5) = 5x^4 + 3x^2 + 10x$$

5. The derivative of a constant times a function is that constant times the derivative of the function. Thus,

$$\frac{d(cu)}{dx} = c\frac{du}{dx}$$

6. The derivative of the quotient of two functions is the denominator times the derivative of the numerator minus the numerator times the derivative of the denominator, all divided by the square of the denominator, that is,

$$\frac{d}{dx}\left(\frac{u}{v}\right) = \frac{v\frac{du}{dx} - u\frac{dv}{dx}}{v^2}$$

$$y = \frac{x^2 + 5}{x + 1}$$

$$\frac{dy}{dx} = \frac{(x + 1)2x - (x^2 + 5)(1)}{(x + 1)^2} = \frac{x^2 + 2x - 5}{x^2 + 2x + 1}$$

7. The derivative of a function may be expressed

$$\frac{dy}{dx} = \frac{dy}{du}\frac{du}{dx}$$

$$y = (x^2 - 3)^{2/3}$$

$$\text{Let } y = u^{2/3}$$

$$\frac{dy}{du} = \frac{2}{3}u^{-1/3} \text{ and } \frac{du}{dx} = 2x$$

$$\frac{dy}{dx} = \frac{dy}{du}\frac{du}{dx} = \frac{2}{3}u^{-1.3}\ 2x = \frac{2}{3}(x^2 - 3)\,2x = \frac{4x}{3}(x^2 - 3)$$

8. The derivative with respect to x of the nth power of a function of x is n times the function to the (n - 1) power times the derivative of the function with respect to x, that is,

$$\frac{d}{dx}(u^n) = nu^{n-1}\frac{du}{dx}$$

$$y = (x^2 + 6)^{3/2}$$

$$\frac{dy}{dx} = \frac{3}{2}(x^2 + 6)^{1/2}\ 2x = 3x(x^2 + 6)^{1/2}$$

PARTIAL DERIVATIVES. Corresponding to the concept of the derivative of a function of one variable, the concept of partial derivatives of a function of several variables may be defined.

If $u = f(x, y)$ and if y is kept fixed, then u becomes a function of x only; its derivative with respect to x is called the partial derivative of u with respect to x and is denoted symbolically

$$\left(\frac{\delta u}{\delta x}\right)_y$$

In the function $u = x^2 + xy + y^2$, the partial derivative with respect to x when y is constant is

$$\left(\frac{\delta u}{\delta x}\right)_y = 2x + y$$

and the partial derivative with respect to y when x is constant is

$$\left(\frac{\delta u}{\delta y}\right)_x = x + 2y.$$

GREEK ALPHABET

Α	α	Alpha	Ν	ν	Nu
Β	β	Beta	Ξ	ξ	Xi
Γ	γ	Gamma	Ο	o	Omicron
Δ	δ	Delta	Π	π	Pi
Ε	ϵ	Epsilon	Ρ	ρ	Rho
Ζ	ζ	Zeta	Σ	σ	Sigma
Η	η	Eta	Τ	τ	Tau
Θ	θ	Theta	Υ	υ	Upsilon
Ι	ι	Iota	Φ	φ	Phi
Κ	κ	Kappa	Χ	χ	Chi
Λ	λ	Lambda	Ψ	ψ	Psi
Μ	μ	Mu	Ω	ω	Omega

GAS CONSTANT

Experimentally, Boyle found that when the temperature remains constant, the volume, v, of a given mass of gas varies inversely as its pressure, p,

$$pv = k_1$$

Gay Lussac and Charles found that at a constant pressure the volume, v, of a gas is directly proportional to its absolute temperature, T,

$$v = k_2T$$

A small change in volume, dv, of a system, produced by changing the temperature and pressure simultaneously, is equal to the sum of two quantities: (a) the change in temperature, dt, multiplied by the rate at which the volume changes with the temperature alone, $\left(\frac{\delta v}{\delta T}\right)_p$, and (b) the change in pressure, dp, multiplied by the rate at which the volume changes with pressure alone, $\left(\frac{\delta v}{\delta p}\right)_T$. Symbolically this may be expressed (see Appendix – Differentiation)

$$dv = \left(\frac{\delta v}{\delta p}\right)_T dp + \left(\frac{\delta v}{\delta T}\right)_p dT$$

Differentiating Boyle's law one obtains

$$\left(\frac{\delta v}{\delta p}\right)_T = -\frac{k_1}{p^2} = -\frac{pv}{p^2} = -\frac{v}{p}$$

and differentiating Guy Lussac-Charles' law one obtains

$$\left(\frac{\delta v}{\delta T}\right)_p = k_2 = \frac{v}{T}$$

Substituting into the expression for a simultaneous temperature and pressure change yields

$$dv = -\frac{v}{p}dp + \frac{v}{T}dT$$

or

$$\frac{dv}{v} + \frac{dp}{p} = \frac{dT}{T}$$

The integrated form of this equation is

$$\ln v + \ln p = \ln T + \ln \text{constant}$$

or

$$pv = \text{constant} \times T.$$

If a volume of 1 mole, V, of a gas is considered the equation becomes

$$pV = RT\cdot$$

and the gas constant, R, may be experimentally determined

$$R = \frac{pV}{T}$$

since at standard conditions (0° and 1 atmosphere) 1 mole of an ideal gas occupies 22.414 liters. Then

$$R = \frac{1 \text{ atm} \times 22.414 \text{ liter}}{273.16^\circ} = 0.08205 \text{ liter-atm degree}^{-1} \text{ mole}^{-1}$$

The gas constant may be express in terms of joules. The pressure in dynes per square centimeter is found by multiplying 76 cm of mercury by the density of mercury and the acceleration of gravity. The pressure in dynes per square centimeter multiplied by the volume in milliliters is the work in ergs. One joule is equal to 10^7 ergs.

$$R = \frac{pV}{T} = \frac{76 \times 13.595 \times 980 \times 22.414}{273.16 \times 10^7} = 8.314 \text{ joules degree}^{-1} \text{ mole}^{-1}$$

As there are 4.184 joules per calorie, the gas constant also equals

$$R = \frac{8.314}{4.184} = 1.987 \text{ cal degree}^{-1} \text{ mole}^{-1}.$$

U.S. STANDARD SIEVES

Size		Sieve Opening	Percent Permissible Variation in Average Opening	Wire Diameter
Micron	Number			
5660	3½	5.66 mm	3	1.28 -1.90 mm
4760	4	4.76	3	1.14 -1.68
4000	5	4.00	3	1.00 -1.47
3360	6	3.36	3	0.87 -1.32
2830	7	2.83	3	0.80 -1.20
2380	8	2.38	3	0.74 -1.10
2000	10	2.00	3	0.68 -1.00
1680	12	1.68	3	0.620-0.90
1410	14	1.41	3	0.56 -0.80
1190	16	1.19	3	0.50 -0.70
1000	18	1.00	5	0.43 -0.62
840	20	0.84	5	0.38 -0.55
710	25	0.71	5	0.33 -0.48
590	30	0.59	5	0.29 -0.42
500	35	0.50	5	0.26 -0.37
420	40	0.42	5	0.23 -0.33
350	45	0.35	5	0.20 -0.29
297	50	0.297	5	0.170-0.253
250	60	0.250	5	0.149-0.220
210	70	0.210	5	0.130-0.187
177	80	0.177	6	0.114-0.154
149	100	0.149	6	0.096-0.125
125	120	0.125	6	0.079-0.103
105	140	0.105	6	0.063-0.087
88	170	0.088	6	0.054-0.073
74	200	0.074	6	0.045-0.061
62	230	0.062	7	0.039-0.052
53	270	0.053	7	0.035-0.046
44	325	0.044	7	0.031-0.040
37	400	0.037	7	0.023-0.035

PARTICLE SIZE

The simplest method of measuring particle size is by the use of standard sieves. In any procedure in which a material is passed through one sieve and retained on another, the size assigned to the retained particles should be clearly defined and used throughout the procedure. The diameter of the particles may be defined as equal to the opening in the larger or smaller sieve, or the arithmetic or geometric mean of the openings of the two sieves.

For example, the size of the particles that pass a 40-mesh sieve and are retained on a 60-mesh sieve might be defined in terms of the larger sieve, i.e., 0.42 mm. The same particles might be expressed as the arithmetic mean of the size of the sieve openings, i.e., (0.42 + 0.25)/2 = 0.335 mm. In general, the arithmetic mean, $\overline{X}$, may be obtained by adding all of the individual items, $\overline{X}$, and dividing the total, ΣX, by the number of items, n, used

$$\overline{X} = \frac{\Sigma(X)}{n}.$$

The geometric mean is the nth root of the product of n items

$$G_m = (X_1 X_2 \ldots X_n)^{1/n}.$$

The particles that pass through a 40-mesh sieve and are retained by a 60-mesh sieve would have a geometric mean

$$G_m = (0.42 \times 0.25)^{1/2} = 0.324 \text{ mm}$$

When a substance is passed through a series of standard sieves and the amount of material retained on each sieve is determined, a weight-size distribution of the material is obtained. Such a size frequency distribution is shown:

Sieve Numbers (passed/retained)	Arithmetic-mean Size of Openings	Weight of Powder Retained on Smaller Sieve	Percent Retained on Smaller Sieve	Weight Size
(1)	(2)	(3)	(4)	(2) X (4)
10/20	1.42 mm	2.11 g	2.21	3.14
20/40	0.63	53.08	55.58	35.015
40/60	0.335	20.01	20.94	7.015
60/80	0.214	17.04	17.84	3.82
80/100	0.163	3.25	3.43	0.56
		95.49	100	49.55

$$\text{Arithmetic Mean} = \frac{49.55}{100} = 0.495 \text{ mm}$$

DISSOCIATION CONSTANTS OF ACIDS IN AQUEOUS SOLUTIONS AT 25° C

Substance	K_a	pK_a
Acetic	1.753×10^{-5}	4.76
Acetylsalicylic	3.27×10^{-4}	3.49
Adipic	3.72×10^{-5}	4.43
α-Alanine	9×10^{-10}	9.05
Aluminum hydroxide	6.3×10^{-13}	12.20
L-Arginine*	3.3×10^{-13}	12.48
Arsenic	5×10^{-3}	2.30
	8.3×10^{-8} (2 H)	7.08
	6×10^{-10} (3 H)	9.22
Arsenious	6×10^{-13}	12.22
L-Aspartic*	1.38×10^{-4}	3.86
	1.51×10^{-10} (2 H)	9.82
Barbituric	1.05×10^{-4}	3.98
Barbituric, allylbenzyl	6.2×10^{-8}	7.21
diallyl	1.6×10^{-8}	7.78
diethyl	1.2×10^{-8}	7.90
ethylisopropyl	1×10^{-8}	8.01
ethyl-1-methylbutyl	8×10^{-9}	8.11
phenylethyl	3.9×10^{-8}	7.41
Benzoic	6.3×10^{-5}	4.20
Boric	5.8×10^{-10}	9.24
n-Butyric	1.506×10^{-5}	4.82
Carbonic	4.31×10^{-7}	6.37
	5.6×10^{-11} (2 H)	10.25
Chloracetic	1.396×10^{-3}	2.86
o-Chlorobenzoic	1.197×10^{-3}	2.92
m-Chlorobenzoic	1.506×10^{-4}	3.82
p-Chlorobenzoic	1.04×10^{-4}	3.98
o-Chlorophenylacetic	8.6×10^{-5}	4.07
m-Chlorophenylacetic	7.24×10^{-5}	4.14
p-Chlorophenylacetic	6.45×10^{-5}	4.19
Chromic	3.2×10^{-7} (2 H)	6.49
Cinnamic (Trans)	3.7×10^{-5}	4.43
(Cis)	1.32×10^{-4}	3.88
Citric	8.7×10^{-4}	3.06
	1.8×10^{-5} (2 H)	4.74
	4×10^{-6} (3 H)	5.40
L-Cystine*	1×10^{-9}	8.00
	5.63×10^{-11} (2 H)	10.25
Dichloracetic	5×10^{-2}	1.3
Diiodo-L-tyrosine*	3.3×10^{-7}	6.48
	1.51×10^{-8} (2 H)	7.82

Formic	1.76×10^{-4}	3.75
Fumaric	9.3×10^{-4}	3.03
	3.4×10^{-5} (2 H)	4.47
Gallic	4×10^{-5}	4.40
L-Glutamic*	8.5×10^{-5}	4.07
	3.4×10^{-10} (2 H)	9.47
Glutaric	4.54×10^{-5}	4.34
Glycerophosphoric	3.4×10^{-2}	1.47
	6.4×10^{-7} (2 H)	6.19
Glycine*	1.67×10^{-10}	9.78
Hippuric	2.3×10^{-4}	3.64
L-Histidine*	6.6×10^{-10}	9.18
Hydrocyanic	7.2×10^{-10}	9.14
Hydroquinone (18°)	1.1×10^{-10}	9.96
Hydrosulfuric	5.7×10^{-8}	7.24
	1.2×10^{-15} (2 H)	14.92
Hydroxy-L-proline*	8.3×10^{-13}	12.08
Hypochlorous	3.5×10^{-8}	7.46
Iodic	1.67×10^{-1}	0.78
p-Iodophenylacetic	6.64×10^{-5}	4.18
Isobutyric	1.55×10^{-5}	4.81
DL-Isoleucine*	1.75×10^{-10}	9.76
Isovaleric	1.68×10^{-5}	4.77
Itaconic	1.46×10^{-4}	3.84
	2.8×10^{-6} (2 H)	5.55
Lactic	1.387×10^{-4}	3.86
DL-Leucine*	1.80×10^{-10}	9.74
L-Lysine*	2.95×10^{-11}	10.53
Maleic	1.0×10^{-2}	2.00
	5.5×10^{-7} (2 H)	6.26
Malic	4×10^{-4}	3.40
	9×10^{-6} (2 H)	5.05
Malonic	1.397×10^{-3}	2.85
	8×10^{-7} (2 H)	6.10
Mandelic	4.29×10^{-4}	3.37
DL-Methionine*	6.17×10^{-10}	9.21
Mucic	6.1×10^{-4}	3.21
α-Naphthonic	2×10^{-4}	3.70
β-Naphthonic	6.9×10^{-5}	4.16
Nicotinic	1.34×10^{-5}	4.87
Nitrous (18°)	4×10^{-4}	3.40
Oxalic	6.5×10^{-2}	1.19
	6.1×10^{-5} (2 H)	4.21
Periodic	2.3×10^{-2}	1.64
Phenol	1.3×10^{-10}	9.89

Phenolphthalein	2×10^{-10}	9.70
Phenylacetic	4.88×10^{-5}	4.31
DL-Phenylalanine*	5.76×10^{-10}	9.24
Phosphoric	7.5×10^{-3}	2.12
	6.2×10^{-8} (2 H)	7.21
	4.8×10^{-13} (3 H)	12.32
Phosphorous	1.6×10^{-2}	1.80
	7×10^{-7} (2 H)	6.15
Phthalic	1.26×10^{-3}	2.89
	3.1×10^{-6} (2 H)	5.51
Picric	4.2×10^{-1}	0.38
L-Proline*	2.5×10^{-11}	10.6
Propionic	1.343×10^{-5}	4.87
Pyromucic (furoic)	7.1×10^{-4}	3.15
Pyrophosphoric	1.4×10^{-1}	0.85
	1.1×10^{-2} (2 H)	1.96
	2.1×10^{-7} (3 H)	6.68
	4.06×10^{-10} (4 H)	9.39
Pyrotartaric	8.5×10^{-5}	4.07
Saccharin	2.5×10^{-2}	1.60
Salicylic	1.06×10^{-3}	2.97
	3.6×10^{-14} (2 H)	13.44
DL-Serine*	7.1×10^{-10}	9.15
Succinic	6.4×10^{-5}	4.19
	2.7×10^{-6}	5.57
Sulfanilic	6.5×10^{-4}	3.19
Sulfuric	1.2×10^{-2} (2 H)	1.92
Sulfurous	1.72×10^{-2}	1.76
	6.24×10^{-8} (2 H)	7.20
Tartaric	9.6×10^{-4}	3.02
	2.9×10^{-5} (2 H)	4.54
Trichloracetic	1.3×10^{-1}	0.89
Tryptophan*	4.06×10^{-10}	9.39
L-Tyrosine*	8×10^{-10}	9.11
Uric	1.3×10^{-4}	3.89
Valeric	1.56×10^{-5}	4.81
DL-Valine*	1.9×10^{-10}	9.72

*Ionization Constant at the Isoelectric Point

DISSOCIATION CONSTANTS OF BASES IN AQUEOUS SOLUTIONS AT 25° C

Substance	K_b		pK_b
Acetanilide (40°)	4.1×10^{-14}		13.39
Aconitine	1.3×10^{-6}		5.89
Ammonium hydroxide	1.8×10^{-5}		4.74
o-Aminobenzoic acid	1.4×10^{-12}		11.85
Anhydroecgonine (15°)	1.4×10^{-11}		10.85
Apomorphine	1.0×10^{-7}		7.00
Arecoline (15°)	1.4×10^{-7}		6.84
Atropine (15°)	4.47×10^{-5}		4.35
Benzocaine (15°)	6×10^{-12}		11.22
Benzoylecgonine (15°)	1.7×10^{-12}		11.77
Berberine (15°)	3.4×10^{-3}		2.47
Brucine	9×10^{-7}		6.05
	2×10^{-12}	(2 OH)	11.7
Caffeine (40°)	4.1×10^{-14}		13.39
Cevadine (15°)	7.1×10^{-6}		5.15
Cinchonidine	1.6×10^{-6}		5.80
	8.4×10^{-11}	(2 OH)	10.08
Cinchonine	1.4×10^{-6}		5.85
	1.1×10^{-10}		9.96
Cocaine	2.6×10^{-6}		5.59
Codeine	9×10^{-7}		6.05
Colchicine	4.5×10^{-13}		12.35
Coniine	1×10^{-3}		3.00
Cupreine	2.7×10^{-7}		6.57
Cytisine	8.3×10^{-7}		6.08
Ecgonine (15°)	6×10^{-12}		11.22
Emetine	1.7×10^{-6}		5.77
	2.3×10^{-7}	(2 OH)	6.64
Ethanolamine	2.77×10^{-5}		4.56
Ethylmorphine (15°)	7.6×10^{-7}		6.12
Glycine	2.26×10^{-12}		11.65
Histidine	1.25×10^{-8}		7.90
Hydrastine	1.7×10^{-8}		7.77
Hydrastinine (15°)	2.4×10^{-3}		2.62
Hydrochinine (15°)	4.7×10^{-6}		5.33
Hydroquinine	4.7×10^{-6}		5.33
Isopilocarpine (15°)	6.76×10^{-8}		7.17
Isoquinoline (15°)	1.1×10^{-9}		8.96

Leucine	2.3×10^{-12}		11.64
Methyl red (18°)	3×10^{-12}		11.52
Morphine	7.4×10^{-7}		6.13
Narceine	2×10^{-11}		10.7
Narcotine	1.5×10^{-8}		7.82
Nicotine	7×10^{-7}		6.15
	1.4×10^{-11}	(2 OH)	10.85
Papaverine	8×10^{-9}		8.10
Pelletierine (15°)	1.78×10^{-5}		4.75
Physostigmine	7.6×10^{-7}		6.12
	5.7×10^{-13}	(2 OH)	12.24
Pilocarpine	7×10^{-8}		7.15
	2×10^{-13}	(2 OH)	12.7
Piperine	1×10^{-14}		14.0
Procaine	7×10^{-6}		5.15
Pseudotropine (15°)	1.59×10^{-4}		3.80
Quinidine	3.5×10^{-6}		5.46
	1×10^{-10}	(2 OH)	10.0
Quinine	1×10^{-6}		6.0
	1.3×10^{-10}	(2 OH)	9.89
Quinoline	6.3×10^{-10}		9.20
Sarcosine	1.8×10^{-12}		11.74
Solanine	2.2×10^{-7}		6.66
Sparteine	5.7×10^{-3}		2.24
	1×10^{-6}		6.0
Strychnine	1×10^{-6}		6.0
	2×10^{-12}	(2 OH)	11.7
Thebaine	9×10^{-7}		6.05
Theobromine (40°)	4.8×10^{-12}		11.48
Theophylline (20°)	1.9×10^{-14}		13.7
Tropacocaine (15°)	4.8×10^{-5}		4.32
Urea	1.5×10^{-14}		13.82
Veratrine	7×10^{-6}		5.15

MOLAL FREEZING POINT DEPRESSION IN WATER AT CONCENTRATIONS APPROXIMATELY ISOTONIC WITH BLOOD SERUM

Antipyrine	1.9
Atropine sulfate	4.3
Boric acid	1.9
Calcium chloride	4.8
Calcium nitrate	4.5
Camphor	1.9
Chloral hydrate	1.9
Chlorobutanol	1.9
Citric acid	2.0
Cocaine hydrochloride	3.4
Dextrose	1.9
Emetine hydrochloride	4.8
Ephedrine hydrochloride	3.4
Ephedrine sulfate	4.3
Epinephrine hydrochloride	3.4
Ethylhydrocupreine hydrochloride	3.4
Ethylmorphine hydrochloride	3.4
Ferric chloride	6.0
Fluorescein sodium	4.3
Homatropine hydrobromide	3.4
Hyoscine hydrobromide	3.4
Hyoscine hydrochloride	3.4
Lactose	1.9
Magnesium chloride	4.9
Magnesium sulfate	2.0
Menthol	1.9
Mercuric chloride	1.8
Mercuric cyanide	1 9
Methenamine	1.9
Metycaine hydrochloride	3.4
Morphine hydrochloride	3.4
Morphine sulfate	4.3
Neosynephrine hydrochloride	3.4
Phenacaine hydrochloride	3.4
Physostigmine salicylate	3.4
Physostigmine sulfate	4.3
Pilocarpine hydrochloride	3.4
Pontocaine hydrochloride	3.4
Potassium bromide	3.4
Potassium chloride	3.4
Potassium iodide	3.4
Potassium phosphate (monobasic)	3.2
Potassium sulfate	4.2
Potassium tetraborate	7.4
Procaine hydrochloride	3.4
Silver nitrate	3.3
Sodium acid phosphate	3.4
Sodium bicarbonate	3.5
Sodium borate	8.0
Sodium bromide	3.4
Sodium chloride	3.4
Sodium citrate	5.2
Sodium iodide	3.6
Sodium phosphate (dibasic)	4.3
Sodium sulfate	4.3
Sodium thiosulfate	4.2
Sugar	1.9
Tartaric acid	2.0
Tutocaine hydrochloride	3.4
Zinc acetate	4.7
Zinc chloride	4.9
Zinc nitrate	4.9
Zinc phenosulfonate	4.8
Zinc sulfate	2.0

SODIUM CHLORIDE EQUIVALENTS

(After E. Hammarlund and K. Pedersen-Bjergaard, J. Am. Pharm. Assoc. Sci. Ed., 47, 107, 1958)

Drug	Experimental Range in Which Sodium Chloride Equivalent Determined	
	1%	3%
Acriflavine	0.10	0.09
Adrenaline hydrochloride	0.27	0.22
Alum (Potassium) N. F.	0.18	0.15
9-Aminoacridine hydrochloride	0.17	----
Aminophylline U. S. P.	0.17	----
Amiodoxyl benzoate	0.20	0.20
Ammonium chloride U. S. P.	1.12	----
Amobarbital sodium U. S. P.	0.25	0.25
Amphetamine phosphate	0.34	0.27
Amphetamine sulfate	0.22	0.21
Amprotropine phosphate	0.18	0.16
Amydricaine hydrochloride	0.24	0.18
Amydricaine nitrate	0.19	0.17
Amylocaine hydrochloride	0.22	0.19
Antazoline hydrochloride	0.23	----
Antazoline phosphate N. F.	0.20	0.17
Antimony potassium tartrate U. S.P.	0.18	0.13
Antipyrine	0.17	0.14
Apomorphine hydrochloride	0.14	----
Aranthol	0.23	0.23
Arecoline hydrobromide	0.27	0.24
Ascorbic acid U. S. P.	0.18	0.18
Atropine methyl nitrate	0.18	0.15
Atropine sulfate U. S. P.	0.13	0.11
Aurothioglucose U. S. P.	0.03	0.03
Bacitracin U. S. P.	0.05	0.04
Barbital sodium	0.30	0.29
Benoxinate hydrochloride	0.18	0.14
Benzalkonium chloride U. S. P.	0.16	0.14
Benzethonium chloride N. F.	0.05	0.02
Benzpyrinium bromide	0.20	0.18
Benzyl alcohol N. F.	0.17	0.15
Bismuth sodium tartrate	0.09	0.06
Boric acid U. S. P.	0.50	----
Bromodiphenhydramine hydrochloride	0.17	0.10
Butacaine sulfate	0.20	0.13
Butethamine formate	0.26	0.21
Butethamine hydrochloride	0.25	----

Caffeine U. S. P.	0.08	----
Caffeine and sodium benzoate	0.26	0.23
Caffeine and sodium salicylate	0.21	0.17
Calcium aminosalicylate N. F.	0.27	0.21
Calcium chloride U. S. P.	0.51	----
Calcium chloride (6 H_2O)	0.35	----
Calcium chloride anhydrous	0.68	----
Calcium gluconate U. S. P.	0.16	0.14
Calcium lactate U. S. P.	0.23	0.21
Calcium levulinate	0.27	0.25
Calcium pantothenate U. S. P.	0.18	0.17
Carbachol U. S. P.	0.36	----
Cetyltrimethyl ammonium	0.09	0.09
Chiniofon	0.13	0.11
Chloramine-T	0.23	0.22
Chlorcyclizine hydrochloride N. F.	0.17	0.09
Chlorobutanol hydrated U. S. P.	0.24	----
Chloresium	0.10	0.06
Chlorpheniramine maleate U. S. P.	0.17	0.12
Chlorpromazine hydrochloride U. S. P.	0.10	0.05
Chlortetracycline sulfate	0.13	0.10
Citric acid U. S. P.	0.18	0.17
Cocaine hydrochloride U. S. P.	0.16	0.15
Codeine hydrochloride	0.15	0.15
Cornecaine	0.18	0.15
Cyclomethycaine sulfate	0.13	0.10
Cyclomethycaine hydrochloride	0.36	----
Cyclopentolate hydrochloride U. S. P.	0.20	0.18
Decamethonium bromide	0.25	0.20
Dextroamphetamine phosphate	0.25	0.25
Dextrose U. S. P.	0.16	0.16
Dextrose, anhydrous	0.18	0.18
Dibucaine hydrochloride N. F.	0.13	0.11
Dibutoline sulfate	0.16	0.15
Dichlorophenarsine hydrochloride	0.55	----
Dicyclomine hydrochloride	0.18	0.17
Dihydrocodeinone enolactate hydrochloride	0.14	0.13
Dihydrohydroxycodeinone	0.14	0.13
Dihydromorphinone hydrochloride N. F.	0.22	0.17
Dihydrostreptomycine sulfate	0.06	0.05
Diphenhydramine hydrochloride U. S. P.	0.28	0.20
Diphenmethanil methylsulfate	0.15	----
Emetine hydrochloride U. S. P.	0.10	0.10
Ephedrine hydrochloride N. F.	0.30	0.28
Ephedrine sulfate U. S. P.	0.23	0.20
Epinephrine bitartrate U. S. P.	0.18	0.16
Epinephrine hydrochloride	0.29	0.26
Ergonovine maleate N. F.	0.16	----
Erythromycin glucoheptonate U. S. P.	0.07	0.07
Ethaverine hydrochloride	0.12	----
Ethylenediamine	0.44	----
Ethylhydrocupreine hydrochloride	0.17	0.11

Ethylmorphine hydrochloride	0.16	0.15
Ethylnorepinephrine hydrochloride	0.32	0.28
Ferrous gluconate N. F.	0.15	0.12
Ferrous lactate	0.21	----
Fluorescein sodium U. S. P.	0.31	0.27
D-Fructose	0.18	0.18
Galactose	0.18	0.18
Gallamine triethiodide	0.08	0.08
D-Glucuronic acid	0.20	0.19
L-Glutamic acid	0.25	----
Glycerin U. S. P.	0.35	----
Glyphylline	0.12	0.10
Guanidine hydrochloride	0.65	----
Heparin sodium U. S. P.	0.08	0.07
Hexamethonium bromide	0.22	0.19
Hexamethonium chloride	0.27	0.27
Hexobarbital sodium	0.26	0.24
Hexylcaine hydrochloride N. F.	0.26	0.22
Hippuran	0.16	0.15
Histalog	0.51	----
Histamine phosphate U. S. P.	0.25	0.23
Histidine monohydrochloride	0.29	0.26
Holocaine hydrochloride	0.20	----
Homatropine hydrobromide U. S. P.	0.17	0.16
Homatropine methylbromide N. F.	0.19	0.15
Hydralazine hydrochloride U. S. P.	0.37	----
Hydrastine hydrochloride	0.15	0.12
Hydroxyamphetamine hydrobromide N. F.	0.26	0.25
Hydroxyquinoline sulfate	0.21	0.14
Hyoscyamine hydrobromide N. F.	0.19	0.16
Hyoscyamine sulfate N. F.	0.14	0.12
Intracaine hydrochloride	0.23	0.20
Iodophthalein sodium	0.17	0.12
Iodopyracet	0.11	0.11
Isoniazid U. S. P.	0.25	0.22
Lactic acid U. S. P.	0.41	----
Lactose U. S. P.	0.07	0.08
Lidocaine hydrochloride U. S. P.	0.22	0.21
Lobeline hydrochloride	0.16	----
Magnesium sulfate U. S. P.	0.17	0.15
Mannitol	0.17	0.17
Menadione diphosphate	0.25	0.22
Menadione sodium bisulfite N. F.	0.20	0.18
Meperidine hydrochloride U. S. P.	0.22	0.20
Mephentermine sulfate N. F.	0.22	0.20
Mephenesin	0.19	----
Merbromin	0.14	0.11

Mercaptomerin sodium U. S. P.	0.18	0.18
Mercuric cyanide	0.15	0.14
Mercurophylline	0.13	0.10
Mercury bichloride	0.13	0.12
Mersalyl	0.12	0.11
Methacholine chloride N. F.	0.32	- - - -
Methadone hydrochloride U. S. P.	0.18	0.14
Methamphetamine hydrochloride	0.37	- - - -
Methantheline bromide N. F.	0.15	0.09
Methapyrilene hydrochloride N. F.	0.19	0.18
Methenamine N. F.	0.23	0.24
Methionine N. F.	0.28	- - - -
Methoxamine hydrochloride U. S. P.	0.26	0.24
Methylatropine bromide	0.14	0.13
Monoethanolamine N. F.	0.53	- - - -
Morphine hydrochloride	0.15	0.14
Morphine nitrate	0.19	0.15
Morphine sulfate U. S. P.	0.14	0.11
Naphazoline hydrochloride N. F.	0.27	0.24
Narcotine hydrochloride	0.10	0.08
Neomycin sulfate U. S. P.	0.11	0.09
Neostigmine bromide U. S. P.	0.22	0.19
Neostigmine methyl sulfate U. S. P.	0.20	0.18
Nicotinamide U. S. P.	0.26	0.21
Nicotinic acid (Niacin) N. F.	0.25	- - - -
Nikethamide	0.18	0.16
Oxytetracycline hydrochloride	0.13	0.08
Papaverine hydrochloride N. F.	0.10	- - - -
Pentobarbital sodium U. S. P.	0.25	0.23
Pentolinium tartrate	0.17	0.15
Pentylenetetrazole	0.22	0.19
Phenindamine tartrate N. F.	0.17	0.12
Pheniramine maleate	0.16	0.14
Phenobarbital sodium U. S. P.	0.24	0.23
Phenol U. S. P.	0.35	- - - -
Phenylephrine hydrochloride U. S. P.	0.32	0.30
Phenylephrine tartrate	0.19	0.16
Phenylpropanolamine hydrochloride	0.38	- - - -
Physostigmine salicylate U. S. P.	0.16	- - - -
Physostigmine sulfate U. S. P.	0.13	0.12
Pilocarpine hydrochloride U. S. P.	0.24	0.22
Pilocarpine nitrate U. S. P.	0.23	0.20
Piperocaine hydrochloride	0.21	0.19
Piridocaine hydrochloride	0.24	- - - -
Polymyxin B sulfate U. S. P.	0.09	0.06
Potassium chloride U. S. P.	0.76	- - - -
Potassium iodide U. S. P.	0.34	- - - -
Potassium nitrate	0.56	- - - -
Potassium penicillin G U. S. P.	0.18	0.17
Potassium phosphate	0.46	- - - -
Potassium phosphate, monobasic	0.44	- - - -

Potassium sulfate	0.44	----
Pramoxine hydrochloride	0.18	0.15
Procainamide hydrochloride U. S. P.	0.22	0.19
Probarbital calcium	0.25	----
Probarbital sodium	0.32	0.29
Procaine hydrochloride U. S. P.	0.21	0.19
Promethazine hydrochloride U. S. P.	0.18	0.10
Propionic acid	0.46	----
Propylene glycol U. S. P.	0.45	----
Pyridoxine hydrochloride U. S. P.	0.37	0.29
Pyrilamine maleate N. F.	0.18	0.11
Quinidine gluconate U. S. P.	0.12	0.10
Quinidine sulfate U. S. P.	0.10	----
Quinine dihydrochloride	0.23	0.19
Quinine hydrochloride	0.14	0.11
Quinine and urea hydrochloride	0.23	0.21
Racephedrine hydrochloride	0.31	0.30
Resorcinol U. S. P.	0.28	0.27
Scopolamine hydrobromide U. S. P.	0.12	0.12
Scopolamine methylnitrate	0.16	0.14
Secobarbital sodium U. S. P.	0.24	0.23
Silver nitrate U. S. P.	0.33	----
Mild silver protein	0.17	0.17
Strong silver protein	0.08	0.05
Sodium acetate, anhydrous	0.77	----
Sodium acetate U. S. P.	0.46	----
Sodium aminosalicylate U. S. P.	0.29	0.28
Sodium ascorbate	0.33	0.30
Sodium benzoate U. S. P.	0.40	----
Soduim bicarbonate U. S. P.	0.65	----
Sodium biphosphate, anhydrous	0.46	----
Sodium biphosphate U. S. P.	0.40	----
Sodium bisulfite U. S. P.	0.61	----
Sodium borate U. S. P.	0.42	----
Sodium cacodylate	0.32	0.28
Sodium carbonate, monohydrated U. S. P.	0.60	----
Sodium chloride U. S. P.	1.00	1.00
Sodium citrate U. S. P.	0.31	0.30
Sodium iodide U. S. P.	0.39	----
Sodium lactate	0.55	----
Sodium metabisulfite	0.67	----
Sodium nitrate	0.68	----
Sodium nitrite U. S. P.	0.84	----
Sodium penicillin G N. F.	0.18	----
Sodium phosphate dried N. F.	0.53	----
Sodium phosphate U. S. P.	0.29	0.27
Sodium phosphate, dibasic (2 H_2O)	0.42	----
Sodium phosphate, dibasic (12 H_2O)	0.22	0.21
Sodium propionate N. F.	0.61	----
Sodium riboflavin phosphate	0.08	0.08
Sodium ricinoleate	0.10	0.09

Sodium salicylate U. S. P.	0.36	----
Sodium sulfate, anhydrous	0.58	----
Sodium sulfate	0.26	0.23
Sodium sulfite, exsiccated	0.65	----
Sodium thiosulfate	0.31	----
Streptomycin calcium chloride complex	0.20	0.19
Streptomycin hydrochloride	0.17	0.16
Streptomycin sulfate U. S. P.	0.07	0.06
Strychnine hydrochloride	0.18	----
Strychnine nitrate	0.12	----
Succinylcholine chloride U. S. P.	0.20	0.20
Sucrose U. S. P.	0.08	0.09
Sulfacetamide sodium U. S. P.	0.23	0.23
Sulfadiazine sodium U. S. P.	0.24	0.22
Sulfamerazine sodium	0.23	0.21
Sulfapyridine sodium	0.23	0.21
Sulfathiazole sodium	0.22	0.20
Sulfisoxazole diethanolamine	0.18	0.15
Sympocaine hydrochloride	0.18	0.15
Synthenate tartarate	0.19	0.17
Tannic acid	0.03	0.03
Tartaric acid N. F.	0.25	0.23
Tetracaine hydrochloride U. S. P.	0.14	0.10
Tetracycline hydrochloride U. S. P.	0.18	0.15
Tetraethylammonium bromide	0.33	0.28
Tetraethylammonium chloride	0.34	----
Tetrahydrozoline hydrochloride U. S. P.	0.28	0.23
Theophylline	0.10	----
Thiamine hydrochloride U. S. P.	0.25	0.22
Thiopental sodium U. S. P.	0.27	0.26
Tolazoline hydrochloride	0.34	0.30
Trasentine hydrochloride	0.22	0.15
Tripelennamine hydrochloride U. S. P.	0.30	0.20
Tropacocaine hydrochloride	0.25	0.20
Tuaminoheptane sulfate N. F.	0.27	0.27
Tubocurarine chloride U. S. P.	0.13	0.10
Urea U. S. P.	0.59	----
Urethan	0.31	----
Vinbarbital sodium	0.26	0.25
Viomycin sulfate	0.08	0.07
Zinc chloride U. S. P.	0.61	----
Zinc phenolsulfonate	0.18	0.17
Zinc sulfanilate	0.21	0.19
Zinc sulfate U. S. P.	0.15	0.13

OPHTHALMIC BUFFER SYSTEMS

ATKINS AND PANTIN

Acid Stock Solution

Boric acid	12.405	g
Sodium chloride	7.50	g
Purified water q. s.	1000	ml

Alkaline Stock Solution

Sodium carbonate, anhydrous	21.2	g
Purified water q. s.	1000	ml

Ml of 0.2M Boric Acid Solution	Ml of 0.2 M Sodium Carbonate Solution	pH
93.8	6.2	7.6
91.7	8.3	7.8
88.8	11.2	8.0
85.0	15.0	8.2
80.7	19.3	8.4
75.7	24.3	8.6
69.5	30.5	8.8
63.0	37.0	9.0
56.4	43.6	9.2
49.7	50.3	9.4
42.9	57.1	9.6
36.0	64.0	9.8
29.1	70.9	10.0
22.1	77.9	10.2
15.4	84.6	10.4
9.8	90.2	10.6
5.7	94.3	10.8
3.5	96.5	11.0

FELDMAN

Acid Stock Solution

Boric acid	12.368 g
Sodium chloride	2.925 g
Purified water q. s.	1000

Alkaline Stock Solution

Sodium borate (10 H_2O)	19.07 g
Purified water q. s.	1000

Ml of Boric Acid Solution	Ml of Sodium Borate Solution	pH
100	0	5.0
100	0.4	6.0
95	5	7.0
94	6	7.1
93	7	7.2
91	9	7.3
89	11	7.4
87	13	7.5
85	15	7.6
82	18	7.7
80	20	7.8
76	24	7.9
73	27	8.0
69	31	8.1
65	35	8.2

GIFFORD

Acid Stock Solution

Boric acid	12.4 g
Potassium chloride	7.4 g
Purified water q. s.	1000

Alkaline Stock Solution

Sodium carbonate (monohydrate)	24.8 g
Purified water q. s.	1000

Ml of Boric Acid Solution	Ml of Sodium Carbonate Solution	pH
30	0.05	6.0
30	0.1	6.2
30	0.2	6.6
30	0.3	6.8
30	0.5	6.9
30	0.6	7.0
30	1.0	7.2
30	1.5	7.4
30	2.0	7.6
30	3.0	7.8
30	4.0	8.0
30	8.0	8.5

PALITZSCH

Acid Stock Solution			Alkaline Stock Solution		
Boric acid	12.404 g		Sodium borate (10 H_2O)	19.108 g	
Purified water q. s.	1000	ml	Purified water q. s.	1000	ml

Ml of 0.2M Boric Acid Solution	Ml of 0.05M Sodium Borate Solution	pH
97	3	6.8
94	6	7.1
90	10	7.4
85	15	7.6
80	20	7.8
75	25	7.9
70	30	8.1
65	35	8.2
55	45	8.4
45	55	8.6
40	60	8.7
30	70	8.8
20	80	9.0
10	90	9.1

SORENSEN MODIFIED PHOSPHATE

Acid Stock Solution		Alkaline Stock Solution		
Sodium biphosphate, anhydrous	8.006 g	Sodium phosphate, anhydrous	9.473 g	
Purified water q. s.	1000	Purified water q. s.	1000	ml

Ml of M/15 Sodium Biphosphate Solution	Ml of M/15 Sodium Phosphate Solution	pH
90	10	5.9
80	20	6.2
70	30	6.5
60	40	6.6
50	50	6.8
40	60	7.0
30	70	7.2
20	80	7.4
10	90	7.7
5	95	8.0

AVERAGE HLB VALUES OF SOME SURFACE-ACTIVE AGENTS

Name	Compound	HLB
Acacia		12.0
Aldol 33[d]	Glyceryl monostearate	3.8
Aldol 28[d]	Glyceryl monostearate (self-emulsifying)	5.5
Arlacel 85[a]	Sorbitan trioleate	1.8
Arlacel 65[a]	Sorbitan tristearate	2.1
Arlacel C[a]	Sorbitan sesquioleate	3.7
Arlacel 83[a]	Sorbitan sesquioleate	3.7
Arlacel 161[a]	Glyceryl monostearate	3.8
Arlacel 80[a]	Sorbitan monooleate	4.3
Arlacel 60[a]	Sorbitan monostearate	4.7
Arlacel 40[a]	Sorbitan monopalmitate	6.7
Arlacel 20[a]	Sorbitan monolaurate	8.6
Atmul 67[a]	Glyceryl monostearate	3.8
Brij 30[a]	Polyoxyethylene lauryl ether	9.5
Brij 35[a]	Polyoxyethylene lauryl ether	16.9
Emcol EO-50[b]	Ethylene glycol fatty acid ester	2.7
Emcol ES-50[b]	Ethylene glycol fatty acid ester	2.7
Emcol PO-50[b]	Propylene glycol fatty acid ester	3.4
Emcol PS-50[b]	Propylene glycol fatty acid ester	3.4
Emcol PP-50[b]	Propylene glycol fatty acid ester	3.7
Emcol PM-50[b]	Propylene glycol fatty acid ester	4.1
Emcol PL-50[b]	Propylene glycol fatty acid ester	4.5
Emcol DO-50[b]	Diethylene glycol fatty acid ester	4.7
Emcol DS-50[b]	Diethylene glycol fatty acid ester	4:7
Emcol DP-50[b]	Diethylene glycol fatty acid ester	5.1
Emcol DM-50[b]	Diethylene glycol fatty acid ester	5.6
Emcol DL-50[b]	Diethylene glycol fatty acid ester	6.1
Emulphor VN-430[c]	Polyoxyethylene fatty acid	9.0
Emulphor El-719[c]	Polyoxyethylene vegetable oil	13.3
Emulphor ON-870[c]	Polyoxyethylene fatty alcohol	15.4
G-1706[a]	Polyoxyethylene sorbitol beeswax derivative	2.0
G-1050[a]	Polyoxyethylene sorbital hexastearate	2.1
G-1704[a]	Polyoxyethylene sorbitol beeswax derivative	3.0
G-922[a]	Propylene glycol monostearate	3.4
G-2158[a]	Propylene glycol monostearate	3.4
G-2859[a]	Polyoxyethylene sorbitol 4.5 oleate	3.7
G-1727[a]	Polyoxyethylene sorbitol beeswax derivative	4.0
G-917[a]	Propylene glycol monolaurate	4.5
G-3851[a]	Propylene glycol monolaurate	4.5
G-2139[a]	Diethylene glycol monooleate	4.7
G-2146[a]	Diethylene glycol monostearate	4.7
G-1702[a]	Polyoxyethylene sorbitol beeswax derivative	5.0
G-1725[a]	Polyoxyethylene sorbitol beeswax derivative	6.0
G-2124[a]	Diethylene glycol monolaurate (soap free)	6.1
G-2242[a]	Polyoxyethylene dioleate	7.5
G-2147[a]	Tetraethylene glycol monostearate	7.7

G-2140[a]	Tetraethylene glycol monooleate	7.7
G-2800[a]	Polyoxypropylene mannitol dioleate	8.0
G-1493[a]	Polyoxyethylene sorbitol lanolin oleate derivative	8.0
G-1425[a]	Polyoxyethylene sorbitol lanolin derivative	8.0
G-3608[a]	Polyoxypropylene stearate	8.0
G-1734[a]	Polyoxyethylene sorbitol beeswax derivative	9.0
G-2111[a]	Polyoxyethylene oxypropylene oleate	9.0
G-2125[a]	Tetraethylene glycol monolaurate	9.4
G-2154[a]	Hexaethylene glycol monostearate	9.6
G-1218[a]	Polyoxyethylene esters of mixed fatty and resin acids	10.2
G-3806[a]	Polyoxyethylene cetyl ether	10.3
G-3705[a]	Polyoxyethylene lauryl ether	10.8
G-2116[a]	Polyoxyethylene oxypropylene oleate	11.0
G-1790[a]	Polyoxyethylene lanolin derivative	11.0
G-2142[a]	Polyoxyethylene monooleate	11.1
G-2141[a]	Polyoxyethylene monooleate	11.4
G-2076[a]	Polyoxyethylene monopalmitate	11.6
G-3300[a]	Alkyl aryl sulfonate	11.7
G-2127[a]	Polyoxyethylene monolaurate	12.8
G-1431[a]	Polyoxyethylene sorbitol lanolin derivative	13.0
G-1690[a]	Polyoxyethylene alkyl aryl ether	13.0
G-2133[a]	Polyoxyethylene lauryl ether	13.1
G-1284[a]	Polyoxyethylene castor oil	13.3
G-1441[a]	Polyoxyethylene sorbitol lanolin derivative	14.0
G-7596J[a]	Polyoxyethylene sorbitan monolaurate	14.9
G-2144[a]	Polyoxyethylene monooleate	15.1
G-3915[a]	Polyoxyethylene oleyl ether	15.3
G-2720[a]	Polyoxyethylene stearyl alcohol	15.3
G-3920[a]	Polyoxyethylene oleyl alcohol	15.4
G-2079[a]	Polyoxyethylene glycol monopalmitate	15.5
G-3820[a]	Polyoxyethylene cetyl alcohol	15.7
G-1471[a]	Polyoxyethylene sorbitol lanolin derivative	16.0
G-7596P[a]	Polyoxyethylene sorbitan monolaurate	16.3
G-2129[a]	Polyoxyethylene monolaurate	16.3
G-3930[a]	Polyoxyethylene oleyl ether	16.7
G-2159[a]	Polyoxyethylene monostearate	18.8
G-263[a]	N-Cetyl N-ethyl morpholinium ethosulfate	25-30
Glaurin[d]	Diethylene glycol monolaurate (soap free)	6.5
Igepal CA-630[c]	Polyoxyethylene alkyl phenol	12.8
Methocel 15 cps[h]	Methylcellulose	10.5
Myrj 45[a]	Polyoxyethylene monostearate	11.1
Myrj 49[a]	Polyoxyethylene monostearate	15.0
Myrj 51[a]	Polyoxyethylene monostearate	16.0
Myrj 52[a]	Polyoxyethylene monostearate	16.9
Myrj 53[a]	Polyoxyethylene monostearate	17.9
P. E. G. 400 monooleate[f, g]	Polyoxyethylene monooleate	11.4
P. E. G. 400 monostearate[f, g]	Polyoxyethylene monostearate	11.6
P. E. G. 400 monolaurate[f]	Polyoxyethylene monolaurate	13.1

Pharmagel B	Gelatin	9.8
Potassium oleate		20.0
Renex 20[a]	Polyoxyethylene esters of mixed fatty and resin acids	13.5
Sodium lauryl sulfate[a]		40
Sodium oleate		18
Span 85[a]	Sorbitan trioleate	1.8
Span 65[a]	Sorbitan tristearate	2.1
Span 80[a]	Sorbitan monooleate	4.3
Span 60[a]	Sorbitan monostearate	4.7
Span 40[a]	Sorbitan monopalmitate	6.7
Span 20[a]	Sorbitan monolaurate	8.6
Tegin 515[e]	Glyceryl monostearate	3.8
Tegin[e]	Glyceryl monostearate (self-emulsifying)	5.5
Tragacanth		12.0
Tween 61[a]	Polyoxyethylene sorbitan monostearate	9.6
Tween 81[a]	Polyoxyethylene sorbitan monooleate	10.0
Tween 65[a]	Polyoxyethylene sorbitan tristearate	10.5
Tween 85[a]	Polyoxyethylene sorbitan trioleate	11.0
Tween 21[a]	Polyoxyethylene sorbitan monolaurate	13.3
Tween 60[a]	Polyoxyethylene sorbitan monostearate	14.9
Tween 80[a]	Polyoxyethylene sorbitan monooleate	15.0
Tween 40[a]	Polyoxyethylene sorbitan monopalmitate	15.6
Tween 20[a]	Polyoxyethylene sorbitan monolaurate	16.7

a = Atlas Powder Company
b = Emulsol Corporation
c = General Aniline & Film Corporation
d = Glyco Products Company, Inc.
e = Goldschmidt Chemical Corporation
f = Kessler Chemical Company, Inc.
g = W. C. Hardesty Company, Inc.
h = Dow Chemical Company

REQUIRED HLB VALUES FOR COMMON EMULSION INGREDIENTS

Ingredient	W/O	O/W	Solubilization
Oleic acid	–	11	–
Stearic acid	6	15	–
Cetyl alcohol	–	15	–
Lauryl alcohol	–	13	–
Myristyl alcohol	–	14	–
Butyl stearate	–	11	–
Isopropyl palmitate	–	10	–
Lanolin, anhydrous	8	10	–
Methyl salicylate	–	14	–
Mineral spirits	–	10	–
Oils			
Castor	–	12	–
Cottonseed	5	12	–
Essential	–	–	15-18
Mineral, paraffinic	–	13	–
Palm (synthetic)	–	13	–
Pine	–	13	–
Silicone	–	11	–
Vitamin (with fats)	–	–	15-18
Vitamin (fat free)	–	–	15-18
Petrolatum	5	12	–
Vitamin esters	–	–	15-18
Waxes			
Beeswax	4	12	–
Carnauba	–	15	–
Ester (synthetic)	4	14	–
Microcrystalline	–	10	–
Paraffin	4	11	–
Polyethylene (oxidized)	–	9	–
Spermaceti	–	9	–

WEIGHTS AND MEASURES

Metric Weights

1 microgram	(γ, mcg, μg)	=	10^{-6} g	
1 milligram	(mg)	=	10^{-3} g	
1 kilogram	(kg)	=	10^{3} g	

Metric Liquid Measure

1 milliliter	(ml)	=	10^{-3} l	

Note–The standard of capacity is the liter, that is the volume of 1 kg of distilled water at 4°.

Metric Linear Measure

1 angstrom	(Å)	=	10^{-8} cm	
1 nanometer	(nm)	=	10^{-7} cm	= 1 millimicron (mμ)
1 micrometer	(μm)	=	10^{-4} cm	= 1 micron (μ)
1 millimeter	(mm)	=	10^{-1} cm	
1 meter	(m)	=	10^{2} cm	

Avoirdupois Weights

1 pound	(lb)	=	16 oz	= 7000 gr
1 ounce	(oz)	=	437.5 gr	

Apothecaries Weights

1 pound	(lb apoth)	=	12℥	= 5760 gr
1 ounce	(℥)	=	8ʒ	= 480 gr
1 dram	(ʒ)	=	3℈	= 60 gr
1 scruple	(℈)	=	20 gr	

Apothecaries Measure

1 gallon	(Cong)	=	8 O	= 128 f℥
1 pint	(O)	=		= 16 f℥
1 fluidounce	(f℥)	=	8 fʒ	= 480 *m*
1 fluidram	(fʒ)	=		= 60 *m*

REFERENCES

Diem, K. and C. Lentner, Eds. 1970. Scientific tables. 7th ed. Ciba-Geigy, Basel. p. 199.

EQUIVALENTS

1 atmosphere	=	14.7 lb in^{-2} = 760 mm mercury
1 centimeter	=	0.3937 in
1 cubic centimeter	=	16.23*m*
1 apothecary fluidram	=	3.697 cc
1 gallon	=	3785 cc
1 grain	=	64.8 mg
1 gram	=	15.432 gr = 980.6 dynes
1 apothecary grain	=	1 avoirdupois grain
1 inch	=	2.540 cm
1 joule	=	10^7 ergs
1 kilogram	=	2.204 lb
1 liter	=	1.05668 qt
1 micron	=	0.0001 cm
1 minim	=	0.059 cc
1 minim of water	=	0.95 gr at 25°
1 apothecary fluidounce	=	480*m* = 29.57 cc
1 apothecary fluidounce of water at 25°	=	454.6 gr
1 apothecary fluid of water at 4°	=	456.4 gr
1 apothecary ounce	=	480 gr = 31.10 g
1 avoirdupois ounce	=	437.5 gr = 28.35 g
1 pint	=	473 cc
1 quart	=	946 cc
C	=	$\frac{5}{9}(F-32)$
F	=	$32 + \frac{9}{5}C$

INDEX